T0342044

*INTRODUCTION TO POPULATION
PHARMACOKINETIC/PHARMACODYNAMIC
ANALYSIS WITH NONLINEAR
MIXED EFFECTS MODELS*

INTRODUCTION TO POPULATION PHARMACOKINETIC / PHARMACODYNAMIC ANALYSIS WITH NONLINEAR MIXED EFFECTS MODELS

JOEL S. OWEN

Professor of Pharmaceutics
Union University, School of Pharmacy
Department of Pharmaceutical Sciences
Jackson, Tennessee

JILL FIEDLER-KELLY

Vice President, Pharmacometric Services & CSO
Cognigen Corporation

Adjunct Associate Professor
University at Buffalo, Department of Pharmaceutical Sciences
Buffalo, New York

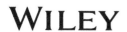

Published by John Wiley & Sons, Inc., Hoboken, New Jersey.
Published simultaneously in Canada.

For general information on our other products and services or for technical support, please contact our
Customer Care Department within the United States at (800) 762-2974, outside the United States at
(317) 572-3993 or fax (317) 572-4002.

Wiley also publishes its books in a variety of electronic formats and by print-on-demand. Not all
content that is available in standard print versions of this book may appear or be packaged in all book
formats. If you have purchased a version of this book that did not include media that is referenced by or
accompanies a standard print version, you may request this media by visiting http://booksupport.wiley.com.
For more information about Wiley products, visit us at www.wiley.com.

Library of Congress Cataloging-in-Publication Data:

Owen, Joel S., author.
 Introduction to population pharmacokinetic/pharmacodynamic analysis with nonlinear
mixed effects models / Joel S. Owen, Jill Fiedler-Kelly.
  p. ; cm.
 Includes bibliographical references and index.
 ISBN 978-0-470-58229-9 (cloth)
I. Fiedler-Kelly, Jill, author. II. Title.
 [DNLM: 1. Pharmacokinetics. 2. Nonlinear Dynamics. 3. Software. QV 38]
 RM301.5
 615.7–dc23
                                                                          2014002869

10 9 8 7 6 5 4 3 2 1

To Melanie, Janie, Matthew, Annette, and Mark for their love and patience. To numerous friends and colleagues at Union University and First Baptist Church, Jackson, Tennessee, for their interest and encouragement.

To Tad, Brynna, and Finn for their love and understanding and without whose support this would not have been possible.

CONTENTS

PREFACE

Nonlinear mixed effects modeling is an analytical approach capable of the efficient use of data to support informed decision making. In drug development and in clinical practice, the culmination of the work of the pharmacometrician is making informed decisions regarding the treatment of patients, either during the development of new treatments or in the clinical care of specific patients. The application of nonlinear mixed effects models to sparse clinical data was a concept brilliantly conceived and implemented via the NONMEM system by Dr. Lewis B. Sheiner and Dr. Stuart L. Beal, supported over the years by Alison J. Boeckmann. The impetus for development of the analytical approach and supporting software was the need to study drugs in the population in which they were to be used, and realization of the direct correlation between the patients who are most vulnerable to pharmacokinetic differences and those who are most difficult to study (Sheiner and Benet 1985). Of course, there have been many additional contributors to the development of this field over the past few decades; their contributions have created an environment where pharmacometric analysis approaches now flourish and contribute significantly to informed decision making.

The realization of the value of the field of pharmacometrics has caused significant demand for new pharmacometricians (Gobburu 2010). In its *Pharmacometrics 2020 Strategic Goals* statement, the FDA set a goal to train 20 pharmacometricians by the year 2020 (FDA 2013). In *Pharmacometrics 2020*, Dr. Gobburu suggests a goal that an additional 500 should be trained in that same time through the support of academia and the pharmaceutical industry (Gobburu 2010). This book is intended to contribute to that effort. It is written at an introductory level to bring clarity to the basic concepts of nonlinear mixed effects modeling for those new to the field. The book is focused on using the NONMEM® software for pharmacometric analysis. This is not to say that other software applications are not useful, but NONMEM was selected in part, because the authors are most familiar with this tool, but also because it is among the most flexible and powerful tools in use today, and because in our estimation, it remains the most often used software for nonlinear mixed effects modeling. There are also clear signs of its continued development and improvement by Dr. Robert J. Bauer and ICON Development Solutions, as evidenced by the release of new versions adding important new estimation algorithms, modernization of the code to improve efficiency, and enhancements to the program output. This book is also written with a particular focus toward drug development applications, but we hope that it will be useful to clinical pharmacists as well, to increase the use of such tools in defining clinical practice and in supporting patient care.

Several researchers have made significant efforts, contributing additional tools to make the application of pharmacometrics more efficient and more attainable to a greater number of people. Tools are now available to assist with the validation of one's NONMEM installation, the production of graphics to assess a dataset and modeling results, the automated implementation of extended processing for applications such as visual predictive checks and bootstrapping, and cataloging and comparing the history of models run during a project. A few of these excellent and generous efforts include the work of Dr. Mats Karlsson and colleagues at Uppsala University through the development and support of the Xpose and Perl Speaks NONMEM (PsN) software applications and the work of Dr. Marc Gastonguay and colleagues at Metrum Institute with the development and support of the nmqual package for validation of NONMEM installation and for their nmfuns set of tools. Wings for NONMEM by Dr. Nick Holford and PLT Tools by Dr. Dennis Fisher also prove to be useful for many. Most of these products are available free of cost but may have licensing fees to access support or additional features. The list of pharmacometric tools available has certainly been enhanced by the work of Dr. Tom Ludden, Dr. Robert Bauer, and colleagues at ICON Development Solutions, through their continued development of NONMEM and their add-on package PDx-POP™. This is by no means an exhaustive list of available tools as many others have made important contributions as well; those listed were simply the programs most familiar to the authors at the time of this writing.

The learning curve for the new pharmacometric analyst is quite substantial. In addition to the theory of the data analytic and statistical methodology, the understanding of experimental design, data collection, quality control, and many other critical components, there are at least three basic types of software with which the analyst must be familiar. These include: (i) a software tool for building the analysis dataset, (ii) software for the pharmacometric analysis itself, and (iii) pre- and postprocessing software for the preparation of graphics which are critical to understanding the data, presenting the results of modeling, and communicating to others the implications of the analysis. It is the latter, effective communication of modeling results and their implications to support critical decision making milestones that makes the significant effort and cost of population modeling worthwhile.

Once the basics of nonlinear mixed effects modeling are understood, one must continue learning new technical skills and gaining additional experience in effectively using the results of models to make informed decisions. And equally important, one must learn to communicate those decisions clearly and authoritatively to others. After mastering this introductory text, continued learning regarding theoretical and technical skills can be enhanced by the study of other texts that deal with the topics of pharmacometrics in more depth, but are perhaps more challenging as an introduction to the field than the present text (Ette and Williams 2007; Bonate 2011). It is our hope that the reader will find the present text a useful introduction to the field, one that may be utilized by graduate students, pharmaceutical scientists, statisticians, pharmacists, engineers, and others interested in gaining a sound, practical foundation in the concepts and techniques relevant to pharmacokinetic-pharmacodynamic modeling applications with NONMEM.

Supplemental content is provided online (http://booksupport.wiley.com) to support use of this text. The content varies across chapters, but includes some datasets, programming code, and questions for application in teaching or further contemplation.

The text includes the topics the authors feel are the most critical building blocks for a comprehensive understanding of population modeling and those that should be considered in most population modeling efforts. Several topics were therefore left behind in favor of increased attention to those included. Those topics not included herein should not be viewed as unimportant, but may require further understanding or background, or the benefit of experience from a project or two. Since we anticipate the potential audience for this text to be quite diverse, we do not assume a particular background or training as a foundation for the concepts herein. Instead, we believe that pharmacometrics involves the unique merging of many disciplines, any one of which might be the initial study of focus during one's academic training. As such, concepts that rely on advanced pharmacokinetic or statistical training (for example) are explained in detail at the level at which understanding is required for the application described. And as they do in their teaching, the authors have attempted to impart as much practical wisdom and consideration of the subject matter as possible, so that the material is tangible for even the most naive student.

The authors' considerable experience in applying modeling and simulation approaches to solve real-world drug development problems comes from more than 20 years of consulting for large and small pharmaceutical and biotechnology companies. The authors' understanding of the researcher or student new to pharmacometrics comes from their personal experience in addition to more than 10 years of teaching introductory courses and workshops in population modeling. This book is written in response to the continual requests and inquiries of such students interested in further or continued study after attending an introductory population modeling workshop or course. For those who have already attended such a course, we hope that this book will fill in any gaps in understanding that may remain as a result of the necessary pace of such a workshop.

ACKNOWLEDGMENTS

The authors are indebted to numerous mentors and colleagues, most either formerly or currently at Cognigen Corporation, with whom scientific discourse over the years has improved our understanding of the field in general and many of the specific topics herein. First and foremost, we wish to thank Ted Grasela for his tremendous influence on our thought processes and whose vision for the ever-increasing importance of quantitative approaches in the future pharmaceutical industry is a natural one to which we subscribe. In addition, we wish to thank several colleagues, including Luann Phillips, David Jaworowicz, and Brenda Cirincione, for sharing generously their wisdom and perspectives over the years. In particular, the authors wish to thank Rebecca Blevins, Amir Youssef, and Lineau Vilson, Jr. for their technical assistance with tables and careful review of the text. Most of all, we are particularly grateful to Elizabeth Ludwig, whose meticulous review and thoughtful editing of this text have resulted in numerous corrections and considerable improvement to the content and message of many passages. Finally, we are grateful for the direction, patience, and professionalism of Jonathan Rose, our Editor at Wiley.

Joel S. Owen
Jill Fiedler-Kelly

REFERENCES

Bonate PL. *Pharmacokinetic-Pharmacodynamic Modeling and Simulation*. 2nd ed. New York: Springer; 2011.

Ette EI, Williams PJ. *Pharmacometrics: The Science of Quantitative Pharmacology*. Hoboken: Wiley-Interscience; 2007.

FDA Division of Pharmacometrics, Office of Clinical Pharmacology, Office of Translational Sciences, Center for Drug Evaluation and Research, Food and Drug Administration. *FDA Pharmacometrics 2020 Strategic Goals*. Available at http://www.fda.gov/AboutFDA/CentersOffices/OfficeofMedicalProductsandTobacco/CDER/ucm167032.htm#FDAPharmacometrics2020StrategicGoals. Accessed July 11, 2013.

Gobburu JVS. Pharmacometrics 2020. J Clin Pharmacol 2010;50:151S–157S.

Sheiner LB, Benet LZ. Premarketing observational studies of population pharmacokinetics of new drugs. Clin Pharmacol Ther 1985;38 (5):481–487.

CHAPTER 1

THE PRACTICE OF PHARMACOMETRICS

1.1 INTRODUCTION

In the course of the development and clinical use of pharmaceutical products, many questions arise that require quantitative answers regarding issues of safety and efficacy, dose selection, and study design and interpretation. The analytical tools available to researchers and clinicians in part define the questions that can be answered. If a useful tool is available, it must have been invented, and there must be a skilled person on hand with the knowledge to use the tool. As we practice the science of pharmacometrics, we employ computer programs as tools to work with mathematical and statistical models to address diverse questions in the pharmaceutical sciences. The pharmacometric tool-kit involves both theoretical modeling constructs as well as analysis software. The would-be analyst must learn the theory and the use of computer software, with its attendant syntax, data format and content requirements, numerical analysis methods, and output of results. Nonlinear mixed effects models have been the primary analysis framework for population-based pharmacometric modeling, and NONMEM (Beal et al. 1989–2011) has been the gold-standard software package for the implementation of these methods. The use of NONMEM in practice requires the development of procedures for efficient and quality-controlled dataset assembly, analysis, model building, hypothesis testing, and model evaluation, as will be discussed in some detail in later chapters of this text.

As pharmacometric tools have developed, the efficiency of use and breadth of applications have also increased. Though these tools have become somewhat easier to use through the development of software packages with graphical user interfaces and ancillary software products such as Perl Speaks NONMEM™ (Lindbom et al. 2004, 2005), PLT Tools (PLTSoft 2013), and MIfuns (Knebel et al. 2008), the learning curve for new pharmacometricians is still quite substantial. This introductory text is written to help with that learning curve for students of these methods.

Perhaps, the key question in regard to the use of a particular drug product is what dosing regimen (i.e., dose and frequency) is safe and effective for use in a patient population, or more specifically, for an individual patient. In the hands of a trained researcher or clinician, pharmacometric analysis can contribute arguably better insight

Introduction to Population Pharmacokinetic / Pharmacodynamic Analysis with Nonlinear Mixed Effects Models, First Edition. Joel S. Owen and Jill Fiedler-Kelly.
© 2014 John Wiley & Sons, Inc. Published 2014 by John Wiley & Sons, Inc.

than any other tool available to answer this question. The development of NONMEM and subsequent programs has dramatically enhanced the ability to evaluate sparse data; to pool data for analysis from different studies, subjects, and experimental conditions; and to simulate new circumstances of drug product use.

In traditional pharmacokinetic (PK) studies, a sufficient number of samples must be collected for the PK analysis to be performed on an individual subject basis, whether that analysis is simply the computation of noncompartmental parameters or it is the estimation of the parameters of a PK model through nonlinear regression or other numerical analysis techniques. Data are considered sparse when an insufficient number of samples are collected in an individual to perform the relevant PK analysis for the individual.

The analysis of sparse data was a prime motivating factor for the development of nonlinear mixed effect model approaches. Those patients from whom it is most difficult to obtain data are frequently the ones for whom the appropriate dose selection is most critical. Neonates and the critically ill are patient groups that are likely to differ in PK disposition from the typical healthy adult volunteers in whom most PK data are obtained. Yet, obtaining enough data for pharmacokinetic modeling on an individual patient basis may be particularly difficult in these patient groups.

Traditional therapeutic drug monitoring (TDM), with dose assessment and adjustment following the collection of one or more drug concentrations, is a simplistic approach to sparse data analysis. TDM methods generally assume a particular, previously identified underlying PK model and are not useful for developing such models. Whether a TDM assessment is made through numerical computations or by use of a nomogram, the approaches are generally limited to answering a single question, and frequently have specific assumptions about the time of the sample collection, the dosing interval of the collection, or simplifying assumptions regarding the underlying model. These approaches are efficient and clinically beneficial in application to individual patient care, but they have very limited flexibility to answer other questions related to patient care that might be better answered with more thorough pharmacometric analysis or to make use of data that might not adhere to the assumptions of the method.

The ability to develop nonlinear mixed effects models of PK data when only a few observations were collected from individuals is a significant contribution to the toolkit of the pharmacometrician. These methods were first formalized and made available through the work of Dr. Lewis Sheiner and Dr. Stuart Beal. These brilliantly creative men have provided the foundation of the field of pharmacometrics as a legacy.

1.2 APPLICATIONS OF SPARSE DATA ANALYSIS

We can consider two broad approaches for the use of sparse PK data. The first is, like the TDM methods described above, to obtain the best description possible for the PKs of a drug in an individual patient. To do so, we assume a prior model with its typical population values and parameter variances and use the patient's observed sparse samples to develop Bayesian estimates of the most likely PK model parameters for this patient. An assessment of the need for dose adjustment is made possible by this knowledge of the most likely estimates of the PK parameters for an individual patient. The patient's data and the prior model are then used to estimate a patient-specific model. The patient-specific model can be used to predict concentrations at different doses to optimize the dosage regimen for the individual. This approach represents a clinical opportunity that is not limited by the simplifying assumptions and requirements of a particular TDM approach. The substantial level of training that is required for a clinical pharmacist or physician to be able to use these tools has severely limited their application in practice. However, improved TDM software based on population PK models and Bayesian analysis continue to be developed to facilitate the knowledge gained from sparse information and to make it more accessible to the clinician (BestDose 2013). Pharmacy school curricula should increase the teaching and use of such tools to improve the ability of clinical pharmacists to individualize therapy and improve patient outcomes.

The second and perhaps most broadly used application of sparse data analysis has occurred in the drug development environment when sparse data from many individuals are pooled for the purpose of population PK model development. Such data may be pooled with or without some subjects contributing full-profile data. Combining sparse concentration–time data from many individuals means the burden of sample collection on each patient is reduced in terms of the number of needle sticks for blood draws, total blood volume collected, and perhaps in the number of clinic visits for PK sample collection. Inclusion of sparse sampling is now commonplace, as recommended by FDA, during the conduct of Phase 3 trials and provides PK data in the patients for whom the drug is intended (Guidance 1999).

Including PK data from many patients lends strength to models that attempt to account for differences in PK model parameters between individuals. Covariates, or observable patient characteristics that correlate with PK parameters, are sought to account for a portion of the differences in parameters between individuals. The greater variety and number of patients included in Phase 3 studies give broader range to the covariates observed and enhance the relevance of the PK findings for future applications of the models in other patients. The ability to analyze sparse data allows this enrichment of covariates without the additional cost required to collect and analyze the large number of samples needed for a traditional PK analysis in each individual.

Although the previous comments considering the role of sparse data analysis were made in the context of PK, these observations equally pertain to pharmacodynamics (PD), which is the study of the effects of drugs. The study of pharmacometrics includes PK, PD, and models that link these in some fashion (i.e., PK/PD models).

A very significant advantage of population approaches in pharmacometric analyses is the ability to pool data from different trials into a single analysis dataset and enrich the data for analysis beyond that which is attained from any single trial. Pooling data in this way enhances the applicability of the resulting models. Through population analysis of pooled study data, we are often able to perform analyses that would not otherwise be feasible. For instance, pooling data from Phase 1, 2, and 3 studies allow the researcher to model data following administration of the broad range of doses included in Phase 1 with the richness of covariates encountered in phases 2 and 3 to develop a more robust dataset for a broader understanding of the properties of a drug.

The development of population PK and PD models during new drug development has become routine. These models serve as a repository of knowledge about the properties of the drug. Depending upon the development plan and the issues that were studied in phase 1, some issues, such as the effect of renal impairment and drug interactions, may be assessed with sparse PK samples from Phase 3 clinical trials. Phase 1 studies may give more conclusive results regarding specific study objectives but from a far smaller group that is less representative of the treatment population. In Phase 3 data, a screening approach can be used to assess whether additional Phase 1 trials are needed to address certain regulatory and clinical PK questions.

Population models may be further used to address important development and regulatory related questions. The knowledge and understanding that may result from a model-based analysis can give insight into new study designs or conditions that can be explored through computer simulations. There is a significant move toward simulating clinical trials before actual study conduct in order to improve the probability of successful outcome through optimization of the trial design (Gobburu 2010).

Simulations can also be used to gain information about drug use in special populations such as patients with renal or hepatic impairment or the elderly. For example, dabigatran etexilate mesylate is labeled to be administered at a dose of 75 mg twice daily in patients with severe renal impairment (creatinine clearance of 15–30 mL/min). This dose was not studied in this patient population but instead resulted from conclusions based on simulations from the population PK model results (Hariharan and Madabushi 2012).

1.3   IMPACT OF PHARMACOMETRICS

The impact of pharmacometrics on regulatory and corporate decision making has been considerable. Pivotal regulatory approval decisions have been made based on pharmacometric modeling and simulation for Toradol®, Remifentanil®, Netrecor®, and Neurontin® (Gobburu 2010). According to an internal FDA survey of 42 NDAs submitted between 2000 and 2004, pharmacometric analysis contributed to both pivotal approval decisions and establishing the product label (Bhattaram et al. 2005). According to this survey, pharmacometric analyses have most commonly influenced language regarding product labeling; however, in 14 of the 42 new drug applications (NDAs) reviewed, pivotal approval decisions were made in part based on the pharmacometrics component of the application. For example, as the result of pharmacometric efforts, a two-step dosing regimen was included in the pediatric section of the product label for busulfan, though this regimen was not tested in a clinical trial. Pharmacometric analysis also influenced language regarding the initial dose recommendation in the label of pasireotide injection for the treatment of Cushing's disease (FDA Briefing Document, Pasireotide 2012).

The number and importance of regulatory decisions made by Food and Drug Administration (FDA) which rely on pharmacometric approaches continues to expand. In a survey of 198 submissions during 2000–2008, pharmacometric analyses influenced drug approval and labeling decisions for more than 60% of submissions, with increasing numbers of submissions and in more therapeutic areas in the later years (Lee et al. 2011). The importance of pharmacometric contributions at the U.S. FDA is also evidenced by the elevation of the Staff of Pharmacometrics to the level of a Division, which occurred in February 2009.

Clinical pharmacology reviewers at the FDA use a question-based review process to review the content of the Clinical Pharmacology summary (Section 2.7.2) of the NDA submission. Questions important to the PK characteristics of a new drug, the influence of intrinsic and extrinsic factors, and the exposure–response relationships for safety and efficacy are included, and the data presented in the NDA are used to answer these questions or to reveal gaps in knowledge. This process is at the heart of an evidence-based review and includes the opportunity for a pharmacometrics review. Pharmacometricians involved in the development of a new drug product need to be able to anticipate the important regulatory questions and provide adequate, quantitative data to address those issues. Such results need to be presented clearly and completely, without ambiguous language, and without errors in the writing, data summaries, or graphical presentations to achieve the appropriate impact.

Pharmacometrics is making a significant impact on corporate development decisions as well, where the support for pharmacometrics in many companies has grown from the ad hoc "clean-up and recovery" applications of the past to planned support for many drug programs (Stone et al. 2010). The majority of pharmacometric modeling activity in the corporate environment takes place in the clinical phases of development. Internal corporate decision making has been influenced by pharmacometrics activities in dose selection and dose modifications, study design, go/no-go decisions, and formulation decisions. Additionally, there has been research and expanding support for areas of decision analysis approaches such as decision models, economic models, comparator models, and utility index applications. New applications such as these will likely move the impact of pharmacometrics forward, beyond the PK and PD modeling support of product labeling. In a recent Pharmaceutical Research and Manufacturers of America (PhRMA) survey on model-based drug development, three companies estimated the financial benefit of pharmacometric activities in 2008 as cost avoidance of $1–5 million, $11–25 million, and $26–100 million (Stone et al. 2010).

Pharmacometric approaches are used to analyze PK and PD data from clinical trials to construct pharmacostatistical models that quantify PK, safety, and efficacy measures and relationships. Pharmacostatistical models differ from the traditional statistics used in drug approval that are historically and routinely performed by statisticians in industry and at FDA for the pivotal assessments of safety and efficacy. There are important differences in the approaches, though there is much benefit to be gained by the groups working together for the efficient and informed development of drug products.

1.4   CLINICAL EXAMPLE

A recent publication details the development of a population PK model for propofol in morbidly obese children and adolescents (Diepstraten et al. 2012), and serves as an example of several important aspects and advantages of the population PK approach. Propofol is commonly used for induction and maintenance of anesthesia in adults and children, but children have demonstrated a higher clearance of propofol than adults on a weight-adjusted basis (Schuttler and Ihmsen 2000).

This study was performed with frequent blood collection for measurement of propofol concentrations in each individual patient, so a traditional PK analysis would have been possible in these patients using a two-stage approach. To use a two-stage approach, one would estimate all the parameters of the model in each patient individually, and then compute the means and variances of the parameters across the individuals. This two-stage method has been shown to inflate the random effects (i.e., the variances and covariances of the parameter estimates) (Sheiner and Beal 1980, 1981, 1983; Steimer et al. 1984; Population PK Guidance 1999). The authors chose to use a population PK approach; however, since one advantage of the population approach is the ability to appropriately model the variance of model parameters across patients.

The population model approach allows the development of a model that accounts for the differences in model parameters between subjects. A covariate model can be developed that explains the intersubject variance in parameters based on a measurable covariate and a random-effect parameter. The random-effect parameter accounts for the portion of the parameter variance that is not explained by the covariate. This method is less biased for the estimates of the variance model than the two-stage approach.

In the propofol example, the authors considered age, total body weight (TBW), lean body weight (LBW), and body mass index (BMI) as predictors, or covariates, of the PK model parameters clearance and volume of the central compartment. Different functional forms were explored to describe the relationship between covariates and model parameters. For example, the relationship between TBW and clearance (Cl) was evaluated with flexible allometric scaling function. The model was expressed as:

$$Cl_i = Cl_{pop} \times \left(\frac{TBW_i}{70} \right)^z$$

where Cl_i is the value of clearance in the ith individual, Cl_{pop} is the population typical value of clearance, and z is the allometric exponent. TBW for the individual subject, TBW_i, is "centered" on the typical weight of 70 kg. The concept of centering will be explained in detail in Chapter 5. Four models were tested that differed in the value of the exponent, z, where $z = 1$, 0.75, 0.8, or y. When $z = 1$, the relationship between propofol clearance and weight is linear. When $z = 0.75$ or 0.8, this is an allometric model with fixed constants, and when $z = y$, this is an allometric model with an estimated allometric scaling exponent. Following a thorough covariate model development process, the selected model included the allometric exponent fixed to a value of 0.8. This was the only covariate parameter retained in the final model. In this example, TBW proved to be a better predictor of propofol clearance in morbidly obese children and adolescents than LBW, age, or BMI. The relationship between propofol clearance and TBW is illustrated in Figure 1.1.

Using this model, a clinician can prospectively individualize the dose for a morbidly obese child or adolescent. Since propofol is dosed by continuous infusion, the anticipated infusion rate, k_0, can be calculated based on the target steady-state concentration, C_{ss} and the individual patient clearance, Cl_i:

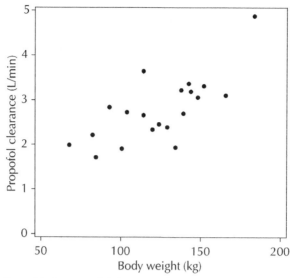

FIGURE 1.1 Propofol clearance (L/min) versus TBW (kg) in morbidly obese children and adolescents ($r = 0.721$) (Adapted from Diepstraten, et al. ADIS. Clin Pharmacokinet 2012; 51(8):547, Figure 1. Adis 2012 Springer International Publishing AG. All rights reserved. Used with kind permission from Springer Science + Business Media B.V.).

$$k_0 = C_{ss} \times Cl_i$$

This individualized dosing rate, derived from the population PK model, gives the best estimate of the anticipated dosing requirement for a patient. This example is intended to illustrate the utility of population PK models in patient care.

Pharmacometric models are built for a purpose. The development of pharmacometric models involves making implicit and explicit assumptions during the model building process. These assumptions may limit the general application of the model to new circumstances, so the user of a model must understand the data on which a model was constructed and the assumptions made in the development of the model (e.g., dose range, linearity, model structure, inter- and intrasubject variability models, patient type, disease state, concomitant medications, method of bioanalytical analysis, or pharmacodynamic measurement). This text is intended to give the reader an introduction to many of the methods and assumptions of pharmacometric model building. The emphasis will be on practical syntax and procedural process for what we believe to be typical modeling practices.

REFERENCES

Beal SL, Sheiner LB, Boeckmann AJ, Bauer RJ, editors. *NONMEM 7.2.0 Users Guides*. (1989–2011). Icon Development Solutions, Hanover, MD. Available at ftp://nonmem.iconplc.com/Public/nonmem720/guides. Accessed December 6, 2013.

BestDose, Laboratory of Applied Pharmacokinetics. 2000–2013. Laboratory of Applied Pharmacokinetics.

Bhattaram VA, Booth BP, Ramchandani RP, Beasley BN, Wang Y, Tandon V, Duan JZ, Baweja RK, Marroum PJ, Uppoor RS, Rahman NA, Sahajwalla CG, Powell JR, Mehta MU, Gobburu JVS. Impact of pharmacometrics on drug approval and labeling decisions: a survey of 42 new drug applications. AAPS J 2005; 7(3):E503–E512.

Diepstraten J, Chidambaran V, Sadhasivam S, Esslinger HR, Cox SL, Inge TH, Knibbe CA, Vinks AA. Propofol clearance in morbidly obese children and adolescents. Clin Pharmacokinet 2012; 51(8):543–551.

FDA Briefing Document, NDA 200677, Pasireotide Injection: 600 mcg, 900 mcg, Endocrinologic and Metabolic Drugs, Advisory Committee Meeting, November 7, 2012. Available at http://www.fda.gov/downloads/AdvisoryCommittees/CommitteesMeetingMaterials/Drugs/Endocrinologicand MetabolicDrugsAdvisoryCommittee/UCM326811.pdf. Accessed January 22, 2013.

Food and Drug Administration, *Guidance for Industry, Population Pharmacokinetics*. Rockville: Food and Drug Administration; 1999.

Gobburu JVS. Pharmacometrics 2020. J Clin Pharmacol 2010; 50:151S–157S.

Hariharan S, Madabushi R. Clinical pharmacology basis of deriving dosing recommendations for dabigatran in patients with severe renal impairment. J Clin Pharmacol 2012; 52:119S–125S.

Knebel K, Bergsma T, Fisher J, Georgalis G, Gibiansky L, Gillespie B, Riggs M, Gastonguay MR. Facilitating the Pharmacometrics Work-Flow with the MItools R Package. Metrum Institute, Tariffville, CT. American Conference on Pharmacometrics, Tuscon, AZ, 2008. Available at http://metruminstitute.org. Accessed December 6, 2013.

Lee JY, Garnett CE, Gobburu JVS, Bhattaram VA, Brar S, Jadhav PR, Krudys K, Lesko LJ, Li F, Liu J, Madabushi R, Marathe A, Mehrotra N, Tomoe C, Wang Y, Zhu H. Impact of pharmacometric analyses on new drug approval and labelling decisions: a review of 198 submissions between 2000 and 2008. Clin Pharmacokinet 2011; 50(10):627–635.

Lindbom L, Ribbing J, Jonsson EN. Perl-speaks-NONMEM (PsN)—a Perl module for NONMEM related programming. Comput Methods Programs Biomed 2004; 75(2):85–94.

Lindbom L, Pihlgren P, Jonsson EN. PsN-Toolkit—a collection of computer intensive statistical methods for non-linear mixed effect modeling using NONMEM. Comput Methods Programs Biomed 2005; 79(3):241–257.

PLT Tools 2013, *PLTSoft*, PLT Tools, San Francisco, CA, 2006–2013. Available at http://www.pltsoft.com. Accessed December 6, 2013.

Schuttler J, Ihmsen H. Population pharmacokinetics of propofol: a multicenter study. Anesthesiology 2000;92 (3):727–738.

Sheiner LB, Beal SL. Evaluation of methods for estimating population pharmacokinetic parameters, I. Michelis-Menten model: routine clinical data. J Pharmacokinet Biopharm 1980; 8:553–571.

Sheiner LB, Beal SL. Evaluation of methods for estimating population pharmacokinetic parameters II. Biexponential model and experimental pharmacokinetic data. J Pharmacokinet Biopharm 1981; 9:635–651.

Sheiner LB, Beal SL. Evaluation of methods for estimating population pharmacokinetic parameters III. Monoexponential model and routine clinical data. J Pharmacokinet Biopharm 1983;11:303–319.

Steimer JL, Mallet A, Golmard JL, Boisvieux JF. Alternative approaches to the estimation of population pharmacokinetic parameters: comparison with the nonlinear mixed effects model. Drug Metab Rev 1984;15:265–292.

Stone J, Banfield C, Pfister M, Tannenbaum S, Wetherington JD, Krishna R, Grasela DM. Model-based drug development survey finds pharmacometrics impacting decision making in the pharmaceutical industry. J Clin Pharmacol 2010; 50(1 Suppl):20S–30S.

CHAPTER 2

POPULATION MODEL CONCEPTS AND TERMINOLOGY

2.1 INTRODUCTION

Pharmacometrics is a science that employs mathematical models in diverse applications of the pharmaceutical sciences. These models are used to concisely summarize the behavior of large quantities of data using a small number of numerical values and mathematical expressions. Models can be used to explore mechanisms or outcomes of a system, whether that is a physiological process, drug action, disease progression, or the economic impact of a particular therapy. Hypotheses may be developed and tested with models, which may lead to changes in behaviors, such as altering a dosing regimen based on an observable or measurable feature of a patient, such as body weight.

Models may be *descriptive* or *predictive* in their applications. Descriptive models are used to characterize existing data. Predictive models enable model-based simulations for testing conditions for which observed data are not available to the researcher. Predictive model applications generally follow and build upon the development of descriptive models. Predictive models may be used for interpolation or extrapolation. Interpolation predicts new values within the range of conditions on which the model was built. For instance, exposures at a dose of 150 mg may be interpolated using a model that was built on data obtained only from doses of 100 and 200 mg. Extrapolation is used to predict values outside the range of conditions on which the model was built. These predictions may include other experimental design characteristics or other patient characteristics. Caution must be used in the extrapolation of models to new circumstances since the assumptions of the model include the nature of the data on which they were built.

The ability to simulate from pharmacometric models is a very powerful tool for informed decision making. A stated goal of the FDA has been that all future clinical trials will be designed using model-based simulations to improve the success rate in clinical trials and to improve the efficiency and probability of obtaining informative results from clinical trials (Gobburu 2010). This goal is intended to improve the historical lack of efficiency of clinical trials and the current development paradigm for new drugs that has dramatically increased research and development spending while producing fewer new drugs (Woodcock and Woosley 2008).

Introduction to Population Pharmacokinetic / Pharmacodynamic Analysis with Nonlinear Mixed Effects Models, First Edition. Joel S. Owen and Jill Fiedler-Kelly.
© 2014 John Wiley & Sons, Inc. Published 2014 by John Wiley & Sons, Inc.

TABLE 2.1 Commonly used
Greek characters in population PK

Name	Uppercase	Lowercase
Delta	Δ	δ
Epsilon	E	ε
Eta	H	η
Kappa	K	κ
Lambda	Λ	λ
Omega	Ω	ω
Sigma	Σ	σ
Theta	Θ	θ

Within the context of this book, we will use the term pharmacokinetics (PK) when discussing models of drug concentrations or amounts; pharmacodynamics (PD) when discussing models of drug effect, whether or not the underlying PKs are included as a component of the model; and PK/PD to explicitly define a joint model of PK and PD, whether that is developed simultaneously or sequentially. We use the term pharmacometrics as an umbrella to cover all models of quantitative pharmacology, including PK, PD, PK/PD, models of normal physiology, models of disease, and even pharmacoeconomics.

Many of the equations used to describe pharmacometric models have adopted letters of the Greek alphabet to represent particular model structures. Some of the more common Greek letters used are listed in Table 2.1.

2.2 MODEL ELEMENTS

A pharmacometric model is a mathematical-statistical construction that defines the relationship between dependent (e.g., concentration) and independent (e.g., time and dose) variables. The function of the model is to describe a system, as observed in a set of data. Models have several required elements: (i) a mathematical-statistical functional form (e.g., a compartmental PK model), (ii) parameters of the model, and (iii) independent variables that improve the ability of the model to describe the data. These three elements are given in the following example:

$$\text{Concentration} = f(\theta, \Omega, \Sigma, \text{weight}, \text{dose}, \text{time})$$

The dependent variable, *concentration*, is related to the prediction of a mathematical function implied by $f(...)$, having parameters, θ, Ω, Σ, and independent variable elements of *weight*, *dose*, and *time*. When we fit a particular model to a collection of data, it is the parameters of the model that we are attempting to estimate.

There are two types of pharmacometric model parameters: fixed-effect and random-effect parameters. These are elements in the mathematical-statistical model. Parameters of both types take on a single numerical value in the model, but they represent different types of *effects* or elements in the model. Fixed-effect parameters are structural parameters that take on a single value that represents the population typical value of the parameter. Random-effect parameters also take on a single value for the population, but this value represents the variance of a distribution of some element of the model. Modeling a parametric distribution requires specification of, or assumptions about, three components of the distribution: (i) the shape of the distribution, (ii) the central tendency (e.g., the median or mean), and (iii) how much the individual values of the distribution vary around the central tendency (i.e., variance). Most applications of NONMEM (Beal et al. 2011) assume that the distribution of random effect terms represented in the model is symmetric, with a central tendency of zero. Parameter distributions that are not symmetric may be modeled through various transformations in the construction of the variance model. Here the underlying elements of the distribution being estimated are symmetric, but a transformation is used to model a distribution that is not symmetric. A common example is the use of a log-linear transformation. More complex transformations may be accomplished through logit, Box–Cox, heavy tailed, or other methods (Petersson et al. 2009).

The first two components of parametric distributions are satisfied by these assumptions and are generally not specifically stated with the model. The adherence of a model to these two assumptions can be tested in the model building process and evaluated from the NONMEM output. The third component is satisfied by estimating the population variance as a random variable.

2.3 INDIVIDUAL SUBJECT MODELS

Traditional PK models for individual subject data define a set of fixed-effect parameters and mathematical structure that relate predicted concentrations to the observed data from an individual and include one level of random effect to account for the variance of the differences between observations and the model predictions (i.e., residual error). These models have a structural part, the PK model, and a statistical part, the variance model for the error between predictions and observations.

For example, the structural model for a one-compartment model with first-order oral absorption, illustrated in Figure 2.1, may be defined as follows:

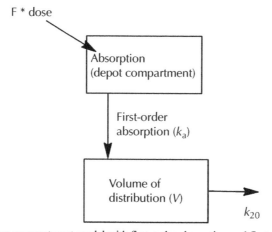

FIGURE 2.1 One-compartment model with first-order absorption and first-order elimination.

$$C_{\text{pred},i} = \frac{k_a F \, \text{Dose}}{V(k_a - k_{20})} (e^{-k_{20}t_i} - e^{k_a t_i})$$

where, k_a is the first-order absorption rate constant, V is the volume of distribution, k_{20} is the first-order elimination rate constant, and F is the fraction of the administered dose that is available for systemic absorption. $C_{\text{pred},i}$ is the model-predicted concentration at the ith timepoint after the administration of a single dose.

In order to fit the model to a set of observed data, a statistical component of the model is needed to address the difference between the predicted and the observed concentrations.

For example, the aforementioned model might be fit to the observed serial concentration data from an individual following a single dose according to the following equation:

$$C_{\text{obs},i} = C_{\text{pred},i} + \varepsilon_i$$

where, $C_{\text{obs},i}$ is the ith observed concentration in the individual, $C_{\text{pred},i}$ is the ith predicted concentration as defined earlier, and ε_i is the difference between the predicted and observed ith concentrations at time t_i. Through the model fitting process, point estimates of parameters are obtained for the structural model components: V/F, k_a, and k_{20}. These estimates define the structural PK model. One additional parameter (Ω for individual models or Σ for population models) is estimated that describes the magnitude of the variance of the ε_i values across the observations of the individual. This parameter represents the statistical component of the model. A variety of statistical error models may be used, each with different assumptions about the nature of the differences between the observed and predicted data. These model components will be discussed more fully in later sections of this chapter.

2.4   POPULATION MODELS

Population approaches in pharmacometric modeling extend traditional individual subject models by adding models that account for the magnitude, and sometimes the sources, of variability in model parameters between individuals. Population models typically include all the model components described earlier but also add parameters and submodels for the variations in structural model parameters between individuals or for variations in those parameters from one occasion to another within an individual. In population models, this leads to nested levels of random effects. The first level is at the parameter level and typically addresses the difference in the model parameters between subjects. The second level is nested within the first. In other words, there may be multiple observations at level two for each instance of the level-one effect. This second level is at the concentration level for PK models. These concepts will be discussed in further detail later in this chapter. The nesting of random effects to account for parameter differences between individuals is the greatest difference between individual and population models.

2.4.1   Fixed-Effect Parameters

Fixed-effect parameters are model elements that take on a particular, or scalar, value. They represent structural elements such as clearance or volume in a PK model. Within NONMEM, the standard nomenclature for a fixed-effect parameter is THETA(n), where n is an integer-valued index variable defining the particular element of the vector of all THETAs in the model. No value of n may be skipped in the definition of model parameters. For instance, there cannot be a THETA(2) in the model without a THETA(1). Writing the control files will be described in detail in Chapter 3, but note here that most code in the control file must generally be written in all uppercase letters. More recent versions of NONMEM allow some exceptions to this, but in this text, we will specify literal NONMEM code using all uppercase letters.

Individual subject models include fixed-effect parameters to describe the structural model (e.g., V_d/F, k_a, and k_{20} in the aforementioned example) for an individual subject's data. For instance, if we define the first-order absorption rate constant, k_a, as the first element of THETA(n), then

```
KA = THETA(1)
```

Here, THETA(1) is the element of the THETA vector used to estimate the typical value of the model parameter, k_a. The index value of THETA, n, is associated with a particular model parameter (e.g., k_a) through the code written in the control file. THETA(1) in one model might be used to model k_a, while in another model, THETA(1) might be used to model clearance.

With population models, fixed-effect parameters of the structural model define the typical values, or central tendencies, of the structural model parameters for the population. Thus, THETA(1) is an estimate of the typical value, or central tendency, of a parameter (e.g., k_a) in the population.

Fixed-effect parameters may also play a role as components of the variance model for a parameter, defining systematic, quantifiable differences in the parameter between individuals. For example, a possible submodel to describe the volume of distribution (V) might be the following:

```
V = THETA(2) + THETA(3)*WTKG
```

Here, THETA(2) defines the typical value of the portion of V that is not related to body weight. THETA(3) defines the typical value of the proportionality constant for that part of the volume that is proportional to body weight expressed in kilograms (WTKG). If this model is appropriate for a set of data, then THETA(3) explains at least some of the systematic difference in V between individuals.

Fixed effects may also be used as components of the residual variability (RV) model or for other modeling techniques. No matter how it is employed in a model, a fixed-effect parameter takes on a single, *fixed* value. This value is updated during the estimation process until convergence is obtained. The final fixed-effect parameter values of the model are those that minimize the objective function or meet other stopping criteria of the estimation method.

2.4.2   Random-Effect Parameters

For population models, random-effect parameters are components of the model that quantify the magnitude of unexplained variability in parameters (Level 1, L1) or error in model predictions (Level 2, L2). In other words, in population models, the L1 parameters quantify the magnitude of the differences of individual parameters from the typical value (i.e., parameter-level random error), and L2 parameters quantify the magnitude of differences between observed dependent variable values and their pre-dicted values from the model (i.e., observation-level random error). For individual subject models, there is only one level of random effect, L1, which describes the observation-level random error. For the remainder of this section, models will be assumed to be population models with two levels of random effects.

Random-effect parameters describe the variance of a parameter, with an assumed mean of zero, as illustrated in Figure 2.2. The distribution of a random var-iable describing the difference between subjects in a parameter (e.g., eta-clearance) is typically assumed to be symmetric but is not required to be normal.

2.4.2.1 L1 Random Effects   For population models, L1 random effects may describe the magnitude of the differences in the values of parameters between subjects (i.e., interindividual variation) or the differences between occasions within a subject (i.e., interoccasion variability).

The vector containing the individual subject estimates of the L1 random-effect parameters is termed the ETA vector (i.e., $\eta_{i,n}$). In principle, $\eta_{i,n}$ is a vector of all the ETAs in the model for an individual, i, with n being an index variable to define the elements of the vector. Each subject will have her own $\eta_{i,n}$ vector. The L1 random-effect parameter that is estimated is the variance of the distribution of $\eta_{i,n}$ values. The standard deviation of the $\eta_{i,n}$ values is ω_n. The variance is the standard deviation squared, ω_n^2. With NONMEM, the variance parameters are output in the omega matrix (Ω). If a population model is constructed with the following fixed and L1 random effects,

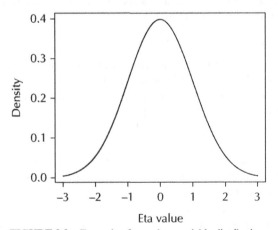

FIGURE 2.2   Example of a random-variable distribution.

```
KA    = THETA(1)*EXP(ETA(1))
K20   = THETA(2)*EXP(ETA(2))
V     = THETA(3)*EXP(ETA(3))
```

then individual subject 1 will have one vector of estimates for $\eta_{1,1}$, $\eta_{1,2}$, and $\eta_{1,3}$. Other subjects in the dataset will have their own unique combination of values of these random effects. Taken together, all of the $\eta_{i,1}$ variables will have a variance that is reported in the omega matrix (Ω) in the diagonal element row=1, column=1 ($\omega_{1,1}^2$). The $\eta_{i,2}$ variables will have a variance that is reported as the (2, 2) element ($\omega_{2,2}^2$), and so on. The omega matrix for this simple example (shown here in lower triangular form) would be given as follows:

$$\Omega = \begin{matrix} \omega_{1,1}^2 & & \\ 0 & \omega_{2,2}^2 & \\ 0 & 0 & \omega_{3,3}^2 \end{matrix}$$

where, $\omega_{1,1}^2$ is the variance of the distribution of $\eta_{i,1}$ values across all subjects and thus describes the variance of k_a for this example. In the more general case, when covariance is estimated between random variables, the values can be understood as:

$$\Omega = \begin{matrix} \text{Variance of } k_a & & \\ \text{Covariance of } k_a \text{ and } k_{20} & \text{Variance of } k_{20} & \\ \text{Covariance of } k_a \text{ and } V & \text{Covariance of } k_{20} \text{ and } V & \text{Variance of } V \end{matrix}$$

Off-diagonal terms (row i, column j) represent the covariance between two parameters, i and j. Thus, $\omega_{2,1}^2$ is the covariance between k_a and k_{20}.

The off-diagonal terms are assumed to be zero unless they are explicitly modeled. To obtain individual subject estimates of the $\eta_{n,i}$ values, a conditional estimation or post hoc Bayesian method must be used, and the individual subject values must be output in a table file in order to be accessible.

2.4.2.2 *L2 Random Effects* L2 random effects describe the magnitude of unexplained differences between the predicted and observed values of the dependent variable. Considering the dependent variable to be plasma concentration, C_p, at time, t, in the ith individual

$$C_p(t)_i = \widehat{C_p(t)}_i \pm \varepsilon_{i,j}$$

$$\text{var}(\varepsilon) = \sigma^2$$

where, $\widehat{C_p(t)}_i$ is the model-predicted value of the concentration. The distribution of differences between the observed and predicted concentrations, ε_i, is called the *residual variability* (RV). That RV is reported as the variance, σ^2. RV may arise due to errors in the measuring or recording of the dependent or independent variables, or due to the use of an inappropriate or incomplete mathematical structure of the model.

For PK data, errors in the values of the dependent variable (i.e., the concentration values) may be due to errors that arise in the sample collection, storage, or bioanalytical processes. The use of adequate quality control in clinical and laboratory procedures is necessary to minimize the magnitude of this source of error. Errors of the independent variables may arise from inaccurate recording of time of dosing or time of sample collection or inaccurate measuring of a covariate such as body weight or height. Quality control efforts in clinical practice are important to reducing errors of this type. Data processing errors that result in the incorrect assembling of analysis datasets can sometimes be a source of error. Quality control procedures in data management are key to reducing these sorts of errors.

The L2 parameters typically estimated are the variance parameters of the RV model(s). With NONMEM, these are output in the sigma matrix (Σ)—a diagonal matrix that includes one term for each random effect in the RV model, for example:

$$\Sigma = \begin{array}{cc} \sigma_1^2 & \\ 0 & \sigma_2^2 \end{array}$$

The sigma matrix is symmetric with the elements of the diagonal being the variances of the distributions of the individual errors, ε_i, and the off-diagonal elements being estimates of the correlation between the elements on the diagonal of the matrix. The aforementioned example sigma matrix is provided in lower triangular form. This correlation is generally assumed to be zero. This assumption can be tested during the model building process.

Table 2.2 shows the relationship of fixed and random effects parameters for n individuals fit by a one-compartment model with first-order absorption. Fixed

TABLE 2.2   Individual parameters of a population PK model for n subjects

	Fixed effects	
	$K_a = \theta_1$	
	$Cl = \theta_2$	
	$V = \theta_3$	

Random effects

Level 1

ID = 1	ID = 2	...	ID = n
$\eta_{1,Ka}, \eta_{1,Cl}, \eta_{1,V}$	$\eta_{2,Ka}, \eta_{2,Cl}, \eta_{2,V}$	...	$\eta_{v,Ka}, \eta_{v,Cl}, \eta_{v,V}$

Level 2

$\varepsilon_{1,1}$	$\varepsilon_{2,1}$	...	$\varepsilon_{i,1}$
$\varepsilon_{1,2}$	$\varepsilon_{2,2}$	...	$\varepsilon_{i,2}$
$\varepsilon_{1,3}$	$\varepsilon_{2,3}$	...	$\varepsilon_{i,3}$
$\varepsilon_{1,4}$	$\varepsilon_{2,4}$	...	$\varepsilon_{i,4}$
...	...	...	...
$\varepsilon_{1,j}$	$\varepsilon_{2,j}$	...	$\varepsilon_{i,j}$

effects take on a single value for the population. L1 random effects take on a single value for the subject, and L2 random effects take on a single value for each observation. This table shows representations of all the parameters of the model. The mathematical relationships that bring them together are the topic of the following sections.

2.5 MODELS OF RANDOM BETWEEN-SUBJECT VARIABILITY (L1)

Since L1 effects describe differences in parameters between subjects, these values are typically constant across the observations of a subject, and thus are *subject-level* effects. Between-subject variability, also called interindividual variability (IIV), is commonly modeled using additive, constant coefficient of variation (CCV), or exponential functions. The variability term enters the model as a component of the expression defining a model parameter, as shown for each model type presented in the following sections.

2.5.1 Additive Variation

Variation in a model parameter may be expressed with an additive function. The individual subject parameter (P_i) is a function of the typical value of the population (P) and the individual specific random effect (η_i), which is drawn from a distribution with a mean of zero and variance of ω^2. This additive model is expressed as:

$$P_i = P + \eta_i$$

A model for the PD parameter that describes the maximum effect of the drug, E_{max}, might be coded with an additive error structure as follows:

```
TVEMAX = THETA(1)          ; Population Typical Value
EMAX = TVEMAX + ETA(1)     ; Individual Specific Value
```

Here, TVEMAX represents the typical value of E_{max} in the population, and EMAX represents the individual specific estimate of E_{max} that includes a *draw* of an η_i element from the distribution of the η_1 values that have a mean of zero and an overall variance of $\omega^2_{E_{max}}$. Each subject has a single, unique value of η_1, and thus a constant value of E_{max} that is unique to the individual.

An additive error model has the same absolute magnitude of variability regardless of the value of the parameter being modeled. In the aforementioned example, small values of E_{max} have comparatively large percent coefficient of variation (%CV) compared to larger values of E_{max}, since,

$$\%CV = \frac{\text{standard deviation}}{\text{mean}} \times 100$$

Since the additive model defines a constant standard deviation at all values of the parameter, when parameters are considered at lower values (i.e., a lower mean), they will have a greater %CV than when parameters are considered at higher values. In other words, the fractional magnitude of variation decreases with increasing values of the parameter. Thus, with this error structure, the %CV is not constant.

2.5.2 Constant Coefficient of Variation

In contrast, a CCV model maintains the same fractional magnitude of variation, but the absolute magnitude increases as the value of the modeled parameter increases. The CCV model may be coded as follows.

```
TVK20=THETA(2)
K20=TVK20+TVK20*ETA(2)
```

or,

```
TVK20=THETA(2)
K20=TVK20*(1+ETA(2))
```

In this model, the standard deviation increases in proportion to increases in the parameter value. Thus, the variation of the parameter has a constant %CV across the range of parameter values.

2.5.3 Exponential Variation

Exponential models for IIV are probably the most commonly used. These models describe variability of the parameter which is log-normally distributed. A model for the $K20$ parameter, with exponential error structure is shown in the following equation. The variance of $K20$ is proportional to TVK20. Actually, $\text{Var}(K20) = \text{TVK20}^2 \times \omega_{K20}^2$.

$$K20_i = \widetilde{K20} \times e^{\eta_i}$$

$\widetilde{K20}$ represents the typical value for the population (a fixed effect), and η_i is a symmetrically distributed, random variable, with a mean of zero and variance ω_{K20}^2. $K20_i$ then is log-normally distributed if the η_i is assumed to be normally distributed. This can be coded as follows:

```
TVK20 = THETA(1)
K20   = TVK20*EXP(ETA(1))
```

In Fortran, EXP(...), is the exponential function raising e (in the case described earlier) to the power $ETA(1)$.

With the first-order estimation method of NONMEM, use of the CCV and exponential-error models result in the same population parameter estimates of the variance terms. However, if post hoc or conditional estimation methods are used, individual parameter estimates will differ, and the exponential structure can be preferable over the CCV structure because it prevents negative parameter estimates.

2.5.4   Modeling Sources of Between-Subject Variation

The value of the L1 random variable (η_i) remains constant within an individual, and thus the model parameter that depends upon it also remains constant within an individual. However, systematic or random changes in the individual subject parameters (e.g., Cl and V) may be modeled. Systematic changes in a parameter over time may represent nonstationarity of a parameter due to factors such as enzyme induction or measurable changes in a covariate that influences the parameter. For example, if the volume of distribution depends on body weight, and the PK of a drug are modeled over an extended period of treatment with a drug effective for the treatment of obesity, the volume parameter might change in a systematic way with changes in body weight.

```
V = (THETA(1)+THETA(2)*WTKG) * EXP(ETA(1))
```

In this example, the value of η_1 remains constant in an individual, but the value of V changes with each recorded change in body weight (WTKG). Random changes in the model parameter between two or more occasions can also be modeled using an occasion-specific random effect for each occasion.

When overall IIV in parameters is small, concentration-time profiles will be similar across patients. Thus, the dose amount required to achieve a certain concentration range will be similar across patients. In this case, a *one dose fits many* approach to dosing guidelines may be appropriate since the common dose will lead to similar exposure across patients.

However, when substantial variation in parameters exists, the administration of a common dosage regimen will result in considerable variation in concentration–time profiles across subjects. To the extent that the variation is systematic and explained by measurable covariates, the dose regimen may be individualized so the desired concentration range is more likely to be attained. If the IIV is large and sources are unexplained, there will be substantial differences in concentration–time profiles between subjects, and the concentration profile in a particular individual cannot be accurately anticipated.

2.6   MODELS OF RANDOM VARIABILITY IN OBSERVATIONS (L2)

The difference between dependent-variable observations (Y) and the corresponding individual specific model predictions (F) defines the residual or unexplained error at the observation level.

$$Y - F = \text{ERROR}$$

One such element of error ($\varepsilon_{i,j}$) is present for each nonmissing dependent variable in the dataset. The distribution of these L2 errors can be modeled based on similar functional forms as the random L1 variables.

2.6.1 Additive Variation

Residual error may be expressed with a single variance that is not dependent upon other factors. Error is simply added to the prediction in order to explain the deviation from the observation, and regardless of the value of the prediction or other factors, the error element (ε_i) is drawn from a distribution with a mean of zero and common variance, σ_1^2.

The additive RV model may be coded in NONMEM as follows:

```
Y = F + ERR(1)        ;appropriate for either individual or
                       population data
```

or,

```
Y = F + ETA(1)        ;appropriate for individual subject data
                       (L1 error)
```

or,

```
Y = F + EPS(1)        ;appropriate for population data (i.e.,
                       L2 error).
```

The common variance across the range of concentrations is shown in Figure 2.3.

This model is frequently appropriate to describe PK or PD data when the range of values of the dependent variable is relatively small (i.e., less than an order of magnitude). This model may be more appropriate than other models when modeling PD data that fluctuate within a small range, or for PK data when the observed concentrations fluctuate within a narrow range, such as a collection of trough values at steady state, or steady-state concentrations during intravenous infusion at a constant rate.

The selection of the appropriate RV model should be evaluated as part of the model development process. Here, we might plot the quantity *DV–F* (i.e., the residual) versus the predicted concentration and evaluate for independence of the variation from

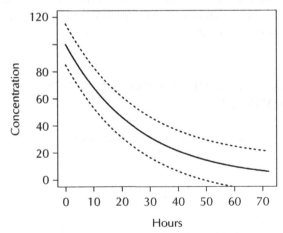

FIGURE 2.3 Concentration independence of the additive residual error model. The error lines are equidistant from the median at all values of time, though the curvature makes them appear to be smaller at higher concentrations.

the predictions. Model diagnostic plots and their interpretation in model selection will be discussed in more detail in Chapter 5.

2.6.2 Constant Coefficient of Variation

When the magnitude of error varies with the magnitude of the prediction, RV may be expressed with a CCV. Other names for this model are proportional or multiplicative RV. The variance of the error is proportional to the current prediction of the model.

This model may be coded in NONMEM as follows:

```
Y = F + F*ERR(1)
```

or,

```
Y = F * (1 + ERR(1))
```

The same alternate expressions using ERR(...), ETA(...), or EPS(...) apply as described previously for additive error.

The magnitude of the difference between the observation and the prediction is dependent upon the current value of the predicted concentration:

$$Y - F = F * \mathrm{ERR}(1)$$

Thus, at lower predicted concentrations the error variance is relatively small, while at higher predicted concentrations the error variance is relatively larger.

In Figure 2.4, the y value (e.g., concentration or effect) is plotted versus time. This example might represent the concentrations of drug following the administration of an intravenous bolus dose of drug. The solid line is the median or typical value prediction, and the dotted lines represent the upper and lower confidence limits which depend on the variance of the observation at a given concentration value.

At early times, the concentrations are greater, and the variance around the typical concentration is greater than when the concentrations are lower at later times.

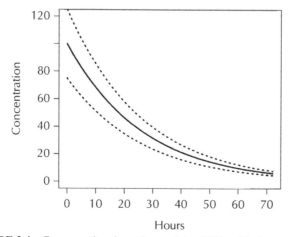

FIGURE 2.4   Concentration dependence of the CCV residual error model.

This model is commonly used to describe the error in PK data that span a wide range of concentrations, particularly when this range is greater than one order of magnitude.

2.6.3 Additive Plus CCV Model

Another model of RV that is commonly used in PK combines the two models described earlier to include an additive component and a proportional component of RV. The additive component dominates the total RV when predicted concentrations are low, while the proportional component of RV is greater as predicted concentrations increase. This model may be expressed most simply using two random variables:

```
Y = F + F*EPS(1) + EPS(2)
```

Here, EPS(1) is the random variable associated with the proportional RV, while EPS(2) is the additive portion of RV. Expressing the total RV as a %CV depends upon the current value of F, and thus is not a constant across the range of predicted values. The %CV will be greatest at the lowest concentrations and will decrease toward a minimum %CV as predicted concentrations increase (minimum %CV $= 100 \cdot \sigma_1$).

The overall %CV can be computed from this model as:

$$\%CV = 100 \times \frac{\sqrt{F^2 \times \sigma_1^2 + \sigma_2^2}}{F}$$

A useful presentation of results from this model is a small table with %CV at low, moderate, and high values of predicted concentration. The magnitude of RV as a %CV across the range of concentrations is then immediately apparent to the reader. For example, if $\sigma_1 = 0.3$ and $\sigma_2 = 10$, the RV results might be presented across a range of concentrations, at least spanning the linear range of the assay, as shown in Table 2.3.

TABLE 2.3 Presentation of residual error (%CV) for an additive plus CCV model

Predicted concentration (F)	%CV
5	202.2
10	104.4
15	73.1
20	58.3
25	50.0
30	44.8
40	39.1
50	36.1
100	31.6
150	30.7
300	30.2
1500	30.0

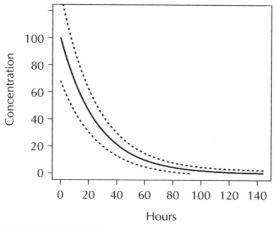

FIGURE 2.5   Residual error for the additive plus CCV model.

Clearly the variance of the additive plus CCV model is greatest as a percentage of the predicted concentration (%CV) when F is low and reaches its minimum at higher concentrations when σ_1 predominates. A plot of the additive plus CCV model is given in Figure 2.5.

Two alternate parameterizations of the additive plus CCV model may be considered. For each of these alternatives, the ratio of the two random effects is expressed using a fixed-effect parameter, thus reducing the number of random variables being estimated. This approach has a couple of advantages. One is that the reduction in the number of random variables may reduce the runtime of the model. A second advantage is that the correct individual weighted residual can be calculated.

If the two random variable expression described earlier is considered, so that σ_1^2 is associated with the proportional RV effect, and σ_2^2 is associated with the additive effect, then we can express the ratio of these two random variables as:

Alternative 1: $\theta_1 = \dfrac{\sigma_1}{\sigma_2}$

or,

Alternative 2: $\theta_1 = \dfrac{\sigma_2}{\sigma_1}$

By estimating one random-effect and one fixed-effect parameter, the additive plus CCV model may be fully specified. For both of the alternatives, a lower bound of zero should be placed on the value of θ_1.

For Alternative 1, the RV at a predicted concentration value may be computed as

$$\%CV = 100 \times \sqrt{\frac{\sigma_2^2}{F^2} + \theta_1^2 \times \sigma_2^2}$$

For Alternative 2, the RV at a predicted concentration value may be computed as

$$\%\text{CV} = 100 \times \sqrt{\sigma_1^2 + \frac{\theta_1^2}{F^2} \times \sigma_1^2}$$

The implementation of additive plus CCV error models using one fixed-effect and one random-effect parameters, as well as an alternative parameterization using two thetas and a single random effect term fixed to a value of 1 is provided in Section 5.6.2.1.

2.6.4   Log-Error Model

While there are other RV models one might consider, the final model we will discuss is the log-error model. This model assumes that the variance of the residual error increases in a log-linear fashion with increases in predicted concentration. The model is implemented using ln-transformed (i.e., natural log transformation) data as the dependent variable. The model is then coded as an additive error with the ln-predicted concentrations:

```
Y = LOG(F) + EPS(1)
```

An important consideration is that one must not attempt to compute $LOG(F)$ when F might be zero or negative since this would return a numerical error. Methods to address this and other model considerations are addressed in Section 3.5.3.1.

2.6.5   Relationship Between RV Expressions and Predicted Concentrations

Consideration of the relationship between predicted values and RV is helpful in selection of the most appropriate RV model for a given application. These relationships are shown in Figure 2.6 for the additive, CCV, additive plus CCV, and log-error models of RV.

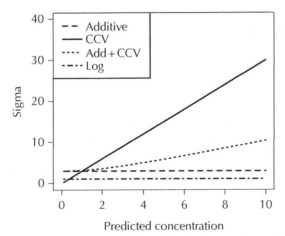

FIGURE 2.6   Relationship of sigma, the SD of the residual variability, with predicted concentration for various residual error models.

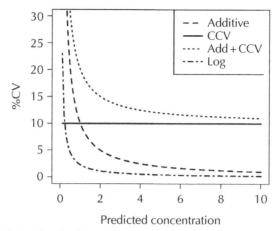

FIGURE 2.7   Relationship of residual variance (%CV) with predicted concentration for various residual error models.

The expression of variability as a standard deviation (sigma) shows a constant variance for the additive and log residual error models, regardless of concentration value. In contrast, the CCV and additive plus CCV models show an increase in sigma with increasing predicted concentration. The major difference between the CCV and additive plus CCV models has to do with their behavior at the lowest concentrations. Note that the CCV model estimate of sigma becomes close to zero as the predicted concentration goes to zero, while the estimate of sigma with the additive plus CCV model levels off at a particular (non-zero) level of sigma at the lowest concentrations, close to zero.

Figure 2.7 demonstrates the relationship between the relative variance (%CV) and concentration for these same models. Expressed as a %CV, the CCV model (as the name implies) is associated with a constant %CV of RV, regardless of predicted concentration. However, each of the other RV models (i.e., the additive, the additive plus CCV, and the log-error model) is associated with a relatively higher %CV of RV at lower concentrations which decreases with increasing predicted concentration and eventually flattens out to a more constant value with high concentrations.

The selection of model depends upon the given set of data. The model building process should include an assessment of the most appropriate model for the given set of data and assumptions.

2.6.6 Significance of the Magnitude of RV

Quantification of the magnitude of RV is an important model development activity since this magnitude accounts for the seemingly random changes in concentrations of a drug in a patient. One impact of RV is illustrated in Figure 2.8.

Concentrations of drug with large RV will not vary in a consistently predictable way across time. A patient may have substantially different concentrations at the same time-after-dose across dosing intervals, even in the presence of a consistent

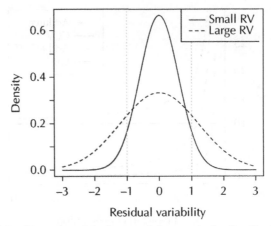

FIGURE 2.8 Illustration of the impact of the magnitude of residual variability.

dosing regimen. Substantial *random* changes in concentration may even occur within a dosing interval. For a drug with a narrow range of therapeutic concentrations, this may preclude the utility of the drug.

In contrast, if RV is small for a drug with linear and stationary PK, concentrations will be relatively consistent at similar time-after-dose across dosing intervals and will follow a more predictable profile within a dosing interval. If RV is low, concentrations will be reasonably predictable on a given dosing regimen, and a stable dosing regimen will keep concentrations within a desired concentration range.

2.7 ESTIMATION METHODS

Construction of pharmacometric models requires the statement of the model in terms of parameters to be estimated both for their value and a measure of uncertainty. The estimation of parameters of nonlinear mixed effects models requires advanced computer applications of numerical analysis techniques. We will not deal with the details of the numerical methods in this introductory text, but will introduce some basic concepts regarding the use of various estimation methods. These are described in Chapter 3.

2.8 OBJECTIVE FUNCTION

The traditional estimation methods of NONMEM use an objective function to compute a numerical value that can be used to guide the process of parameter estimation and to compare models in a sequential model building process. In some fashion, the objective function quantifies the fit of the model to the data. Changes in the value of the objective function following iterative changes in parameter values provides a stopping criterion, identifying the point at which changes to model parameters no longer lead to substantive improvement in model fit. The objective function is computed with each iteration of the parameter estimation and continues until a minimum value of the objective function is reached. These concepts will be discussed more in Chapters 5 and 6.

2.9 BAYESIAN ESTIMATION

Bayesian estimation is an approach to analyzing data that can combine prior knowledge (e.g., a population PK model and its parameters) with present data to improve the understanding of the modeled process in individuals. This is achieved by computing the most likely parameter values appropriate to the individual, given her data and the assumed prior population model. Individual parameter estimates can be used for many purposes that include guiding clinical treatment decisions, providing exposure estimates for PK/PD modeling applications, assessing exposure in individuals from whom only limited concentration data are available, and many others. Applications of individual parameter estimates will be discussed separately in Chapter 7.

REFERENCES

Beal SL, Sheiner LB, Boeckmann AJ, Bauer RJ, editors. *NONMEM 7.2.0 Users Guides (1989–2011)*. Icon Development Solutions, Hanover, MD; 2001. Available at ftp://nonmem.iconplc.com/Public/nonmem720/guides. Accessed December 13, 2013.

Gobburu JVS. Pharmacometrics 2020. J Clin Pharm 2010;50:151S–157S.

Petersson KJF, Hanze E, Savic RM, Karlsson MO. Semiparametric distributions with estimated shape parameters. Pharm Res 2009;26 (9):2174–2185.

Woodcock J, Woosley R. The FDA critical path initiative and its influence on new drug development. Annu Rev Med 2008;59:1–12.

CHAPTER 3

NONMEM OVERVIEW AND WRITING AN NM-TRAN CONTROL STREAM

3.1 INTRODUCTION

After describing the main components of the NONMEM system, this chapter will provide a detailed explanation of the essential elements of coding an NM-TRAN control stream. Since NONMEM is run in batch mode (i.e., programs or control streams are written and submitted for execution all at once and not line-by-line), the coding of the NM-TRAN control stream is the fundamental building block upon which the rest of the system is built. Therefore, a solid understanding of how to code simple control streams is required before building up to more and more advanced and complicated examples. This chapter will describe many of the common control stream records, explain the various options that may be used with each, and provide examples of typical control stream statements.

3.2 COMPONENTS OF THE NONMEM SYSTEM

The NONMEM system consists of three major program components: NM-TRAN, the NonMem TRANslator; PREDPP, subroutines for the PREDiction of Population Pharmacokinetic models and parameters; and NONMEM, the engine for the estimation of NONlinear Mixed Effect Models. NONMEM, the heart of the program, consists of FORTRAN subroutines that govern the estimation of parameters of nonlinear mixed effects models. As such, NONMEM is by no means limited in its application to population and individual pharmacokinetic (PK) and pharmacokinetic/pharmacodynamic (PK/PD) applications. That being said, the PREDPP library of specific subroutines provides the pharmacometrician with access to multiple prewritten subroutines for many common and typical PK models, all of which can be *customized* to meet the individual needs of a particular compound to facilitate model development. The *language* we as modelers use is provided in NM-TRAN, the

Introduction to Population Pharmacokinetic / Pharmacodynamic Analysis with Nonlinear Mixed Effects Models, First Edition. Joel S. Owen and Jill Fiedler-Kelly.
© 2014 John Wiley & Sons, Inc. Published 2014 by John Wiley & Sons, Inc.

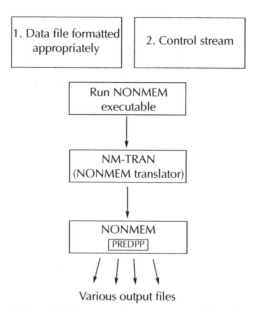

FIGURE 3.1   Schematic illustrating the components of the NONMEM system.

framework for the specification of the models, as well as the interaction with the system as a whole (Beal et al. 1989).

While many interfaces and *helper* programs have been developed over the years to facilitate interactions with NONMEM, the NONMEM system itself can be thought of as a batch programming language. An NM-TRAN control stream is written and executed by the modeler. This control stream, in turn, calls the NONMEM dataset file (described in detail in Chapter 4) and the appropriate subroutines to complete execution of the specified model and return various files for review. There is no graphical user interface to *open* and no windows or drop-down boxes available from which to select model features or options. For this reason, the learning curve for proficiency with the use of NONMEM is a bit steeper than for many other programs that allow for a trial-and-error clicking approach. This text is intended to help ease that learning curve.

Figure 3.1 graphically depicts the interactions of some of the main components of the NONMEM system. The NM-TRAN control stream, along with a separate data file, is created by the user. Typically, when the NONMEM executable is called, the user files are passed through NM-TRAN first, which parses each for syntax and formatting issues and then converts each file to a version appropriate for NONMEM. NM-TRAN also calls the appropriate FORTRAN subroutines, based on the specification of the model, and sends them to the FORTRAN compiler for compiling and loading. If PREDPP is also called (based on the control stream specifications), the generated PK and ERROR subroutines, along with the NONMEM-ready control file and data file, are then passed through NONMEM for estimation or other steps based on additional specifications in the control stream. Various NONMEM output files are generated, some by default and others optionally, again based on the specifications in the control stream (Beal et al. 1989).

The focus of the remainder of this chapter will be on the development of the NM-TRAN control stream, the program or instruction file, in which the model and various options for its estimation and requested output are specified. The reader is referred to User's Guide IV: NM-TRAN or the online help files for additional information about each of the records and options described herein (Beal et al. 1989). The information provided in this chapter will aim to provide the novice user with the essential information needed to understand how to write a typical NM-TRAN control stream for the estimation of a simple PK model.

3.3   GENERAL RULES

The NM-TRAN control stream file is an ASCII text file, usually written with an available text editing tool, such as Microsoft WordPad®, Notepad, emacs, vi, or other NONMEM-friendly text-editing applications. Since the file must be saved as a plain ASCII text file, editing in a word processing program, such as Microsoft Word®, is possible, but not recommended, as the modeler must always remember to change the save settings in order to save to a plain (DOS) text file. The NM-TRAN control stream file is made up of a series of defined records and blocks of code, each of which starts with a particular string of characters following a dollar sign ("$"), which denotes the start of a new record or block of code to the program. For all record identifiers, a shorthand version of the record identifier name is available, consisting of at least the first three characters of the record or block name (e.g., $PROBLEM can be abbreviated to $PROB or even $PRO). Within the control stream file, blank spaces are allowed both between records and between options within a particular record. Although more recent versions of NONMEM now allow the use of tab characters in certain circumstances (where previously not allowed), it has been the author's experience that it is safer to simply avoid the use of tabs in control streams (or data files). In the cases where syntax rules and options have changed over time with subsequent versions of NONMEM, it will be specifically noted.

Each record in the control stream can be a maximum of 160 characters in length. For versions of NONMEM prior to 6.2, records of no more than 80 characters in length were allowed. Records that must extend beyond the allowable limit can continue after pressing the enter key. This rule also applies to the individual lines of code within a block statement, such as the $PK or $ERROR block. In these sections of code, equations must be broken up into parts, each less than the allowable line length and then combined together, as appropriate, in a separate equation(s). With NONMEM version 7.2 and higher, mixed case (a combination of upper and lower case) is permitted within the control stream. With versions prior to 7.2, however, all portions of the control stream, with the exception of file names, must be in all upper-case letters. Comments are permitted anywhere within the control stream, and are prefaced with a semicolon. Any text between a semicolon and the end of the line is considered a comment and not read by NM-TRAN. For early versions of NONMEM (prior to 7.0), a return was required after the last character in the control stream in order for the last record to be recognized.

A control stream is provided in the following example for reference and to visualize the file elements to be discussed throughout this chapter. As described earlier, the statements in this example are not all-inclusive, nor are all the options specified in the records shown; this is merely an example of a typical PK model specification using NM-TRAN.

Example NM-TRAN control stream for a simple one-compartment PK model

```
$PROBLEM Example NM-TRAN Control Stream for a 1-cmt Model
$DATA /home/pathtomydatsaset/datafilename.dat   IGNORE=#
$INPUT ID TIME AMT DV CMT EVID MDV
$SUBROUTINES ADVAN2 TRANS2
$PK

TVCL = THETA(1)
CL = TVCL * EXP(ETA(1))
TVV = THETA(2)
V = TVV * EXP(ETA(2))
TVKA = THETA(3)
KA = TVKA

; scale predictions based on dose (mg) and Cp (ng/mL)
S2 = V/1000

$ERROR

Y = F*(1 + EPS(1))

$THETA    (0, 3.9)          ; Clearance (L/h)
          (0, 52.1)         ; Volume (L)
          (0, 0.987)        ; Absorption Rate (1/h)

$OMEGA    (0.09)     ; IIV on CL (use 30%CV as init est)
          (0.16)     ; IIV on V  (use 40%CV as init est)

$SIGMA    (0.04)     ; RV (use 20%CV as init est)

; Use conditional estimation with interaction
$EST METHOD=1 INTER MAXEVAL=9999 PRINT=5 MSFO=example.msf
$COVAR PRINT=E

$TABLE ID IME AMT CMT ONEHEADER NOPRINT FILE=example.tbl
```

3.4 REQUIRED CONTROL STREAM COMPONENTS

3.4.1 $PROBLEM Record

Typically, the first record of an NM-TRAN control stream, the $PROBLEM record, is a required record that serves as an identifier for the control stream as a whole, allowing the user a space to label the file descriptively for later reference and identification purposes. The text that the user writes following the $PROBLEM record identifier is copied to the output file as a title, of sorts, for that file and to link together the problem specification and the results. If your practice is to modify or edit your most recent control stream to the specifications of the new model you wish to run (as opposed to starting with a blank page for each new control stream you write), it is good practice to train yourself to always start with modification of the $PROBLEM record to match your new purpose, before going on to the other required changes. A systematic method for describing models and naming files is helpful in maintaining some sense of organization as you add more and more complexity to your models. Another good practice involves adding a more complete header using commented text (i.e., following a semicolon ";") to the top of each new control stream, to be filled in before saving and running the file; such a header might include the control stream author's name, a date/time stamp, a section where the author can describe the purpose of the control stream, and the data file to be used.

3.4.2 The $DATA Record

The $DATA record is used to indicate to NM-TRAN where to find the associated data file for the problem. The relative or complete filepath is provided, along with the data file name. Note that the appropriate specification of the filepath is based on operating system/environment-dependent syntax. The examples in this text use the forward slash "/" symbol to denote the separation between various subdirectories, as would be appropriate for a UNIX- or Linux-based system. Many Windows-based systems will use a backward slash "\" for this purpose and filepath specifications will begin with the drive (e.g., *C:\My Documents*...). See the example control stream in Section 3.3 for a typical $DATA record specification.

3.4.2.1 Subsetting the Dataset with $DATA Additional options (i.e., IGNORE and ACCEPT) for subsetting the data for use with a particular model are also available with the $DATA record. The simplest method of subsetting the dataset requires modification to the data file itself, in conjunction with the use of a particular version of the IGNORE option of $DATA. To use this particular feature of the IGNORE option, a character is inserted in the left-most position of a particular dataset record intended for exclusion. The inserted character value (most ASCII characters are fine to use, except ";") is placed on only those records selected for exclusion, and the records not selected for exclusion are left unchanged. Typically a "#," "@," or "C" is used for this purpose. If the "#" is used, NM-TRAN's default behavior is to exclude those records containing this value in the first column and no extra option on $DATA is required. However, if a different character is used (e.g., "@"), the $DATA record would read:

```
$DATA mydatafilepath_and_name IGNORE=@
```

where "@" would be whatever character was used in the dataset to indicate such exclusions. In this case, as NM-TRAN reads in the datafile, all records with an "@" in the first column will be skipped over and not retained in the NONMEM version of the datafile used for processing and estimation of the model at hand. Such exclusions from the datafile can be confirmed by viewing the FDATA output file and also by checking the number of records, subjects, and observation records reported in the report file output (see Chapter 6 for additional information on where to find this information in the output file).

If the exclusions to be tested are recognized at the time of dataset creation, the inclusion of an additional column or columns containing exclusion indicator flags may be considered. Suppose a variable called EXCL is created with values of 0, 1, and 2, where 0 indicates that the record should not be excluded, and 1 and 2 indicate different reasons for possible exclusion. To take advantage of this data field, another type of IGNORE option is available whereby the $DATA record may be written as follows:

```
$DATA mydatafilepath_and_name IGNORE=(EXCL.EQ.1)
```

or

```
$DATA mydatafilepath_and_name IGNORE=(EXCL.EQ.2)
```

or

```
$DATA mydatafilepath_and_name IGNORE=(EXCL.GE.1)
```

This type of conditional IGNORE option may be used in conjunction with the IGNORE=# type of exclusion described previously to exclude both records with a "#" in the first column in addition to those records that meet the criteria contained within the parentheses in the aforementioned examples. In this case, the IGNORE option would be included twice, perhaps as follows:

```
$DATA mydatafilepath and name IGNORE=# IGNORE=(EXCL.EQ.1)
```

While these options are clearly quite useful to the modeler, the real advantage lies in the fact that the dataset need not be altered to accomplish this latter type of subsetting, allowing different subsets of the data to be specified quite simply with different control stream statements. The conditional IGNORE option may be used with any variable or variables (i.e., data items) read in on $INPUT, including those not specifically created to deal with possible exclusions (in addition to those dropped with the "=DROP" option, see Section 3.4.3). In this way, the data file may be subset to include, for example, only those subjects from a particular study, only those subjects weighing more than a certain value, or even to exclude those subjects with a particular level of disease severity. Another important use of this feature is to temporarily exclude one or more observations in order to assess their influence on the model fit, as when a small number of concentrations are associated with high weighted residuals during model development. To use a single conditional argument, the syntax is as described earlier:

```
$DATA mydatafilepath_and_name IGNORE=(STDY.GE.2000)
```

NONMEM also allows more than one conditional argument to be used to express more complicated exclusion criteria with the IGNORE option; however, if more than one conditional argument is used, the conditions are assumed to be connected by an ".OR." operator. No other operator may be specified with this option. Therefore, if one wishes to exclude those records where a subject's weight is greater than or equal

TABLE 3.1 Desired inclusions and exclusions of data, based on study number and disease severity

		Study	
		101	Not 101
Disease	<2		
severity	≥2	■■■	

to 100 kg OR a subject is from Study 301 from the dataset for estimation, the $DATA record may be specified as follows:

```
$DATA mydatafilepath_and_name IGNORE=(WTKG.GE.100,
    STDY.EQ.301)
```

Note that the additional conditional statement is specified within the same set of parentheses, followed by a comma. In fact, up to 100 different conditional arguments may be specified in this same way with a single IGNORE option.

The converse of the IGNORE option is also available—the ACCEPT option. ACCEPT may be specified with conditional arguments in the same way as IGNORE, also assuming an ".OR." operator when multiple conditions are specified. Similar to IGNORE, the ACCEPT option may be used in conjunction with the IGNORE="#" option, but may NOT be used in conjunction with an IGNORE option specifying conditional arguments. To illustrate the use of this option, if one wishes to include only those records where weight is less than 100 kg OR the study is not 301 in the dataset for estimation, while still excluding those records with a "#" in the first column, the $DATA record may be specified as follows:

```
$DATA mydatafilepath_and_name IGNORE=#
    ACCEPT=(WTKG.LT.100, STDY.NE.301)
```

Now, there may be situations where the easiest and most intuitive way to envision the subsetting rules is with an ".AND." operator. In those cases, consider the following helpful trick to coding an implied ".AND." using the available implied ".OR." If one wishes to *exclude* the subjects in Study 101 AND with disease severity greater than or equal to level 2 (i.e., exclude STDY.EQ.101.AND.DXSV.GE.2—a statement that would not be allowed by NONMEM in an IGNORE option due to the ".AND."), as shown in Table 3.1 where the desired exclusion is indicated in black, this may be coded with the following $DATA record:

```
$DATA mydatafilepath_and_name ACCEPT=(STDY.NE.101,
    DXSV.LT.2)
```

3.4.2.2 $DATA CHECKOUT Option Another option some users may find helpful with $DATA is the CHECKOUT option. When this option is specified on the $DATA record, the CHECKOUT option indicates that the user desires to simply perform a check of the dataset based on the corresponding data file, $INPUT, and other records in the control stream. With this option, no tasks in the control stream other than $TABLE and $SCAT are performed (see Section 3.9). Furthermore, items requested in $SCAT should not include WRES which will not be computed with such a checkout run. Using the dataset only, table files and scatterplots will be produced, if requested, in order to allow the user to confirm the appropriateness of the dataset contents with regard to how it is read into NONMEM via $INPUT.

3.4.3 The $INPUT Record

The $INPUT record is used to indicate how to read the data file, by specifying what variables are to be found in the dataset and in what order. After $INPUT, the list of variables is specified, corresponding to each column of the dataset, using reserved names for variables where appropriate (see Chapter 4 for a complete description of the required variables for NONMEM and PREDPP). The list of variables to be read can include no more than 50 data items; with NONMEM versions 6 and earlier, only up to 20 data items were allowed in $INPUT. Since it is not uncommon to create a master dataset containing all of the relevant variables for modeling as well as many others that may be needed only to comply with regulatory submission standards, datasets may often contain more than the 50 (or 20) allowable fields. However, there is an $INPUT record feature that can be employed to accommodate this situation. If the data file includes more than the allowable maximum number of variables, certain variables not needed for the particular model estimation may be dropped by specifying their name in the list with an "=DROP" modifier after the variable name. So, if the dataset contains many demographic variables, only a small handful of which are to be used in a given model, the others in the list may be specified with the "=DROP" feature. Any conditional subsetting requested via the IGNORE or ACCEPT options of $DATA is performed prior to dropping variables via $INPUT, so even those variables intended to be dropped may be used to specify data subsets to NM-TRAN.

In a similar way, if a name other than the reserved variable name is preferred for a particular variable (e.g., DOSE instead of the reserved term AMT), the nickname feature used to drop variables can also be used to assign an alternate variable name; in this case, the variable AMT would be specified as AMT=DOSE. Use of this feature ensures that the variable is read in correctly with the reserved name and that the alternate name is used in any output referring to this field. Furthermore, if characters such as "/" or "-" are used within a date format, the DATE variable must be read in with the "=DROP" modifier, although it will, in fact, *not* be dropped at all, but read by NM-TRAN and used in conjunction with the TIME variable to compute the relative time of events. The specific options for reading in date and time information are discussed in detail in Chapter 4.

3.5 SPECIFYING THE MODEL IN NM-TRAN

3.5.1 Calling PREDPP Subroutines for Specific PK Models

When PK models are to be specified, the library of specific subroutines available in PREDPP may be utilized. The $SUBROUTINES record in the NM-TRAN control stream identifies to PREDPP which subroutines to use based on the model structure and desired parameterization. A typical $SUBROUTINES record consists of the choice of a particular ADVAN and a particular TRANS subroutine, each identified by number. For example, the ADVAN1 subroutine contains the appropriate equations for a one-compartment model with first-order elimination, the ADVAN2 subroutine contains the appropriate equations for a one-compartment model with first-order absorption and elimination (thus allowing for oral or subcutaneous dosing), the ADVAN3 subroutine contains the appropriate equations for a two-compartment model with first-order elimination, the ADVAN4 subroutine contains the appropriate equations for a two-compartment model with first-order absorption and elimination, the ADVAN11 subroutine (numbered so because it was added to the PREDPP library years after the core set of ADVANs1–10 were developed) contains the appropriate equations for a three-compartment model with first-order elimination, and the ADVAN12 subroutine contains the appropriate equations for a three-compartment model with first-order absorption and elimination. While this chapter focuses on the specific ADVANs, the more general linear and nonlinear ADVANs are discussed in Chapter 9. Here, the reader is referred to User's Guide VI: PREDPP or the online help files for more detailed and specific information about each of the available subroutines in the PREDPP library (Beal et al. 1989).

While the specific ADVAN routines define the particular model to be employed, the corresponding TRANS subroutines indicate how the parameters of the models should be transformed, or in other words, which parameterization of the model is preferred. TRANS1 subroutines, which may be used with any of the specific ADVAN routines discussed earlier, parameterize the models in terms of rate constants for the first-order transfer of drug from compartment to compartment, or k_{10}, k_{12}, k_{13} types of parameters. TRANS2 subroutines, also available with any of the specific ADVAN subroutines described so far, parameterize the models in terms of clearance and volume terms. Alternative TRANS subroutines are available for select ADVANs, offering additional options for parameterizations in terms of clearance and volume parameters or exponents (i.e., α, β, γ, and so on).

It is this combination of the selected ADVAN and TRANS subroutines on the $SUBROUTINES record that determines which required parameters must be defined, and which additional parameters are recognized and also available for estimation. Table 3.2 provides the required and additional parameters available for select ADVAN and TRANS combinations. For example, with the ADVAN2 and TRANS2 subroutines selected on the $SUBROUTINES record, the required parameters include *CL*, *V*, and *KA*. Additional parameters including *F1*, *S2*, *ALAG1*, and others are also available and may be assigned and estimated, if appropriate. If the ADVAN3 TRANS4 combination is specified in $SUBROUTINES, then *CL*, *V2*, *Q*, and *V3* parameters would be the required parameters and a variety of additional optional parameters would be available as well. As described in Section 3.5.2, equations must then be written to define each of the required parameters and any additional parameters used. The reader is referred again to User's Guide VI: PREDPP or the online help files for the relationships between the required parameters of each of the ADVAN and TRANS subroutines (Beal et al. 1989).

TABLE 3.2 Required and additional parameters for select ADVAN and TRANS subroutine combinations

ADVAN subroutine	TRANS subroutine	Required parameters	Select additional parameters
ADVAN1	TRANS1	K	S1, S2, F1, R1, D1, ALAG1
	TRANS2	CL, V	
ADVAN2	TRANS1	K, KA	S1, S2, S3, F1, F2, R1, R2, D1, D2, ALAG1, ALAG2
	TRANS2	CL, V, KA	
ADVAN3	TRANS1	K, K12, K21	S1, S2, S3, F1, F2, R1, R2, D1, D2, ALAG1, ALAG2
	TRANS3	CL, V, Q, VSS	
	TRANS4	CL, V1, Q, V2	
	TRANS5	AOB, ALPHA, BETA	
	TRANS6	ALPHA, BETA, K21	
ADVAN4	TRANS1	K, K23, K, KA	S1, S2, S3, S4, F1, F2, F3, R1, R2, R3, D1, D2, D3,
	TRANS3	CL, V, Q, VSS, KA	ALAG1, ALAG2, ALAG3
	TRANS4	CL, V2, Q, V3, KA	
	TRANS5	AOB, ALPHA, BETA, KA	
	TRANS6	ALPHA, BETA, K32, KA	
ADVAN10	TRANS1	VM, KM	S1, S2, F1, R1, D1, ALAG1
ADVAN11	TRANS1	K, K12, K21, K13, K31	S1, S2, S3, S4, F1, F2, F3, R1, R2, R3, D1, D2, D3,
	TRANS4	CL, V1, Q2, V2, Q3, V3	ALAG1, ALAG2, ALAG3
	TRANS6	ALPHA, BETA, GAMMA, K21, K31	
ADVAN12	TRANS1	K, K23, K32, K24, K42, KA	S1, S2, S3, S4, S5, F1, F2, F3, F4, R1, R2, R3, R4, D1,
	TRANS4	CL, V2, Q3, V3, Q4, V4, KA	D2, D3, D4, ALAG1, ALAG2, ALAG3, ALAG4
	TRANS6	ALPHA, BETA, GAMMA, K32, K42, KA	

3.5.2   Specifying the Model in the $PK Block

3.5.2.1 Defining Required Parameters   With the appropriate subroutines called, the variables of the model are the next item to be specified in the control stream. This includes the assignment of thetas and etas to the required (and additional) parameters based upon the selected ADVAN and TRANS subroutine combination, and the random-effect terms for interindividual variability in PK parameters. These are specified and assigned within the $PK block. The $PK block (and other block statements to be discussed subsequently) differs from the NM-TRAN records described thus far in that following the block identifier ($PK, in this case), a block of code or series of program statements is expected before the next record or block identifier. With NM-TRAN record statements (such as $PROB, $DATA, and $INPUT), multiple statements are not allowed prior to the next record or block, although a single record may sometimes continue onto multiple lines, as is often the case with $INPUT. New variables may also be created and initialized within the $PK block and may be based upon those data items read in with the $INPUT record and found in the dataset specified in the $DATA record. Within the block, FORTRAN syntax is used for IF-THEN coding, variable assignment statements, and so forth.

In the section of code from the $PK block in the following example, the typical value of each parameter is specified, and in a separate statement, the interindividual variability (IIV) is specified for estimation on the drug clearance and the volume of distribution. A common notation has been adopted by many pharmacometricians to denote typical value parameters and to distinguish them from individual subject-specific estimates. The variable name used to denote a typical value parameter is the parameter name, prefaced by the letters *TV*. Therefore, the variable name denoting the typical value of clearance would commonly be referred to as *TVCL*, whereas *CL* would denote the individual-specific value. Similarly, the typical value of volume would commonly be referred to by the variable name *TVV*. It is important to note, however, that such typical value parameter names are not recognized by NM-TRAN as referring to any specific predefined value (as a reserved name variable does) but are merely a convention used by many NONMEM modelers.

Example partial $PK block

```
$PK

TVCL = THETA(1)
CL = TVCL * EXP(ETA(1))

TVV = THETA(2)
V = TVV * EXP(ETA(2))
```

Clearly, these clearance and volume assignments could have been more simply stated as:

```
CL = THETA(1) * EXP(ETA(1))
V = THETA(2) * EXP(ETA(2))
```

The reason for utilizing a separate statement to define the typical value parameter (as in the *Example partial $PK block*) is twofold: (i) by defining TVCL and TVV as parameters, estimated values of each parameter (for each subject) are now available for printing to a table output file for use in graphing or other postprocessing of the results of this model and (ii) setting up the code in this standard way allows for easier modification as the equations for TVCL and TVV become more complicated with the addition of covariate effects. For example, to extend the model for clearance to include the effect of weight, one might simply edit the equation for TVCL to

```
TVCL = THETA(1) * (WTKG/70)**THETA(3)
```

3.5.2.2 Defining Additional Parameters
With each ADVAN TRANS subroutine combination, a variety of additional parameters may be defined, if relevant, given the model and dataset content. The additional parameters typically include an absorption lag time, a relative bioavailability fraction, a rate parameter for zero-order input, a duration parameter of that input, and a scaling parameter. With all additional parameters, the parameter name is followed by a number, indicating the compartment to which the parameter applies. Given the model, certain parameters are, therefore, allowed (or definable) in certain compartments and not in others. Table 3.2 provides a detailed description of which additional parameters are defined for each of the common model structures.

If ADVAN2, ADVAN4, or ADVAN12 are selected, allowing for input of drug into a depot compartment, an absorption lag time parameter may also be defined and estimated. With these subroutines, a variable, *ALAG1*, may be specified within the $PK block, defined as the time (in units of time consistent with the TIME variable in the dataset) before which drug absorption begins from the depot or first compartment. If the time of the first sample is well beyond the expected absorption lag time, this parameter may also be fixed to a certain value instead of being estimated.

A relative bioavailability fraction may be estimated for most model compartments, defining the fraction of drug that is absorbed, transferred to, or available in a given compartment. This parameter is denoted *F1*, *F2*, or *F3*, and, although typically constrained to be between 0 and 1, may be estimated to be greater than 1, if appropriate and defined relative to another fraction (see the following example). The default value for this parameter is 1.

```
F1 = 1                          ; initialize F1 to 1 in all
                                subjects/doses (although
                                technically not necessary
                                since 1 is the default value)

IF (DOSE.LE.5) F1 = THETA(4)    ; for doses less than or
                                equal to 5, estimate a
                                relative bioavailability
                                fraction using THETA(4),
                                which may be constrained
                                to be between 0 and 1, if
                                appropriate, or allowed to
                                be estimated to be greater
                                than 1 (for this example,
                                the estimate of THETA(4) is
                                considered relative to the
                                F1 of 1 for doses greater
                                than 5)
```

Rate $(R1)$ and duration $(D1)$ parameters may be estimated or fixed to certain values when necessary to describe zero-order input processes. If input is into a compartment other than the first compartment, the numerical index value is changed to the appropriate compartment number (e.g., $R2$ and $D2$ would describe input into the second compartment).

Scaling parameters are required to obtain predictions in units consistent with observed values, based on dose amount and parameter units. As such, scaling parameters are very important to understand and set correctly.

Model predicted concentrations result from dividing the mass amount of drug in a compartment by the volume of distribution, V, of that compartment, or a scaled volume that is discussed here. The mass units of the amount of drug in the nth compartment are the same as the units used to express the dose in the AMT data item in the dataset. In addition, there may be a desire to obtain the estimate of volume in certain units, for example, liters. This can be expressed as follows in Equation 3.1:

$$\text{Concentration}(\text{cmt}\_n) = \frac{\text{amount}}{V} \tag{3.1}$$

If the units of the predicted concentrations are different than those of the dependent variable (DV), that is, the observed concentrations, they must be normalized, or scaled, for the correct computation of residuals during the estimation process. One cannot properly subtract predicted from observed concentrations to compute the residual, if both values are not expressed in the same units.

One can define a scale parameter that can be used to normalize the units of the predicted concentrations with the observed concentrations. The scale parameter, Sn, serves to reconcile: (i) the mass units of the dose and concentration values and, simultaneously, (ii) the volume units of the volume of distribution parameter and the units of the observed concentrations. Here n is the compartment number in which the concentrations are observed.

The scale parameter, Sn, is defined as the product of the volume of distribution and a unitless scalar value needed to reconcile the units of predicted and observed concentrations.

For this exercise, let the unitless scalar value be usv as shown in Equation 3.2. Then,

$$Sn = V \times \text{usv} \tag{3.2}$$

We should define usv, such that when V is replaced by Sn in Equation 3.1, the predicted and observed concentrations have the same units. Thus, the predicted concentration in the nth compartment is as shown in Equation 3.3:

$$\text{Concentration}(\text{cmt}\_n) = \frac{\text{amount}}{Sn} = \frac{\text{amount}}{V \times \text{usv}} \tag{3.3}$$

The predicted concentration must have equivalent units to the DV recorded in the DV data item of the dataset. If the concentrations of the observed values are thought of in units of $\text{DV}_{\text{mass}}/\text{DV}_{\text{Vol}}$, then the units should be balanced by the following relationship, as shown in Equation 3.4:

$$\frac{\text{Amount}}{V \times \text{usv}} = \frac{\text{DV}_{\text{mass}}}{\text{DV}_{\text{Vol}}} \tag{3.4}$$

Substituting in the units for each term, one may solve for the value of usv.

Consider the following example. Suppose the dose units are *mg*, the volume of distribution parameter is expressed in *L*, and the observed concentration units are *ng/mL*. Then, substituting these values into Equation 3.4, we get:

$$\frac{\text{mg}}{\text{L} \times \text{usv}} = \frac{\text{ng}}{\text{mL}} \tag{3.5}$$

The ng/mL units of DV are 1000 times smaller than mg/L units, so the numerical value of an equivalent concentration is 1000 times larger for ng/mL (e.g., 1 mg/L = 1000 ng/mL). Thus, we need to multiply the left-hand side by 1000 to get the same numerical value in the same units as the right-hand side. The value of usv in this case can be reasoned to be 1/1000, and the $PK code used to implement this scaling would be as shown in Equation 3.6:

$$S2 = \frac{V2}{1000} \tag{3.6}$$

Steps to compute this value are also shown here. For this example, starting with Equation 3.5, we wish to use usv to achieve equivalence with ng/mL on the right-hand side of the equation.

$$\frac{\text{mg}}{\text{L}} \times \frac{10^6 \, \text{ng}}{1 \, \text{mg}} \times \frac{1 \, \text{L}}{10^3 \, \text{mL}} = 10^3 \times \frac{\text{mg}}{\text{L}} = \frac{\text{ng}}{\text{mL}} \tag{3.7}$$

Since we want to express the scale factor in terms of volume, we can rearrange the relationship given earlier to see that:

$$Sn = \frac{\text{L}}{10^3} \tag{3.8}$$

balances the units of mg × mL/ng.

Here usv = 1/1000, which, when substituted in the $PK expression of the scale parameter *Sn*, for example, S2 = V2/1000, will normalize the units of predicted and observed concentrations.

This method for determining an appropriate scale factor can be easily applied to situations with differing dose and/or concentration units. It is important to remember, however, that the variable name for the appropriate volume parameter is determined by the ADVAN TRANS combination selected for the model and should be set accordingly.

3.5.2.3 *Estimating Interindividual Variability (IIV)*   In the Example Partial $PK Block provided in Section 3.5.2.1, an exponential function (i.e., EXP(x) in FORTRAN) is used to introduce IIV on clearance and volume. In terms of the

population estimate obtained for the ETA, this model is equivalent to modeling IIV with the constant coefficient of variation (CCV) or proportional error model (described in more detail in Chapter 2) when first-order (i.e., *classical*) estimation methods are implemented. This is because, when the first-order Taylor series approximation is applied to models using these parameterizations [× (EXP(ETA(x)) and × (1 + ETA(x))], the result is the same. However, the advantage of the exponential function for IIV (over the CCV or proportional function) is that the PK parameter is inherently constrained to be positive if the fixed effects are constrained to be positive. For the simple case, when the typical value of the PK parameter is defined to be an element of THETA with a lower bound of 0, the incorporation of IIV using the exponential notation will always result in a positive value for the subject-specific estimate of the PK parameter, even with extremely small and negative values of ETA(1). On the other hand, with the CCV notation, negative values of ETA(1) may result in a negative individual PK parameter estimate even when the fixed-effect parameter is constrained to be positive. Other options for modeling IIV would be coded as follows:

Additive (homoscedastic or constant variance) model

```
TVCL = THETA(1)
CL = TVCL + ETA(1)
```

Note that this parameterization is also subject to the possibility of negative individual parameter values (CL_i) when the ETA(1) is negative. This possibility is typically of concern for PK parameters but may be very reasonable for certain PD parameters (e.g., parameters measuring a change from baseline scale which could either increase or decrease). The resulting distribution of individual PK parameter values is normally distributed with the additive model for IIV.

Proportional or constant coefficient of variation (CCV) model

```
TVCL = THETA(1)
CL = TVCL * (1 + ETA(1))
```

Similar to the exponential model for IIV, this parameterization results in a log-normal distribution of the individual PK parameter values. Here, the variance is proportional to the square of the typical parameter value.

Logit transform model for adding IIV to parameters constrained between 0 and 1

```
TVF1 = THETA(1)
TMP = THETA(1) / (1 - THETA(1))
LGT = LOG(TMP)
TRX = LGT + ETA(1)
X = EXP(TRX) / (1 + EXP(TRX))
```

With this model, the typical value, THETA(1), may be constrained between 0 and 1 (via initial estimates), resulting in TMP being constrained between 0 and +∞, and LGT and TRX being "constrained" between −∞ and +∞. The variable, X (which can be thought of like a probability, but including IIV) is also constrained between 0 and 1, and it is the individual subject estimate of bioavailability, $F1$.

3.5.2.4 Defining and Initializing New Variables
At times, new variables are required and these may be initialized and defined within the $PK block. It is important to always initialize a new variable, that is, define it to be a certain value prior to any conditional statements which may alter its value for some subjects or conditions, to ensure proper functioning of any code that depends on the values of this variable. A simple way to initialize new variables is to use the type of coding provided in the following example:

```
NEWVAR = 0
IF (conditional statement based on existing variables(s))
NEWVAR = 1
```

Some of the more common situations where new variables are required include the following: when a variable needs to be recoded for easier interpretation of a covariate effect or when multiple indicator variables need to be created from a single multichotomous variable. Both of these examples are illustrated as follows.

To recode a gender variable from the existing SEXM (0=female, 1=male) to a new variable, SEXF (0=male, 1=female), first create and initialize the new variable:

```
SEXF = 0                    ; new variable SEXF created
                            and initialized to 0 for all
                            subjects
IF (SEXM.EQ.0) SEXF = 1     ; when existing variable
                            SEXM=0 (subject is female),
                            set new variable SEXF equal
                            to 1
```

To create multiple indicator variables for race from a single multichotomous nominal variable (i.e., RACE, where 1=Caucasian, 2=Black/African American, 3=Asian, 4=Pacific Islander, 5=Other):

```
RACB = 0                    ; new variable RACB created
                            and initialized to 0 for all
                            subjects
IF (RACE.EQ.2) RACB = 1     ; when existing variable
                            RACE=2 (subject is Black),
                            set new variable RACB=1
RACA = 0                    ; etc.
IF (RACE.EQ.3) RACA = 1
RACP = 0
IF (RACE.EQ.4) RACP = 1
RACO = 0
IF (RACE.EQ.5) RACO = 1
```

Note that with this coding method, a total of only $n-1$ indicator variables are necessary, where $n=$ the number of levels or categories of the original multichotomous variable. In this case, the original RACE variable had a total of five levels, and four indicator variables (RACB, RACA, RACP, and RACO) were created. A fifth new variable to define race=Caucasian (the only remaining group) is not necessary because this group can be uniquely identified by the new dichotomous variables, when all are=0; this indicates that the subject is not *positive* for any of the other categories, and therefore, must be Caucasian. The category without a specific indicator variable is thus, considered the reference group or population for this covariate effect. Although the selection of the particular group to set as the reference can be based on desired interpretability of the parameters, choosing the group with the largest frequency can also be considered a reasonable strategy for model stability and to ensure a reasonable degree of precision of the parameter estimates.

3.5.2.5 IF–THEN Structures   At times, it may be necessary or convenient to define parameters differently for portions of the analysis population. In those situations, it may be useful to code the model using an IF–THEN conditional structure. There are several ways to implement such a structure and several examples follow.

Example 3.1
Estimation of relative bioavailability for data collected following the administration of doses by a particular route of administration (RTE=1)

```
IF (RTE.EQ.1) F1 = 1
ELSE F1 = THETA(6)
```

Note that this assignment could also have been accomplished with coding similar to the initialization code provided previously:

```
F1 = 1
IF (RTE.NE.1) F1 = THETA(6)
```

There are often multiple ways to code the same structure using NM-TRAN.

Example 3.2
Estimation of differing magnitudes of between-subject variability in clearance for males (ω_1^2) and females (ω_2^2)

```
TVCL = THETA(1)
IF (SEXF.EQ.0) THEN
CL = TVCL*EXP(ETA(1))
ELSE
CL = TVCL*EXP(ETA(2))
ENDIF
```

Example 3.3
Estimation of differing typical values of ka and differing magnitudes of between-subject variability in ka for dose amounts less than or equal to 5, as compared to higher dose amounts

```
IF (RTE.EQ.1) THEN
     IF (DOSE.LE.5.0) THEN
          KA = THETA(1)*EXP(ETA(1))
     ELSE
          KA = THETA(2)*EXP(ETA(2))
     ENDIF
ENDIF
```

Example 3.4

Estimation of differing typical values of E_{max} for doses greater than 10 and having a flag set to 1, as compared to others

```
TVEMAX = THETA(1)
IF (FLAG.EQ.1.AND.DOSE.GT.10) TVEMAX = THETA(2)
EMAX = TVEMAX*EXP(ETA(1))
```

3.5.3   Specifying Residual Variability in the $ERROR Block

Up to this point, the coding discussed for the specification of the model in the $PK block has dealt with defining the required and additional PK parameters and describing IIV in one or more of these parameters. The remaining random residual variability has not yet been specified. This is accomplished in the $ERROR block. The $ERROR block, much like the $PK block, is a block of code where a particular functional form is used to describe a random variable, in this case residual error. Within the $ERROR block, new variables can also be defined and initialized, if appropriate. In addition to epsilons from the SIGMA matrix, the variables relevant to the specification of residual variability and available to the user in the $ERROR block are F, the individual predicted concentration (the model-based prediction for the concentration based on the individual-specific values of the PK parameters; more on this in Chapter 5), and Y, a variable denoting the true value of the measured concentration (or the value in the DV column of the dataset). Several examples for coding residual variability were introduced in Chapter 2 and are provided in the following subsections.

3.5.3.1   Typical Functional Forms for Residual Variability   Residual variability is a composite of within-subject intraindividual variability, assay variability, model misspecification, and errors in the data contributing additional random variability in particular measurements. In order to express residual variability, various functional forms are available and can be coded within the $ERROR block.

Additive (homoscedastic) residual variability

```
$ERROR
Y = F + EPS(1)
```

Proportional or CCV residual variability

```
$ERROR
Y = F * (1 + EPS(1))
```

Exponential residual variability

```
$ERROR
Y = F * EXP(EPS(1))
```

Additive plus CCV residual variability (also known as additive plus proportional or slope-intercept residual variability)

```
$ERROR
Y = F + EPS(1) + F*EPS(2)
```

An alternative structure for residual variability is the so-called log-error model. This model is equivalent to the exponential model, in that log transformation of the concentrations and the exponential model structure resolves to the structure we will define here for the log-error model. This structure is also referred to as the *log-transform both sides* approach. Use of this model involves first, natural log-transforming the concentrations (DV) in the dataset and reading in these transformed values as the DV. A good practice to consider involves always including a column in the dataset containing the natural log-transformed values of the concentrations for those situations when the use of a log residual variability model is warranted and/or for use in exploratory graphics. This can save valuable time when the new error model is to be tried but it also obviates the need for a new dataset and documentation of same. Coding for this model is provided as follows.

Log residual variability model

If the original $INPUT was:

```
$INPUT ID TIME AMT DV LNDV EVID MDV AGE WTKG
```

where DV = the concentrations on their raw, untransformed, original units and LNDV = the natural log-transformed concentration values.

In the control stream in which a log-error model structure is to be tested, change $INPUT to read in LNDV as DV:

```
$INPUT ID TIME AMT ODV=DROP DV=LNDV EVID MDV AGE WTKG
```

(Note that two columns may not both be named DV, even if one is dropped. Therefore, the original DV column must be renamed and in this example, the variable name ODV is used as a new label for the DV column, in its original units.)

Then, after $PK:

```
$ERROR (OBSERVATIONS ONLY)
Y= LOG(F) + EPS(1)
```

Or alternatively:

```
$ERROR
CALLFL=0
Y=LOG(F) + EPS(1)
```

Or alternatively:

```
$ERROR
FLAG = 0
IF (F.EQ.0) FLAG = 1
Y = (1-FLAG)*LOG(F+FLAG) + EPS(1)
```

Notice that the DV column in original units was renamed to *ODV* before dropping it. This particular variable name is arbitrary, but is used to replace DV, which could not have been dropped and then redefined in the next column, as it is a NONMEM-required dataset variable. Next, note that an option is available on the $ERROR block called *(OBSERVATIONS ONLY)*. This option tells NONMEM to apply the error block coding on observation records only (i.e., not on dosing or other event records). The alternative coding option using *CALLFL = 0* also indicates to NONMEM that the ERROR subroutine should be called only with observation records. The reason for such qualifications is to avoid certain mathematical errors that would result from attempting to log-transform the expected values of 0 for *F*, the individual predicted concentration, on dosing records. Be advised, however, that individual predicted values of 0 are possible at times other than dosing times (e.g., at times very long after dosing) and even with the *(OBSERVATIONS ONLY)* or *CALLFL = 0* options, these predictions will still result in a mathematical error and will need to be dealt with in another way. Finally, note that the coding for the log residual variability model uses an additive error structure with the log transformed value of *F*. Also, the LOG() function in FORTRAN is, in fact, the natural log function and the $\log_{10}$ function is specified with LOG10(). Finally, in the third and perhaps safest variation given earlier, an indicator variable called FLAG is initialized and used. The coding provided should result in the avoidance of any calculations of LOG(0) (on dose or other records) which would generate an error message and halt the minimization of the model.

Additional detail regarding alternative coding of various residual variability models is provided in Section 5.6.2.1.

3.5.3.2 *More Complex Residual Variability Structures*   Much more complexity can be introduced into the residual variability model, if warranted, based on the particular study designs and/or analysis dataset. For example, if the analysis dataset consists of the data from several different studies pooled together, it may not be unexpected that some studies used a particular assay method, while others used a different method. Recalling that residual variability in our population models is a composite of assay variability, true intrasubject variability, model misspecification, and errors in the data, allowing the data measured with a certain technique to be estimated with a different extent of residual variability than the data measured with the alternative technique may be warranted. To accomplish this, a variable is needed to indicate which assay methodology was applied to each concentration. If the variable does not already exist in the dataset, but can be defined in terms of other existing variables, such as study or ID number, the new assay variable can be created and initialized within the $ERROR block as we have

illustrated previously. Assuming that an indicator variable, ASAY, is defined with a value of 0 for method #1 and 1 for method #2, the following coding provides a way of estimating different amounts of residual variability associated with each method.

```
$ERROR
Y = F + F*EPS(1)*(1 - ASAY) + F*EPS(2)*ASAY
```

Because the ASAY indicator is coded with values of 0 or 1, the equation resolves to $Y = F + F*EPS(1)$ when $ASAY = 0$, and $Y = F + F*EPS(2)$ when $ASAY = 1$. Thus, the estimate of EPS(1), with a variance of σ_1^2, reflects the residual variability associated with method #1 and the estimate of EPS(2), with a variance of σ_2^2, reflects the residual variability associated with method #2.

Similarly, when data from studies conducted during different phases of drug development are pooled together, it may be reasonable to expect that residual variability would not only be of different magnitudes in the different phases but also that the functional form representing that variability may differ given the expected differences in sampling schemes across development phases as well. In order to allow for such differences, again, an indicator variable denoting the different phases needs to be utilized. Assuming such a variable does not exist, but can easily be created based on study number, an existing variable in the dataset, the following code allows for such a differentiation.

```
$ERROR

P1 = 0
IF (STDY.LE.110) P1 = 1
P3 = 0
IF (STDY.GE.300) P3 = 1
Y = F + EPS(1)*P1 + F*EPS(2)*P1 + F*EPS(3)*(1-P1)*(1-P3) +
    F*EPS(4)*P3
```

Given the coding of the Phase 1 (P1) and Phase 3 (P3) indicator variables, any data associated with a value of STDY between 110 and 300 would be part of the reference population, where P1 and P3 are both set to 0, in this case, indicating that the data were from Phase 2. So, in this case, for the data from Phase 1 studies, the equation resolves to $Y = F + EPS(1) + F*EPS(2)$, and for the data from Phase 2 studies, the equation resolves to $Y = F + F*EPS(3)$ because both P1 and P3 = 0. For the data from Phase 3 studies, the equation resolves to $Y = F + F*EPS(4)$. Notice that the constant F term is present in all models because it is not multiplied by either of the indicator variables and that the term intended to represent Phase 2 residual variability is multiplied by both $(1 - P1)$ and $(1 - P3)$ such that the entire term resolves to 0 for either Phase 1 or Phase 3 data and stays in when both P1 and P3 are 0. Also note that the functional forms differ between phases; the Phase 1 data are represented by a combination additive plus CCV residual variability model (σ_1^2 and σ_2^2) while the Phase 2 and 3 data are each represented by CCV error models, with differing variance estimates, σ_3^2 and σ_4^2, respectively.

For additional information on alternative coding options for residual variability, please refer to Section 5.6.2.1.

3.5.4   Specifying Models Using the $PRED Block

When NONMEM is to be utilized to develop a model that does not involve PK equations or does not require utilization of the PREDPP library, an alternative structure is used in place of the $SUBROUTINES record, $PK, and $ERROR blocks. The $PRED block is inserted in the control stream after the $INPUT and $DATA records and essentially provides a section of code whereby the model is specified using multiple equations, culminating with an equation for Y in terms of a predicted response and one or more epsilons. Because the prewritten subroutines are not called, there are no required or additional parameters, and parameters can take on just about any name the user desires. An example $PRED block for a simple E_{max} equation as a function of dose is provided in the following.

```
$PRED

BSLN  = THETA(3)  + ETA(3)
TVEMX = THETA(1)
EMAX  = TVEMX*EXP(ETA(2))
TVD50 = THETA(2)
ED50  = TVD50*EXP(ETA(1))

NUM = EMAX*DOSE
DEN = ED50 + DOSE
RESP = BSLN * (1 + NUM/DEN)

Y = RESP + EPS(1)
```

This section of code illustrates one example of how such a model might be written using the $PRED block. Another concept that is illustrated with this code fragment is that the elements of the THETA vector and the OMEGA (and SIGMA) matrix need not be introduced in a particular order within the control stream. As shown in this example, the first theta and eta that appear in the code are THETA(3) and ETA(3). Similarly, the elements of THETA and OMEGA need not correspond to each other in subscript; THETA(1) may be paired with ETA(2) or any other eta; and there is no requirement that it be paired with an eta of the same subscript. Note also that in this example, the individual predicted response is defined with the variable, RESP, and then the final equation for Y is written in terms of this RESP and EPS(1).

Another important feature of models specified using $PRED is that many of the dataset requirements relating to PREDPP are not applicable. The notion of separate dosing and observation records is one of those requirements. Furthermore, since in the aforementioned example, a value for DOSE is required to predict RESP, DOSE must be present on all records in the dataset. In fact, if DOSE were missing on a particular record, the predicted RESP for that record would be equal to BSLN since DOSE would be assumed to be equal to 0.

3.6   SPECIFYING INITIAL ESTIMATES WITH $THETA, $OMEGA, AND $SIGMA

As with most nonlinear regression packages, in order to estimate the parameters of the model in NONMEM, initial guesses must be provided for each one. These initial estimates are provided for each fixed- and random-effect parameter via the $THETA, $OMEGA, and $SIGMA records. For each type of parameter, an initial estimate may be provided for each individual element of the vector or matrix. For fixed-effect parameters, lower and upper bounds may also be set for each parameter. These bounds serve to limit the search space utilized by the estimation routine in searching for the global minimum for that parameter. As such, unless the bounds used are system related, implementation comes with some risk of preventing the search from locating the global minimum and the use of bounds should be approached with appropriate caution and understanding of this risk.

An example of a $THETA record is provided in the following and then explained.

```
$THETA (3.9) (52) (0.7)
```

In this record, initial estimates are provided for three parameters, listed in order, by subscript: 3.9 represents the initial estimate for THETA(1), 52 is the initial estimate for THETA(2), and the initial estimate for THETA(3) is 0.7. The parentheses around each estimate are not necessary with this statement but provide a bit of organization around the values when bounds are used. An equally valid $THETA record including lower bounds of 0 for all parameters would be:

```
$THETA (0, 3.9) (0, 52) (0, 0.7)
```

Within the parentheses relating to each element of THETA, bounds may be specified as follows: lower bound, initial estimate, and upper bound. Both the lower and upper bounds are optional, but when two values are provided within the parentheses, as in the aforementioned example, they are interpreted as the lower bound and the initial estimate. If only the initial estimate and the upper bound were desired, both estimates would need to be preceded by a comma, as follows: (,3.9, 100); this implies that no lower bound is set, the initial estimate is 3.9, and an upper bound of 100 is to be utilized. The absence of a lower or upper bound implies a bound of negative or positive infinity, respectively. To explicitly provide such a bound, the syntax would be (−INF, 5, +INF).

If a particular parameter is not to be estimated, but fixed to a specific value, this can be accomplished within the $THETA record using the FIXED option. For the aforementioned example, if THETA(3) were to be fixed to the estimate provided, then no lower or upper bound would be utilized for that parameter and the syntax would be as follows:

```
$THETA (0, 3.9) (0, 52) (0.7 FIXED)
```

Alternatively, fixing a parameter to a specific value can also be accomplished directly within the $PK block by not assigning a theta to the fixed parameter and using the fixed value directly in the equation. An example of this method of fixing a parameter is provided in the following for KA, the absorption rate constant:

```
$PK

TVCL = THETA(1)
CL = TVCL*EXP(ETA(1))
TVV = THETA(2)
V = TVV*EXP(ETA(2))
KA = 0.7

S2 = V/1000
```

Initial estimates for elements of the OMEGA and SIGMA matrices are also required. It is important to remember that these matrices are variance–covariance matrices, where the default assumption is that they are diagonal matrices with all off-diagonal elements assumed to be 0. Given this structure, the initial estimates that are to be provided for each ETA and EPS represent variance terms and NOT the mean or median of the individual ETA or EPS values (which are assumed to be 0 or at least near 0).

Default OMEGA matrix for three ETAs (expressed as the lower diagonal form):

$$
\begin{matrix}
\omega_{1,1}^2 & & \\
0 & \omega_{2,2}^2 & \\
0 & 0 & \omega_{3,3}^2
\end{matrix}
$$

Default SIGMA matrix for two EPSILONs:

$$
\begin{matrix}
\sigma_{1,1}^2 & \\
0 & \sigma_{2,2}^2
\end{matrix}
$$

Thus, initial estimates for OMEGA and SIGMA are provided via the $OMEGA and $SIGMA records as in the following example:

```
$OMEGA    0.25    0.25    0.49
$SIGMA    0.04    0.0625
```

These statements provide initial estimates for $\omega_{1,1}^2$ and $\omega_{2,2}^2$, interindividual variances in (for example, the) clearance and volume of distribution of 0.25 for each, and an initial estimate of 0.49 for $\omega_{3,3}^2$, interindividual variance in (for example) the absorption rate constant. Similarly, initial estimates of 0.04 and 0.0625 are provided for $\sigma_{1,1}^2$ and $\sigma_{2,2}^2$, respectively. Note that the use of $OMEGA and $SIGMA followed by a series of initial estimates is the equivalent of using $OMEGA DIAGONAL(x) or $SIGMA DIAGONAL(x) where x is equal to the size of the matrix (the number of matrix elements, in terms of rows, columns, or diagonal elements).

In certain estimation and/or simulation situations, it may be of interest to fix the variance of one of the components of OMEGA or SIGMA to a particular value. When $OMEGA or $OMEGA DIAG is used and the term *FIXED* appears anywhere within the record, the block is assumed by NONMEM to consist of separate blocks, each of dimension one.

```
    $OMEGA      0.25 FIXED    0.25     (FIXED 0.49)
```

In this example, the variances of both ETA(1) and ETA(3) are fixed, while the variance of ETA(2) is estimated and an initial estimate of 0.25 is provided.

If the term *FIXED* appears anywhere within the list of initial estimates of an $OMEGA BLOCK record (to be described in additional detail in a later example), the entire block is assumed to be fixed. A value of 0 may not be used in $OMEGA or $SIGMA unless it is FIXED to this value.

Since it can be a bit difficult to determine appropriate initial estimates of variance terms, the following derivation of a %CV for residual variability (using a proportional error model) is provided.

Starting with:

$$Y = F \times (1 + EPS(1))$$

This is equivalent to:

$$Y = F + F \times EPS(1)$$

Now, taking the variance of both sides, we get:

$$var(Y) = var(F) + var(F \times \varepsilon_1)$$

or:

$$var(Y) = 0 + F^2 \times var(\varepsilon_1)$$

since F is constant (with var(F)=0) and the variance of a constant value (i.e., F) times a random variable (i.e., ε_1) is equal to the square of the constant value multiplied by the variance of the random variable.

Simplifying this, given that the variance of EPS(1) is σ_1^2, we get:

$$var(Y) = F^2 \times \sigma_1^2$$

Then, to find the SD:

$$SD(Y) = \sqrt{(F^2 \times \sigma_1^2)}$$

Since the CV = SD/mean:

$$\frac{SD(Y)}{mean} = \frac{\sqrt{(F^2 \times \sigma_1^2)}}{F}$$

because F, the individual predicted concentration can be thought of as the mean or expected value. Further simplifying this, we get:

$$\frac{(F \times \sigma_1)}{F} = \sigma_1$$

Finally, to calculate the %CV, we multiply the CV by 100, as follows:

$$\%CV = \sigma_1 \times 100\%$$

Based on this derivation, and using the result that the $\%CV = \sigma_1 \times 100\%$, if we start with an initial estimate for residual variability in %CV terms, by back-transforming, the variance estimate can be obtained from $(\%CV/100)^2 = \sigma^2$. This same method, can of course, be used to derive initial estimates for elements of the OMEGA matrix, based on initial guesses for IIV in %CV units. Thus, if we think IIV in clearance may be around 30%CV and a bit higher, or around 45%CV for volume, we would use the following initial estimates for $OMEGA:

$$\left(\frac{\%CV}{100}\right)^2 = \left(\frac{30}{100}\right)^2 = 0.09 \text{ for CL}$$

$$\left(\frac{\%CV}{100}\right)^2 = \left(\frac{45}{100}\right)^2 = 0.2025 \text{ for V}$$

```
$OMEGA   0.09   0.2025
```

If the default assumption that the off-diagonal elements of the OMEGA or SIGMA matrices are equal to 0 is either not appropriate or is to be tested for appropriateness, one can choose to estimate these matrix elements. By specifying $OMEGA BLOCK(x) or $SIGMA BLOCK(x), initial estimates can be provided for all on- and off-diagonal elements of the OMEGA or SIGMA matrices (in a specific way). Without the diagonal matrix assumption, the OMEGA matrix appears as follows:

$$
\begin{matrix}
\omega_{1,1}^2 & \omega_{1,2} & \omega_{1,3} \\
\omega_{2,1} & \omega_{2,2}^2 & \omega_{2,3} \\
\omega_{3,1} & \omega_{3,2} & \omega_{3,3}^2
\end{matrix}
$$

Note that the matrix is still a symmetric matrix where, by definition, $\omega_{2,1} = \omega_{1,2}$, $\omega_{3,1} = \omega_{1,3}$, and $\omega_{3,2} = \omega_{2,3}$. Therefore, specification of initial estimates for such a matrix is required for only the lower triangular matrix or the elements in bold given earlier. The estimates are listed in the $OMEGA record in order, by reading across each row of the matrix, starting at the top. For example, initial estimates for the aforementioned matrix would be specified in the following specific order:

$$\$OMEGA \ BLOCK(3) \ \omega_{1,1}^2 \ \omega_{2,1} \ \omega_{2,2}^2 \ \omega_{3,1} \ \omega_{3,2} \ \omega_{3,3}^2$$

Remember that these off-diagonal elements represent the covariance between the corresponding variance terms, i.e., $\omega_{2,1} = \text{cov}(\omega_{1,1}^2, \omega_{2,2}^2)$. Therefore, to select an appropriate initial estimate for these off-diagonal OMEGA matrix elements, one might consider constructing pair-wise plots of the individual ETA estimates (as shown in Figure 3.2 for a pair of ETAs with an apparent correlation). Such plots not only give insight as to the appropriateness or lack of appropriateness of the default assumption

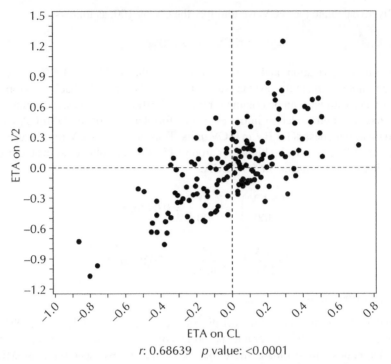

r: 0.68639   p value: <0.0001

FIGURE 3.2 Representative eta biplot: scatterplot of the ETA on clearance (CL) versus the ETA on volume (V2).

of no covariance but may also be useful in considering initial estimates for the estimation of off-diagonal terms. As a corollary to these plots, correlation coefficients representing the degree of linear correlation between two elements of OMEGA can be easily calculated. From a correlation coefficient (i.e., r^2), an estimate of covariance can easily be derived based on the following formula:

$$\text{Correlation coefficient } (\rho_{1,2}) = \frac{\text{cov}(\omega_{1,1}^2, \omega_{2,2}^2)}{\left[\sqrt{\omega_{1,1}^2} \times \sqrt{\omega_{2,2}^2}\right]} \quad \text{or} \quad \frac{\omega_{2,1}}{\left[\sqrt{\omega_{1,1}^2} \times \sqrt{\omega_{2,2}^2}\right]}$$

Thus,

$$\rho_{1,2} \times \left[\sqrt{\omega_{1,1}^2} \times \sqrt{\omega_{2,2}^2}\right] = \omega_{2,1}$$

There are certain limitations, imposed by NONMEM, with regard to the estimation of nondiagonal OMEGA and SIGMA matrices. When a nondiagonal OMEGA or SIGMA matrix is specified within a particular $OMEGA record (using $OMEGA BLOCK(n) as shown in the following example), all off-diagonal elements must be estimated (see exception for BAND matrices). As an example, assume that the pairwise plots of ETAs based on a two-compartment model with first-order absorption indicate that a trend exists between η_{CL} and η_Q, η_{V2} and η_{V3}, η_{V3} and η_{ka}, and η_{V2} and η_{ka}, where the elements of OMEGA, in order from 1 to 5, are $CL(\eta_1)$, $V2(\eta_2)$, $Q(\eta_3)$, $V3(\eta_4)$, and $ka(\eta_5)$. A full OMEGA block specification would require the estimation of several terms that may not be of interest: for example, the covariances between η_1 and η_2, η_2 and η_3, η_1 and η_4, η_1 and η_5, η_3 and η_4, and η_3 and η_5. One simple way to avoid the estimation of off-diagonal elements that are not of interest would be to reorder the elements of OMEGA; in this example, switching the order of η_2 and η_3 would be required. With η_2 redefined as the IIV on Q, and η_3 redefined as the IIV on V2, the estimation of uninteresting or unnecessary off-diagonal elements of OMEGA can be avoided. The following two $OMEGA records, used in conjunction, allow the user to specify initial estimates for only those elements of interest in this example:

$$\text{\$OMEGA BLOCK(2)}\ \omega_{1,1}^2\ \omega_{2,1}\ \omega_{2,2}^2$$

$$\text{\$OMEGA BLOCK(3)}\ \omega_{3,3}^2\ \omega_{4,3}\ \omega_{4,4}^2\ \omega_{5,3}\ \omega_{5,4}\ \omega_{5,5}^2$$

In matrix notation, this is the equivalent of the following matrix:

$$
\begin{matrix}
\omega_{1,1}^2 & \omega_{1,2} & 0 & 0 & 0 \\
\omega_{2,1} & \omega_{2,2}^2 & 0 & 0 & 0 \\
0 & 0 & \omega_{3,3}^2 & \omega_{3,4} & \omega_{3,5} \\
0 & 0 & \omega_{4,3} & \omega_{4,4}^2 & \omega_{4,5} \\
0 & 0 & \omega_{5,3} & \omega_{5,4} & \omega_{5,5}^2
\end{matrix}
$$

Similarly, if the covariance between two elements of an OMEGA matrix of size 3 is to be estimated while the covariances between the third element and the other two are assumed to be 0, one may order the elements to correspond with the matrix in the following and use the provided $OMEGA records:

$$
\begin{matrix}
\omega_{1,1}^2 & \omega_{1,2} & 0 \\
\omega_{2,1} & \omega_{2,2}^2 & 0 \\
0 & 0 & \omega_{3,3}^2
\end{matrix}
$$

```
$OMEGA BLOCK(2)
0.3
0.01      0.3
$OMEGA    0.4
```

It is important to note that if the term *FIXED* is detected anywhere within an $OMEGA BLOCK(n) statement, the entire block is assumed to be fixed to the values provided. A special case matrix type (and exception to the rule of not using an initial estimate of 0 within a BLOCK OMEGA structure) which can also be specified using $OMEGA and $SIGMA is the BAND matrix. In this case, the initial estimate of one or more elements of a BLOCK OMEGA structure may be specified (effectively fixed) as 0, indicating that no covariance between these elements is to be estimated or simulated, depending on the problem. The elements available for fixing to 0 are limited to those in the matrix which fall in the lower triangular portion, whereby the resulting matrix appears as a band. For example, the following matrix illustrates the use of a BAND structure:

$$
\begin{array}{ccccc}
\omega_{1,1}^2 & \omega_{1,2} & \omega_{1,3} & 0 & 0 \\
\omega_{2,1} & \omega_{2,2}^2 & \omega_{2,3} & \omega_{2,4} & 0 \\
\omega_{3,1} & \omega_{3,2} & \omega_{3,3}^2 & \omega_{3,4} & \omega_{3,5} \\
0 & \omega_{4,2} & \omega_{4,3} & \omega_{4,4}^2 & \omega_{4,5} \\
0 & 0 & \omega_{5,3} & \omega_{5,4} & \omega_{5,5}^2
\end{array}
$$

And the corresponding $OMEGA statement for this structure might read as follows, for example:

```
$OMEGA BLOCK(5)
0.3
0.01    0.3
0.01    0.01    0.3
0       0.01    0.01    0.3
0       0       0.01    0.01    0.3
```

This coding fixes the estimates of $\omega_{4,1}$, $\omega_{5,1}$, and $\omega_{5,2}$ to 0 while allowing the remaining off-diagonal and diagonal terms to be estimated with the initial estimates provided.

3.7 REQUESTING ESTIMATION AND RELATED OPTIONS

Working our way through the control stream, we have now specified the problem, read in the data, called appropriate subroutines, specified the structural model, including interindividual and residual variability, and provided initial estimates for all parameters. At this point, one of the important remaining steps involves requesting that estimation be performed, along with relevant options that tell NONMEM which type of estimation to do and how to provide the output from estimation. These steps are accomplished via the $ESTIMATION record.

Several different methods of estimation are available in NONMEM, allowing great flexibility to the user in terms of accomplishing different types of analysis with one tool as well as comparing the results obtained with different methods. The default method is the first one that was developed and implemented with NONMEM—the so-called first-order or FO method. The method is so-named because of the first-order Taylor series approximation used to perform the linearization of the model for the predicted concentration at a given time with respect to the etas (and epsilons), of which at least the etas are most often introduced into the model in a nonlinear way. The first-order method provides only population mean (typical value) estimates of all parameters; an optional second step (of the estimation method) is required to obtain individual-specific estimates of parameters. This subsequent step is referred to as POSTHOC estimation since it is accomplished with the POSTHOC option on $ESTIMATION and is performed after the first step of determining the population (typical value) estimates. Other classical estimation method options include the first-order conditional estimation (FOCE) method, the hybrid method, and the Laplacian estimation method. The first-order conditional estimation method estimates population parameters as well as individual-specific parameters in a single step, via conditioning on the individual-specific estimates of ETA terms during the minimization process. With the exception of run time, there are many advantages to the FOCE method over the FO method.

The hybrid method, as the name implies, is a hybrid of the first-order and FOCE methods, allowing the user flexibility in the selection of estimation method on a parameter-by-parameter basis within the same model run. The Laplacian method, also a conditional estimation method, requires even more time in estimation than the FOCE method, as it utilizes the second derivatives with respect to each ETA during minimization. The Laplacian estimation method is the most appropriate option for the analysis of categorical endpoint data (sometimes referred to as odd-type data), such as dichotomous endpoints analyzed with logistic regression models, ordered categorical data analyzed with proportional odds models, or time-to-event data analyzed with survival-type models.

Specification of the various estimation methods via the $ESTIMATION record is accomplished as follows:

```
$ESTIMATION POSTHOC      ; this requests FO (the default)
                           method PLUS requests POSTHOC
                           estimates of individual-specific
                           parameters
$ESTIMATION METHOD=1     ; this requests FOCE method
$ESTIMATION METHOD=COND  ; this is an alternative to
                           METHOD=1 which also requests the
                           FOCE method
$ESTIMATION METHOD=1 LAPLACIAN  ; this requests Laplacian
                                  estimation
$ESTIMATION METHOD=HYBRID ZERO=(1, 3)  ; this requests
                                   hybrid estimation, with FO
                                   estimation for ETA1 and
                                   ETA3, and FOCE for all
                                   other ETA terms
```

The INTERACTION option may be specified on the $ESTIMATION record with any of the estimation methods described earlier. This option requests that NONMEM preserve the dependence of the model for intraindividual random error on the ETAs during the computation of the objective function. Without this option (and by default), the ETA-EPS interaction term, which comes to be calculated during the objective function computation, is ignored. This option is specified on the $ESTIMATION record after the estimation method choice with INTERACTION, INTER, or INT. Oftentimes, a particular NONMEM estimation method will be referred to in shorthand notation as FOCEI, indicating the first-order conditional estimation method with the INTERACTION option.

Although the vast majority of the NONMEM literature to date has utilized FO or FOCE (i.e., the classical methods), with the release of NONMEM version 7, the arsenal of estimation methods available within the NONMEM system expanded dramatically. The new methods include the iterative two-stage method, the Monte Carlo Importance Sampling EM method (also, assisted by Mode A Posteriori estimation), the Stochastic Approximation Expectation Maximization (SAEM) method, and a Full Markov Chain Monte Carlo (MCMC) Bayesian Analysis method.

As further experience with these methods is published via case studies and simulation studies comparing the performance and various features of the different methods, guidance regarding the optimal use of each of these methods in different circumstances will also likely emerge. At the time of this writing, it is clear that the developers of NONMEM have invested in the inclusion of the many alternative estimation methods within the NONMEM system in an effort to remain current with the plethora of new and emerging software options for estimation and simulation of nonlinear mixed effects models.

Several other options are available on the $ESTIMATION record, including those for specifying the maximum number of allowable function evaluations, the iterations from which to print detailed results during minimization, and the number of significant digits requested in the final estimates. Furthermore, a specific option for implementing THETA recovery is also specified on $ESTIMATION and an option may be specified to capture the minimization results in a special binary file useful for further NONMEM processing. Additional detail on each of these options follows.

The maximum number of function evaluations allowed during a given estimation can be set with the MAXEVAL=x option on $ESTIMATION, where x is the selected value. Values between 0 and 99,999,999, inclusive, may be used for this option with NONMEM versions 6.2 and higher (previously 9,999), in an effort to limit the progress of the estimation routine. This may be useful, in the earliest stages of model development, when attempting to limit time wasted on model forms not likely to produce meaningful output. If a value of 0 is set, this is the equivalent of requesting that estimation not be performed; in this case, the values specified in $THETA, $OMEGA, and $SIGMA or alternatively, those implied with an $MSFI record, are used in the computation of the objective function, predictions, and residuals. Other uses for MAXEVAL=0-type runs are discussed in Chapter 5. If the MAXEVAL option is not specified at all on $ESTIMATION, a maximum value will be selected by the program. It is entirely possible that the value selected by the program may be too small, and the progress of the run will be halted due to exceeding this value. A specific error message is produced in this situation, which can be remedied in a subsequent run, by setting the value to a number considerably higher than that selected by NONMEM. A similar course of action is recommended when the value set by the user is exceeded, unless it is anticipated that the model is unlikely to converge, even after allowing for additional function evaluations.

The PRINT=n option on $ESTIMATION requests that detailed output from the estimation routine be printed to the report file with every nth iteration. A typical setting for this option may be PRINT=5, but smaller or larger values may be used to request more or less information, respectively. If the PRINT=n option is not specified, the default behavior is to print the 0th and the last iteration from the minimization routine; these iterations are, in fact, printed in the report file regardless of the number requested with the PRINT option. The information that is provided by default with this option consists of the minimization search output: the objective function value, the value of each parameter in its original units (listed with the row heading of *NPARAMETR* in versions 7.2.0 and higher), the transformed, scaled value of each parameter (called the unconstrained parameters, or UCPs, which scale each parameter to an initial estimate of 0.1; these are provided with the row heading of *PARAMETER* in versions 7.2.0 and higher) at that particular step in the minimization, along with the gradient with respect to that parameter. This output is particularly useful to track in real-time for models with extremely long run times to confirm that continuing progress is being made in obtaining a minimum value of the objective function. Tracking of the gradients of the response surface with respect to each parameter may also be useful as a means of ensuring that no gradient has arrived at a value of exactly 0: an indication that the parameter is no longer contributing information to the objective function and minimization process.

The values of each gradient should be checked for 0 values at the 0th iteration in particular, as well as during the search and at the last iteration. A gradient value of exactly 0 with the 0th iteration indicates that the associated parameter is not contributing anything to the model or the objective function calculation. There are several reasons why this may be so, but in some cases, this situation can arise without any other syntax errors or indications of problems. Suppose, for instance, that after utilization of IGNORE and/or ACCEPT options on the $DATA record, all female subjects have been excluded from the dataset available to NONMEM. Furthermore, suppose that, unaware of this effect of the dataset exclusions, the user wishes to estimate the influence of gender on drug clearance by testing the following model within the $PK block:

```
TVCL = THETA(1)  +  THETA(2)*SEXF
CL = TVCL  *  EXP(ETA(1))
```

Since the variable SEXF still exists in the dataset, no syntax errors will arise when the variable is called within $PK, but clearly no information would be available in the dataset with which to estimate a possible gender effect on clearance (since all values of SEXF=0). In this situation, the gradient associated with THETA(2) would be 0 at the 0th iteration, regardless of the initial estimate used for it. For any additional iterations that may be obtained, the gradient for THETA(2) will remain exactly 0. On the other hand, if we had inadvertently referred to the SEXF variable as SEXG in $PK, after reading it in as SEXF in $INPUT, a syntax error would of course arise, indicating that the variable SEXG is undefined. Additional detail regarding the interpretation of the output is given in Chapter 6.

The desired number of significant figures to be obtained in the final parameter estimates may be specified using the SIGDIGITS=n option on the $ESTIMATION record. If this option is not specified, the default number of significant digits is 3. If either greater or fewer significant figures are desired in a particular model, the user would simply substitute a larger or smaller integer for the n value in the option. When

NONMEM is unable to obtain the specified number of significant figures in the final parameter estimates upon minimization, the run may result in a failure due to rounding errors. However, in this situation, when either the overall number of significant figures or the smallest number obtained with a given parameter is quite similar to the requested number (e.g., if 3 are requested and 2.9 are obtained), one may choose to accept the results of this run, bearing in mind this minor deviation in significant figures in comparisons with other models. Alternatively, if one wishes to obtain a successful minimization with the requested options, changing the value of the SIGDIGITS option to a smaller number of significant figures may very well result in a minimization without errors or warnings. Interestingly, although not particularly intuitive, requesting a larger number of significant figures may also result in a successful minimization, at times and in some cases; this is because this variation in the estimation options will cause the minimization to follow a different path in finding the lowest point in the response surface (associated with the minimum value of the objective function).

The NOABORT option on the $ESTIMATION record is another useful option. This option requests that THETA-recovery be implemented at any time when the estimates of THETA attempted during minimization result in a PRED error return code of 1; this is an indication that the PRED subroutine is unable to compute for some reason. (A return code of 2 is more serious and indicates to NONMEM that the run should be aborted.) According to the NONMEM help files, with the use of the NOABORT option, terminations of the minimization process due to a nonpositive Hessian matrix for some individual in the dataset are also minimized. When NOABORT is requested on $EST and is invoked by some condition during the minimization, a warning is provided near the end of the report file, indicating that there are error messages in the PRDERR file. The analyst may find it useful to examine the contents of this file, when it is generated, and to scrutinize situations or subjects requiring that this recovery be invoked, for clues as to possible errors in the data, sources of problems, or information concerning model instabilities.

Another controllable option on $ESTIMATION has to do with a warning which often arises as a result of poorly chosen initial estimates. When the final estimate obtained by NONMEM for a particular parameter is more than two orders of magnitude different from the corresponding initial estimate, a warning is obtained indicating the following:

```
PARAMETER ESTIMATE IS NEAR ITS BOUNDARY THIS MUST BE
ADDRESSED BEFORE THE COVARIANCE STEP CAN BE IMPLEMENTED
```

As described in the warning message, this situation results in a COVAR step failure. This error can also be obtained when elements of the CORRELATION matrix are very close to 0 or 1. In order to suppress this message, and allow the covariance step to proceed without regard to these checks, the following options may be included on the $ESTIMATION record: NOTBT NOOBT NOSBT, which are shorthand for NOTHETABOUNDTEST NOOMEGABOUNDTEST NOSIGMABOUNDTEST (which may be specified if one prefers the explicit version). Thus, separate options are available for each type of parameter and any or all of these options may be used, as desired. Specifying these options, in effect, turns off this default *boundary* test, which may be desirable in situations where the initial estimates are not known with a great deal of certainty, especially early in model development.

Another option available on $ESTIMATION requests that the individual contributions to the objective function be sorted prior to summation. It has been shown that summing the objective function values from smallest to largest (as opposed to the order in which the subjects appear in the dataset, which is the default) can result in a more stable minimization for some datasets and models with perhaps less likelihood of rounding errors. To request such a sort be performed, the user would simply specify the option SORT anywhere on the $ESTIMATION record. In this and other situations, even when sorting is not performed, it may be of interest to examine these individual contributions to the objective function for the purpose of exploring which subjects contribute the most to this value. In this case, a subject contributing to the overall objective function value to a substantially greater degree relative to other subjects is an indication of either a poorly fit subject or a subject whose data do not tend to support the proposed model. In NONMEM version 7 and higher, the *.phi output file provides these individual objective function values by default.

A special type of output file may be requested on the $ESTIMATION record: the MSF or model specification file. This file attempts to capture information regarding the model estimated, the options used for estimation, and the results of the minimization in a small binary file. This file is requested through the MSFO= option on $ESTIMATION as shown in the following example:

```
$ESTIMATION MAXEVAL=9999 PRINT=5 METHOD=COND MSFO=run49.msf
```

If the run terminates successfully, a model specification file, called *run49.msf* will be available for subsequent use. There are many uses of such a model specification file. First, the existence of such a file may save valuable time if postprocessing steps are required, such as requesting a $COVARIANCE step if one was not requested with the original estimation, requesting additional table files or changes to table file output, or even requesting estimation with an alternative estimation method. With the availability of UPS's (uninterrupted power supplies) and other sophisticated systems and technology for NONMEM processing on grid systems and with cloud computing, issues with power failures during a minimization are no longer as devastating as they once were. However, even in the event of a power or hardware failure during an extremely long NONMEM run time for a given model, a model specification file can save the analyst valuable time, as the subsequent run, which would request input from the model specification file (feature to be illustrated in the following example) will essentially pick up where the last run left off instead of starting back at the beginning of the problem. In addition to these uses, model specification files can be very useful in simulation problem settings, where the need to type in and verify each of the parameter estimates to be used as starting or true values can be eliminated.

To read in an existing model specification file, one would simply replace the $THETA, $OMEGA, and $SIGMA records with the following statement:

```
$MSFI run49.msf
```

The new run will then use the information captured in the model specification file as the starting point. Please note that a model specification file may only be used in conjunction with the identical model specification in $PK ($PRED) and $ERROR as the original run. If changes are made to the model statements, additional parameters are added or existing parameters removed or changed in some way, the run will terminate with errors. Therefore, the uses of such a file are limited to implementation of the postprocessing steps ($COVARIANCE, $TABLE, and $SCATTERPLOT records to be described in detail in subsequent sections) and in a limited way to testing alternative estimation options.

3.8 REQUESTING ESTIMATES OF THE PRECISION OF PARAMETER ESTIMATES

The existence of the $COVARIANCE record in a control stream including estimation indicates to NONMEM that additional postprocessing of the estimation output is to be performed after the minimization routine is complete. The typical COVARIANCE step output consists of the standard errors for each estimated parameter, the complete variance–covariance matrix of the estimates, the corresponding correlation matrix of the estimates, and the inverse of the variance–covariance matrix. These matrices are provided in the NONMEM report file immediately following the final parameter estimates.

The default computation method is used when the $COVARIANCE record is specified without further options related to computation. This default is the $R^{-1}SR^{-1}$ or so-called sandwich matrix computation. Use of either the R or S matrices may also be requested by specifying MATRIX=R or MATRIX=S as an option after $COVARIANCE. For certain problems, such as the estimation of models using a categorical DV, an alternative computation of the COVARIANCE matrix (such as the S matrix) is recommended. In addition to these options, the COMPRESS option specifies that the output from the COVARIANCE step be printed in a compressed format in the NONMEM output file. This saves many lines of output, as the results are no longer printed in a matrix structure, but are instead printed in simple rows and columns with each element specifically identified.

Another useful option available on the $COVARIANCE record, PRINT=E, allows the user to request that the eigenvalues of the variance–covariance matrix be printed to the NONMEM output file in addition to the other typical COVARIANCE step output. The eigenvalues are commonly used to compute a condition number for the model, by dividing the largest eigenvalue (the last one in the list) by the smallest eigenvalue (the first one in the list). The ratio of these two values is considered the condition number of the run and provides some insight as to the status and characteristics of the model. Although different sources cite widely different cut-off values to consider *high* or noteworthy, in general, a high condition number (>200, >1,000, or >10,000) is considered an indication that the model is ill conditioned (Bonate 2006). Ill-conditioning occurs when many possible sets of parameter values are nearly as good. This situation may arise when a model is over-parameterized, or in other words, has too many parameters relative to the amount of data being fit. In this case, simplification of the model may remove the ill conditioning and result in a better conditioned (and more stable) model.

Finally, another potentially useful option of the $COV record allows for the computation of the covariance step output regardless of the status of the estimation step termination. The default option (*CONDITIONAL*) of $COV requests that the covariance step is implemented only when the estimation step terminates successfully. The *UNCONDITIONAL* option specifically requests the covariance step output regardless of the estimation step success.

3.9   CONTROLLING THE OUTPUT

Besides the standard and typical information regarding the results of a particular model which are included in the NONMEM report file, and the various other output files by default, NM-TRAN allows the user two additional mechanisms by which to control the specific output obtained from a given model. These include the $TABLE record and the $SCATTERPLOT record. With these statements, the user can request tables of output containing the detailed individual- and observation-specific results as well as simple ASCII scatterplots of results.

The $TABLE record allows the user to request one or more tables of output containing the specified fields. A list of the requested fields is specified along with various options for table format and display. The following example record illustrates the use of several of these options:

```
$TABLE ID TIME DOSE CL V KA ETA1 ETA2 IPRED NOPRINT
   ONEHEADER FILE=run23.tbl
```

In this $TABLE record, the user is requesting that the table file be excluded from the NONMEM report file (NOPRINT option), be output to a separate external file called *run23.tbl* (FILE=option), and contain one single header row providing the names of each of the variables included in the file (ONEHEADER). Without the NOPRINT and FILE= options, the table file output would be printed within the NONMEM report file. Without the ONEHEADER option, the table file would contain a header (series of additional rows identifying the table number, corresponding rows in the dataset, and listing the names of the variables in each column) at the top of the file and then after every 900 records. Sending the contents to a separate file allows for easier processing of that file by other helper programs. Other options related to the format of the table file include NOHEADER, FIRSTONLY, and NOAPPEND. The NOHEADER option requests that no header information be included in the table file at all, requiring that the user read the fields from the control stream $TABLE record or the list reported in the NONMEM output file. The FIRSTONLY option requests that the table file contain a single row of output for each subject in the dataset (i.e., only the first record for each subject). This option is useful when outputting a table file containing variables that would not change within an individual subject's records (e.g., empirical Bayesian estimates of parameters or etas and stationary covariates). Finally, the NOAPPEND option requests that NONMEM not append the following four fields that are appended as additional columns of every NONMEM table file by default: DV, PRED (the population prediction), RES (the population residual or difference between DV and PRED), and WRES (the population weighted residual value).

The $SCATTERPLOT option, once a useful mechanism to obtain *quick-and-dirty* plots of model results is a limited feature for most NONMEM users with access to other more elaborate and sophisticated graphing programs. Typically, users will now read the table file output into another program, such as R (R Core Team 2013), SAS® (SAS Institute 2008), or Xpose (Jonsson and Karlsson 1999), where a prescripted program can be written to take the results and return the standard and typical goodness-of-fit type diagnostic plots. Nonetheless, without such a mechanism in place, the user can request some basic scatterplots from NONMEM which are included at the end of the NONMEM output file. Few options are available to improve the look of these ASCII scatterplots, whose x axis is presented at the top of the graph, and whose content is limited to 900 records in a single plot. With careful interpretation (especially if the dataset contains more than 900 records), the scatterplots provided by NONMEM do, however, provide a rough idea of the relationships between requested variables. Examples of typical $SCATTERPLOT records are provided followed by a brief explanation of the options:

```
$SCAT DV VS PRED UNIT
$SCAT (RES WRES) VS PRED
$SCAT DV VS IPRED UNIT FROM 1 TO 900
$SCAT DV VS IPRED UNIT FROM 901 TO 1800
$SCAT DV VS IPRED UNIT FROM 1801
$SCAT CL VS WTKG FIRSTONLY
```

The format of the scatterplot record is to provide the variables to be plotted as X versus Y. The UNIT option on the first example requests that a line of unity (unit slope line) be superimposed on the requested scatterplot. In the second example, parentheses are specified around a list of X variables, requesting that each be plotted versus the specified Y variable in separate plots. The next list of plots also include unit slope lines, but allow for an examination of all of the data in the dataset, even for datasets containing more than 900 records, albeit in separate plots. The first of the list of requested plots of the DV versus the individual predicted value includes the first 900 records of the dataset, while the second plot contains the next 900 records, and the third contains records 1801 through the end of the dataset, assuming it is less than 900 more records. If, in fact, the dataset contained well over 2700 records, the third plot in this series would simply be truncated to include only the records between 1801 and 2700. The points represented by record numbers greater than 2700 would not be shown. This behavior is the same for all $SCATTERPLOT records which do not specify a range of record values with the *FROM X TO Y* option—if no option is specified, only the first 900 records are shown. For large datasets, if this option is not specified, extreme care must be taken to not overinterpret the findings or patterns that may be present in plots of the first 900 records. The final example $SCATTERPLOT record illustrates the use of the FIRSTONLY option, requesting (exactly as with the $TABLE option) that only the first record within each individual's records be plotted.

REFERENCES

Beal SL, Sheiner LB, Boeckmann AJ, Bauer RJ, editors. 1989 *NONMEM 7.2.0 Users Guides (1989–2011)*. Icon Development Solutions, Hanover. Available at ftp://nonmem.iconplc.com/Public/nonmem720/ guides. Accessed December 13, 2013.

Bonate PL. *Pharmacokinetic-Pharmacodynamic Modeling and Simulation*. New York: Springer Science + Business Media, LLC; 2006. p 65–69.

Jonsson EN, Karlsson MO. Xpose—an S-PLUS based population pharmacokinetic/pharmacodynamic model building aid for NONMEM. Comput Methods Programs Biomed 1999;58 (1):51–64.

R Core Team. *R: A Language and Environment for Statistical Computing*. 2013. R Foundation for Statistical Computing, Vienna. Available at http://www.R-project.org. Accessed December 13, 2013.

SAS Institute Inc., *SAS User's Guides, Version 9*, 1st ed., volumes 1–3. Cary: SAS Institute Inc.; 2008.

CHAPTER 4

DATASETS

4.1 INTRODUCTION

Analysis of pharmacometric datasets intended for population analysis requires a potentially complex arrangement of information in a format upon which the analysis program can act. Pharmacometric datasets are generally time-ordered arrangements of records representing the time course of events related to drug administration, resulting plasma concentrations, and/or pharmacodynamic (PD) responses occurring within the individuals enrolled in a clinical trial or in a particular patient. The complexity of the dataset is dependent upon the complexity of the features of the system being modeled.

Discussions of dataset construction are sometimes overlooked when the modeling process is considered. Dataset construction can be tedious work that must be done before the *interesting* work of modeling can begin. Datasets are a critical component of modeling; therefore, the importance of skills in constructing datasets should not be underestimated. The task of dataset construction is not trivial, especially when large datasets are assembled from multiple studies or *messy* clinical trial data, such as when covariates are recorded in mixed units (e.g., weight in pounds and kilograms for different individuals) or the time and date information for concomitant medication usage needs to be sequenced with study drug administration and blood sample collection in the analysis dataset. The amount of time and effort required to construct a complex dataset can sometimes rival the amounts required to perform the modeling. Quality control is critical in constructing datasets that reflect the events that gave rise to the data. If errors in stating the times of doses or concentrations are made, the analysis becomes flawed by the errors in the data. Documentation of that quality control process is especially important when models are to be used for regulatory and/or decision-making purposes. The activities of good quality control add to the effort of constructing datasets.

Modeling pharmacokinetic (PK) data generally requires specification of the occurrence of doses (dosing events) in a study, the values of independent variables (e.g., time, body weight, age), and the values of the dependent variable (DV) (i.e., concentrations of drug). The model is then fit to, or is used to simulate, the time course of drug concentrations resulting from those doses.

Datasets for PD models may or may not include dosing events in the dataset, depending upon the structure of the system being modeled, whether the data represent the biological process of disease progression or placebo effects, and whether drug concentrations are included in the model. Additionally, some PD models may not require that the data be structured according to time-ordered events, as in the simple linear or nonlinear regression of QTc versus peak drug concentration. Models that do not use time-ordered data do not use PREDPP and are expressed in a user-supplied PRED routine. Datasets for these analyses associate independent variable(s) and DV on a record within an individual, but are not necessarily time ordered and do not contain separate dose records. Models implemented using PREDPP require that the data be time oriented.

When modeling the time course of changes in the concentration of endogenous compounds, or whenever the initial conditions of the system are not zero, the initial circulating amount or concentration of the compound must be input into the system. Similarly, if the baseline values of a PD response variable are nonzero, then an initial nonzero value must be specified for modeling the response variable. Baseline values may be entered in the dataset or assigned through certain options in the control file.

In general, the pharmacometric dataset will have elements of *input mass*, time, covariates, and the observations of events which the model is intended to describe. In addition, there are NONMEM-required variables that allow NONMEM to appropriately interpret and process the data in the manner intended by the analyst.

The data file can be generated using many different data management packages, spreadsheets, programming languages, or text editors. The use of programming languages such as R (R Development Core Team 2013) or SAS Institute Inc. (2002–2010) has significant advantages in processing data in a consistent, repeatable, and verifiable manner. However, the use of such systems requires skill with the language. Using a spreadsheet for data assembly and formatting may be easier when working with small datasets or for a novice but is prone to errors that are not easily discovered, such as a key being unintentionally pressed that leads to unintended changes. Such errors are not easily found since spreadsheets do not keep a record of changes made in a file. Federal regulation 21 CFR Part 11 requires accountability of data and a record of any changes made, which cannot easily be done in a spreadsheet that doesn't keep a log of all changes. When built using a spreadsheet, validation of the analysis dataset would require 100% verification against the source data. The use of a programming language to construct datasets allows one to track every change made to the dataset. Spreadsheets might be considered for the analysis of simple data from a small number of individuals or from a single Phase 1 study; however, when the analysis includes more complex dosing histories, merging data from multiple Phase 1 and 2 studies, or data from a Phase 3 study, use of a programming language becomes essential. Dataset assembly according to regulatory standards is best accomplished by the use of a programming language in order to comply with quality management requirements.

For most platform configurations, the data file could not contain embedded tabs when using older versions of NONMEM. In current versions, column delimiters such as spaces, commas, or tabs are acceptable.

4.2 ARRANGEMENT OF THE DATASET

The NONMEM (NM-TRAN) system has certain structural requirements of analysis datasets. Data must be present in a text (i.e., ASCII) format *flat file* with appropriate delimiters. The data file has a two-dimensional arrangement of data in rows and columns. All NONMEM data should be numerical except for certain formats of DATE and TIME, which may include alphabetic characters.

A data *record* refers to a line, or row, of data, as shown in Table 4.1.

The record contains a specific collection of associated data elements. When modeling a time-dependent system, the record is the collection of concurrent values of data and variables at a specific point in time.

The terms variable, field, or data item are used to refer to the information contained in a column of a space-delimited file or a specific position within a record of a comma-delimited file. A space-delimited file uses one or more spaces to separate data items in each row of the dataset. Space-delimited files with data arranged in columns have the advantage of readability to the analyst. If problems arise in fitting the data of a particular individual, or an error is reported in processing the data on a particular record, data arranged in space-delimited columns are easier for the analyst to review than data in comma-delimited files.

Each dataset record must contain the same number of variables. The order of variables is arbitrary but must be consistent across all records (within a subject and across subjects). Missing values should have a placeholder such as "." or "0"; blanks are not acceptable for missing data in space-delimited files. While it is not always required, it may be advisable to keep the format of a variable consistent across all records. NONMEM will allow some mixed format entry of some variables, but for clarity to the analyst and prevention of unanticipated errors, consistency might be of value. Consider the example in Table 4.2. TIME could be expressed as hh:mm for one record and as a real number (elapsed time) for another record. If the analyst intended

TABLE 4.1 Example of a data record

ID	Time	AMT
01	10:00	100 ←

Record = a row

TABLE 4.2 Example of data records in unlike units that lead to an error in analysis

ID	TIME
001	8:00
001	0.5

8:00 to be time zero and 0.5 hours to be the time of an event occurring one-half hour later, the records in Table 4.2 would result in a data error in the NONMEM report file stating that *ELAPSED TIME MAY NOT BE NEGATIVE*. The values that NONMEM assigns to TIME for each record can be reviewed in the FDATA file. In this case, the event at 0.5 hours would evaluate to −7.5 hours. The first record time of 8:00 is assigned the TIME=0 in FDATA, but the 0.5 record is converted to −7.5 hours.

If other variables such as covariates were included in the dataset using different units, one would need to capture the differences and convert them to like units within the control stream file. For example, if estimated creatinine clearance (CrCl) was expressed in common clinical units of mL/min for data from one study and SI units of mL/s from another study, the control stream would need to adjust the units of one or the other form before CrCl is used in a covariate model equation. In the authors' experience, constructing the analysis dataset to have like units is best achieved through programmatic adjustments during the construction of the analysis dataset. In general, good documentation and consistency can lead to reduced errors during analysis.

The maximum number of variables (data items) that can be read into and used for any one model run in NONMEM 7 is 50. A greater number of items may be contained in the dataset, but some of them must be ignored on each execution using the DROP option on the $INPUT statement. This allows NM-TRAN to process a dataset with more than the maximum number of variables by simply ignoring or dropping some of the variables not currently being used. Earlier versions of NONMEM allowed a maximum of only 20 data items and were thus quite limited in this regard.

The control file includes a $INPUT statement to specify to NONMEM the order of variables in the dataset record. Variable names (data labels) in this statement may be up to 20 characters long in NONMEM 7 but in prior versions must have been between 1 and 4 characters in length. This variable name will be used in the control file to identify the data read from the dataset.

Certain variable names are reserved in NONMEM (and PREDPP) and must be used in accordance with the reserved definitions. The following are examples of reserved variable names: ID, DATE, DAT1, DAT2, DAT3, TIME, DV, AMT, RATE, steady state (SS), interdose interval (II), ADDL, event identification (EVID), missing dependent variable (MDV), CMT, prediction compartment (PCMT), CALL, CONT, $L1$, and $L2$. In addition, PK parameter names have reserved definitions in accordance with the ADVAN subroutine being used. For example, KA, CL, V, $F1$, $F2$, ALAG1, ALAG2, $S1$, and $S2$ are reserved for ADVAN2.

Unlike some other analysis programs, the PREDPP routines of NONMEM require the use of an *event-type* structure to the records of the dataset. Each record contains information about a particular event. In the case of some dosing options, the dose record may imply the occurrence of other past or future events as well. Events may be of the following types: (i) dosing event, (ii) observation event, or (iii) *other*-type event.

Dosing events introduce an amount (recorded in the variable AMT) of the DV (e.g., drug mass or response variable in the case of PD models) into the system at a particular time. Observation events (recorded in the variable DV) record the concentration or effect measure at a particular time. *Other*-type events record a

TABLE 4.3 Example of incorrect expression of simultaneous events in the analysis dataset

ID	TIME	AMT	DV
001	0.0	100	35.4
001	0.5	.	12.6
001	1.0	.	8.6

Not allowed

TABLE 4.4 Example of correct expression of simultaneous events in the analysis dataset

ID	TIME	AMT	DV
001	0.0	100	.
001	0.0	.	35.4
001	0.5	.	12.6
001	1.0	.	8.6

change in some other system parameter such as a physiological condition like a change in body weight or the administration of a concomitant medication. *Other*-type events may also be included as part of a dose or observation record. However, administered doses cannot be present on the same record as an observed concentration or effect measure. Similarly, observation data cannot appear on the same record with an administered dose. Either AMT or DV, or both, must be missing on each record. Values other than 0 or "." for these variables cannot appear together on the same record, as shown in Table 4.3.

Sometimes two events, such as a dose and an observation, need to be recorded at the same time in an individual. When this is needed, as illustrated in Table 4.4, the two events should be reported in separate, consecutive records with the same value for TIME.

Data items that report descriptive information (covariates) about a patient, for example, age or body weight, should be nonmissing on all records (dose, observation, and other events). If these items are used in the model, they must be present on every record as it is processed. If the value of a covariate is missing, the model will be evaluated with the missing value (interpreted by NM-TRAN as 0), and numerical errors or unanticipated erroneous results may occur.

Datasets for models not using PREDPP do not use all the elements of the event-type structure. Some such datasets are used for a variety of PD models, and each record is an observation event. In these datasets, there is generally no concept of a *dose record*. These datasets are set up for a specific nonlinear regression approach and must be constructed in a fashion consistent with the model to be applied.

4.3   VARIABLES OF THE DATASET

Some of the efficiency and flexibility of NONMEM comes through the dataset construction. A variety of data items are available to communicate the events to be modeled with NONMEM and PREDPP. Some data items are required by NONMEM for all population models (e.g., ID and DV), while others are required only in certain circumstances and may be optional in other situations. When using PREDPP, TIME and AMT are required for all datasets. Some data items that have specific requirements for use are outlined in the following sections.

4.3.1   TIME

In a time-oriented dataset (intended for use with PREDPP), the value of TIME must be nonmissing and non-negative on all records. All records within an individual must be arranged in increasing (or equal) values of TIME, unless there is a record indicating the occurrence of a *reset event* that allows the elapsed time interval to restart.

   The value of TIME may be formatted as clock time (e.g., 13:30) or decimal-valued time (13.5) but should be of the same type on all records. If a clock time format for TIME is selected, however, it is critical that times be recorded using military time to prevent a syntax error from NM-TRAN regarding a potential nonconsecutive time sequence for values recorded past noon. Decimal-valued time represents the elapsed time since some initial event; however, there is no requirement that the first record for each subject has a TIME value of zero.

4.3.2   DATE

The DATE data item is not required, but may be useful in constructing the sequence of events in time. It is used in conjunction with TIME to construct the time sequence of event records. The DATE data item may be expressed as an integer (e.g., representing the study day) or as a calendar date. Several variables are available for expressing date values as calendar dates using different formats, as shown in Table 4.5.

   Using these formats, the year can be expressed using from 1 to 4 digits (e.g., 9, 09, or 2009). If the year is specified using 1–2 digits, then the LAST20=n option should be specified on the $DATA line in the control file, where n is an integer from 0 to 99. The value of n determines which century is implied for the year. The default value of n is 50. When the value of year (YY) is greater than n, the year is assumed

TABLE 4.5   Date formats for input of calendar dates

Variable name	Format
DATE	MM/DD/YY or MM-DD-YY
DAT1	DD/MM/YY or DD-MM-YY
DAT2	YY/MM/DD or YY-MM-YY
DAT3	YY/DD/MM or YY-DD-MM

TABLE 4.6   Example of correct use of TIME and calendar date

DATE	TIME
1/2/13	12

TABLE 4.7   Example of incorrect use of TIME and calendar date

DATE	TIME
1/1/13	36

to be 19YY, and when YY $\leq n$, it is assumed to be 20YY. For example, if $n = 50$ and YY = 9 or YY = 09, the year is interpreted as 2009.

Whenever DATE is formatted as a calendar date (i.e., using "/" or "-" as a delimiter), $INPUT must specify DATE=DROP. In this case, the data preprocessor will use the DATE item to compute the relative time of events but will drop the item from the dataset. Since DATE is dropped, its value cannot be output to the $TABLE file.

Whenever the DATE variable is used in the dataset, values of TIME are restricted to a range from 0 to 24 hours. To specify a greater TIME interval than 24 hours, the DATE must be incremented by the appropriate amount so that the value of TIME will fall within 0–24 hours, for example, if a dose is given at 0:00 on 1/1/2013 and a sample is collected 36 hours later. The sample record could be coded as shown in Table 4.6 but not be recorded as shown in Table 4.7.

The data preprocessor will use DATE and TIME together to compute the relative or elapsed time of events since the first record within the individual. It is important to note that if TIME is output to the $TABLE file, the value output will be the relative time, not the TIME value specified in the original data file.

If a DATE data item is not used, then TIME must be defined as the elapsed time since the first event. Events spanning more than 1 day will have time values greater than 24 hours.

Even when the time sequence of events is defined using TIME and DATE, we have often found it useful to include a time variable that describes the elapsed time of all events within a subject. We frequently refer to this as the *time since first dose* (TSFD). A second time value that is frequently useful is the time since the most recent dose was administered, or *time after dose* (TAD). These values of time are often useful for graphing the data, producing goodness-of-fit plots, and as a merge key for certain data handling operations.

4.3.3   ID

For population data, the dataset must have an ID variable, which is the subject identifier. All records for a single subject must be contiguous and, for PREDPP, sorted in order of increasing time. If records from a particular subject are separated in the dataset by those of another ID number, the separated records will be treated by NONMEM as separate individuals (even though they have the same ID value). As such, an ID number could be *recycled* and seen as different subjects, but this is generally not a good practice and could lead to unexpected errors when plotting, sorting, counting individuals, or otherwise handling the dataset.

One practice we have found helpful is to create a unique patient identifier variable for the analysis dataset. This value can be particularly useful when data are to be combined from multiple studies. In this case, the unique ID number value may be generated by concatenating unique information from the clinical study number and the subject number in the study. For instance, subject 126 from Study 10 might have a new ID value of 10126. In this way, subject 126 in Study 10 would not be confused with subject 126 in Study 7 (whose ID would be 7126). This reassignment of ID occurs during the process of building the analysis dataset, and of course, accurate documentation of the assignment process is required so that identification of every subject in the dataset can be maintained with the source data.

With NONMEM 7, ID values can be up to 14 digits in length. However, using a value with greater than 5 digits in length may create an unanticipated problem in the table files. NONMEM will read the analysis dataset correctly with up to 14 digits in the ID field. However, with the default settings, the table file will report the value of ID with only 5 unique digits. The default table format for all fields is s1PE11.4. This format allows a total width of 11 characters, including sign and decimal places. Four decimal places are used, with one digit to the left of the decimal place. An example default value is as follows: $-2.4567E+01$. Therefore, 5 unique digits are the most that will show by the default settings. Two consecutive subjects in a dataset with the ID values of 12345678901234 and 12345678901235 would be seen by NONMEM as different individuals, and model estimation would be performed as anticipated. However, the ID value output in the table would be $1.2346E+13$ for both individuals. Thus, when postprocessing for summary values, plots, or tables, the records from the two individuals would be seen as arising from a single subject. Longer ID records, or any other data item, can be accommodated by changing the output format used in the table file. The LFORMAT and RFORMAT options can be used to accomplish this, using FORTRAN syntax. For example, the following code could be used to generate table file in which the ID numbers given earlier could be distinguished:

```
$TABLE ID DOSE WT TIME NOPRINT
FILE=./filename.tbl
RFORMAT="(F15.0,"
RFORMAT="7(s1PE11.4))"
```

This example gives a real number output of the 14-character ID, plus one space for a decimal, and uses the default format for the remaining 7-item output in the table file (3 named items, plus 4 items automatically appended to the table file). The reader is referred to the user's manuals and help files for more details on the use of LFORMAT and RFORMAT.

4.3.4 DV

DV is the *dependent variable* data item. The values in this field represent the observations to be modeled. These observations could be drug concentrations for a PK model and drug effects for a PD model, or the DV field might contain observations of both PK and PD types in a PK/PD model. The DV item is used in conjunction with the compartment (CMT) data item, which specifies the model compartment in which the observation was made to the program.

The value of DV must be missing on all dose records. It would also be missing on *other*-type event records. However, if an *other* event and DV appear on the same record, the record would be understood by NONMEM to be an observation record with DV equal to a nonmissing value that also includes a change in another variable (e.g., weight).

4.3.5 MDV

The MDV data item allows the user to inform NONMEM whether or not the value in the DV field is missing. MDV is a logical variable, so MDV should have a value of 1 (i.e., true) on records for which DV is missing, such as on dosing records. MDV should have a value of 0 (i.e., false) on observation records where DV is not missing. If DV is missing on an observation record and MDV is not specified or MDV = 0, then an error will be reported.

MDV is not a required data item. NM-TRAN will assign a value from the context of the dataset if it is not included. We find it a good practice, however, to assign the value of MDV in the construction of the dataset, in order to be certain that the behavior is what we expect.

4.3.6 CMT

The compartment number data item (CMT) specifies in which compartment a dosing or observation event is occurring. CMT is not a required item in some models, where the dosing and observations are occurring in the default compartments for those events. PREDPP models, such as those using ADVAN1 through ADVAN4, ADVAN11, and ADVAN12, have default dose and observation compartments defined, so CMT is not required in these. CMT is a required item in situations where the user defines the model or where doses or observations are occurring in compartments other than the defaults. The default dose and observation compartments associated with certain ADVAN subroutines are described in Table 4.8.

When CMT is included, its value in the dataset is an integer corresponding to the compartment number in which the event described by the record is occurring. On *other*-type event records, CMT is generally set to the value of missing (e.g., ".").

CMT is a necessary component of models describing two types of data, such as models of parent and metabolite concentrations or of PK and PD observations. Observations of different types are modeled using specific compartments, and CMT is used to instruct NONMEM of the type of observation recorded with a given record. CMT is also required when using ADVAN2 or ADVAN4 when intravenous (IV) doses

TABLE 4.8   Default dose and observation compartment assignments for the specific ADVAN routines

ADVAN	Default dose compartment	Default observation compartment
1	1	1
2	1	2
3	1	1
4	1	2
10	1	1
11	1	1
12	1	2

are given in addition to the doses administered into the absorption compartment (e.g., when an IV loading dose is followed by oral maintenance therapy or data from IV and oral administration studies are pooled). With these models, the default dose compartment is CMT=1, the absorption compartment. An IV dose is administered directly into the central compartment, avoiding the absorption process, so the value of CMT=2 is required on these dosing records. This use of CMT to indicate the compartment invoked in a particular record provides a great deal of flexibility to the event handling capabilities for modeling with NONMEM. In the past, certain advanced *tricks* have been employed using an extra compartment as a switch for the current state of a system. The need for such techniques has been reduced by the implementation of such features as model event time (MTIME) variables in NONMEM. MTIME is a model event time variable that can be estimated by NONMEM. Use of the MTIME variable will be described briefly in Chapter 9.

4.3.7   EVID

The EVID data item is an explicit declaration to NONMEM of the *type* of the current record. As with MDV, this is frequently not a required data item, but we have found it a good practice to define the item in the dataset. Values of EVID are integers 0, 1, 2, 3, or 4.

EVID=0 defines the record as an observation event. EVID=1 defines the record as a dose event. EVID=2 defines the record as an *other*-type event record. EVID=3 or 4 are values that *reset* the conditions of the system, with EVID=4 indicating a combination of an EVID=3 (reset only) and an EVID=1 (dosing) event, whereby there is a reset immediately prior to the administration of a dose at the time of the record. By *reset*, we mean that the values of mass or concentration in the various compartments of the model are all reset to zero (i.e., the compartments are emptied). This is a way of allowing NONMEM to keep track of the individual between two disjoint periods of time, where the concentrations of the first period do not affect the concentrations of the second period (i.e., there is no superpositioning of concentrations across the two periods). An example of the utility of this might be a crossover study in which sufficient time is allowed for all concentrations from the first period to be eliminated before dosing and sample collection in a subsequent period. The use of a reset event

TABLE 4.9 General requirements for DV and AMT variable values
on the various types of EVID records

EVID	DV	AMT
0	Generally nonmissing	Required to be missing
1	Required to be missing	Required to be nonmissing
2	Required to be missing	Required to be missing
3	Required to be missing	Required to be missing
4	Required to be missing	Required to be nonmissing

keeps the records of the individual together, so NONMEM will keep the same random-effect parameter values for the individual and allows the restarting of TIME within the individual without an error message.

The use of EVID in certain circumstances implies certain conditions of the value of AMT and DV on the same record. Differences exist in the implications based on whether the model is being used to fit a dataset and the DV values in the dataset are nonmissing or whether the model is being used to simulate a new dataset based on a defined model and set of parameters and the data in the DV column are all missing. These distinctions will be covered in more detail later in this text. As shown in Table 4.9, when fitting a dataset, the following conditions are implied:

In addition to dosing and observation records, some event records may be included that have a missing DV value, MDV=1, and EVID=2. The observation records without missing values (EVID=0) are used in the fitting process. The observation records with missing DV values (EVID=2) are useful for returning a model-predicted value at particular timepoints. These predicted values may be useful for other purposes such as reconstructing the entire PK profile for an individual, matching a predicted concentration value with a simultaneous PD record, or for producing plots of predicted observations.

A related item is the optional *PCMT* data item. This item allows one to state the compartment for which a predicted value will be computed on nonobservation records such as dose records, other-type events, and reset events. If PCMT is not included, then the prediction on these records will be in the default observation compartment. With an EVID=1 (dose) or 2 (other type) record, the value of PCMT may specify the compartment from which the predicted value F is obtained. This provides a way to retrieve a prediction in a compartment other than the default observation compartment on these types of records. Of note, the PCMT value is ignored on observation records (EVID=0), since CMT defines the PCMT for observation records.

4.3.8 AMT

The amount of administered doses (AMT) is recorded in the AMT variable item on dosing records. While not specified in the dataset, all dose amounts must be expressed as values with consistent units on all dosing records. As with all data items, since character data are not generally allowed in the NONMEM dataset, no data item is included to express the units of the dose, unless that item is dropped on $INPUT statement. The value of AMT must be missing on all observation and *other*-type records. AMT gives the amount of the administered dose, regardless of the route (e.g., oral administration, bolus, or infusion).

The dose record may have other variables that give additional information about doses. These include RATE, ADDL, SS, II, and/or some variable capturing the duration of an infusion. Records containing these additional types of qualifiers must still include the total dose amount specified in AMT.

4.3.9 RATE

For drug administration by infusion, or any zero-order input models, the rate of drug administration may be defined using the RATE data item. Rate defines the amount of drug administered per unit time. Use of the RATE data item is required for specifying doses administered via infusion, though it may not always include the rate of the infusion. There are several options for using the RATE item to define the infusion process. The rate of infusion may be included as a data item, or it may be modeled using rate as a parameter to be estimated. In either case, the RATE data item must be included in the dataset. The value for RATE in the data determines the way in which the rate of the infusion is handled in NONMEM.

In the dataset, RATE may have values of 0, –1, –2, or a real number greater than zero. When RATE=0 on a dosing record, the dose is not considered an infusion. For example, in a dataset where both bolus and infusion doses are given, the value of RATE on the bolus doses is set to zero.

RATE may have a real number value greater than zero. In this case, the value of RATE specifies the rate of the infusion as mass per unit time. The mass is the dose given in AMT, and time, or the duration of the infusion, is determined by AMT/RATE.

The time course of the infusion may also be modeled in one of two alternative ways. In either case, the total amount of drug administered is defined in AMT. One option for modeling the time course of the infusion is to include the rate of infusion as a parameter in the model, and the other option is to include the duration of the infusion in the model as a parameter.

When RATE=–1 in the dataset, the rate of infusion is defined as a parameter of the model. The control stream must therefore define the additional parameter Rn, where *n* is the number of the compartment into which the infusion is administered. Including RATE=–1 in the dataset records and $R1 = \text{THETA}(1)$ in the control stream, instructs NONMEM that the dose given on the record is an infusion, and it is defined by the value of AMT and the rate of infusion that is estimated by NONMEM as a parameter in the model.

A similar approach exists for modeling the infusion in terms of duration. When RATE=–2, the duration of the infusion is defined to be a parameter of the model. In this case, *Dn* must be defined in the control stream, where *n* is the number of the compartment into which the infusion is administered. With RATE=–2 in the dataset, $D1 = \text{THETA}(1)$ would define that an infusion is administered into the first compartment, and it is defined by the value of AMT and the duration of the infusion that is to be estimated by NONMEM. THETA(1) specifies the fixed-effect parameter for duration. Random effects could also be added to the definition to obtain individual subject estimates of $D1$, the infusion length.

Oftentimes, however, case report forms used for clinical trials will be designed to capture the exact length of the infusion for each subject by recording the exact start and stop times of the infusion. Infusions intended to be administered over 30 minutes may, in reality, vary considerably in length due to varying conditions during the trial. If data are available indicating the length of the infusion for each subject, specific values of the duration may be included as an item in the dataset. In this case, the $INPUT would specify a variable containing the duration of the infusion (e.g., DUR), and the $PK block would include a statement setting the duration parameter (e.g., $D1$) equal to this duration variable (i.e., the individual-specific lengths of infusion). This is illustrated below:

```
$INPUT ID TIME ... ... AMT DUR RATE ... ... ...
$PK
...
D1 = DUR
```

Here, the dataset includes the exact duration of infusion dose that might be computed by taking the difference between the time of the end of infusion and the time of the start of infusion. In this case, the infusion process is fully specified, and no parameter needs to be estimated to define the infusion.

To invoke either option of specifying the infusion in terms of the duration of the infusion, RATE is included in the dataset with a value of −2 on the infusion dosing records. The value of RATE must be missing on observation and *other*-type event records.

4.3.10   ADDL

We have described the explicit inclusion of dosing records in the dataset. NONMEM also offers the ability to consolidate the expression of multiple dosing records when additional doses are given in the same amount and with the same II of time. The imputation of additional doses is achieved using the ADDL data item. The value of ADDL is greater than zero on a dosing record when one wants to inform the system about a number of additional doses given at times subsequent to the current record time, with the interval of time specified in II (to be described in Section 4.3.11). If a total of N doses are administered, ADDL is given the value "$N-1$" since the dosing record explicitly gives the occurrence of the sequence of doses.

For example, if study subject 10010 received 5 days' dosing of 100 mg administered twice daily, all of the doses could be specified with a single dosing record with the variable values shown in Table 4.10.

TABLE 4.10   Example of a single dosing record describing multiple additional doses

ID	TIME	AMT	ADDL	II	EVID	MDV
10010	0	100	9	12	1	1

TABLE 4.11   Expanded table of the individual dosing records specified by
the ADDL example given before

ID	TIME	AMT	ADDL	II	EVID	MDV
10010	0	100	.	.	1	1
10010	12	100	.	.	1	1
10010	24	100	.	.	1	1
10010	36	100	.	.	1	1
10010	48	100	.	.	1	1
10010	60	100	.	.	1	1
10010	72	100	.	.	1	1
10010	84	100	.	.	1	1
10010	96	100	.	.	1	1
10010	108	100	.	.	1	1

This record explicitly specifies a 100-mg dose at time equal to 0 and implicitly defines 9 additional doses administered at exactly 12 hour intervals thereafter. At the beginning of processing the records for the individual, NONMEM sets up an array in memory with the implied doses. As any additional records for the subject are processed, these implied doses are inserted in time sequence to the overall record set for the individual. The event sequence implied by this record would be the same as the 10 individual dosing records given in Table 4.11.

One can see the efficiency and power of the ADDL item for simplifying the construction of datasets, as long as the II can be assumed to be constant and the dose remains constant.

4.3.11   II

As just described, the II data item defines the length of time between doses. II is used in conjunction with ADDL or an SS item, to be discussed in the next section. Since the II must remain constant to use the II item, the specification of some dosing regimens using ADDL and II might not be feasible. There is a work-around for drug regimens with varying time intervals between the doses to be administered on a given day. Consider the case where a 100-mg dose is given for 10 days at regular mealtimes, for example, 8:00 A.M., 12:00 P.M., and 6:00 P.M. The II within the day would be 4, 6, and 14 hours. Since the II are not uniform, the ADDL and II items cannot be used with a single record to define the dosing history. However, one could consider this regimen as three once-daily regimens given at the appropriate times. With this construct, the dosing history can be specified using ADDL and II with only three separate dosing records as shown in Table 4.12.

This example demonstrates a small degree of the flexibility in specifying complex event histories that is possible with NONMEM. With a little creativity, a variety of complex situations may be described with relative simplicity. Of course, it is very important to understand how NONMEM is utilizing the data records and to ensure that what was intended is what is achieved.

TABLE 4.12 Example of dosing records for repeated, irregular dosing patterns

ID	TIME	AMT	ADDL	II	EVID	MDV
10010	8:00	100	9	24	1	1
10010	12:00	100	9	24	1	1
10010	18:00	100	9	24	1	1

When using II, the interval of time must be expressed in the same units as time in the TIME variable. II can be formatted as either a real number or as clock time (hh:mm). The value of II must be missing on observation and *other* event records.

4.3.12   SS

Like ADDL, the SS data item implies the state of the system with regard to past and current dosing. SS is a data item that may take on integer values of 0, 1, or 2.

When SS = 0 on a dosing record, the record does not specifically assume the system is at SS. If a dosing record includes SS = 1, the dose is assumed to be an SS dose, and the record resets the amounts in the compartments to SS condition, ignoring the contribution of any previous dosing records for the individual. Since the attainment of SS conditions is dependent upon the dosing interval, a nonmissing value of II must always be included on a dosing record with an SS value greater than 0.

When SS = 2, the current record is assumed to be an SS dose, but prior recorded doses are not ignored because there is no reset of the system. Concentrations from both sources are added using superpositioning principles to determine the time course of concentration values.

The variable SS must have a missing value on observation records and *other*-type event records.

4.4   CONSTRUCTING DATASETS WITH FLEXIBILITY TO APPLY ALTERNATE MODELS

In some circumstances, when a range of models might be explored, which might require different structures of the data, it is advantageous to define multiple values of some data items such as CMT within a single dataset. Thus, a single dataset can be built, rather than separate datasets for each model approach. In the dataset, one might have two CMT columns, each using the appropriate definition of CMT for a particular modeling approach that might be tried. Then in the application of a particular control stream that defines a particular model, the desired CMT values would be selected on the $INPUT statement by putting the reserved variable name, CMT, in the correct position on that statement. The position of the other CMT column would be given a different, nonreserved variable name, and the item may be dropped, for example, CMT2 = DROP.

4.5 EXAMPLES OF EVENT RECORDS

4.5.1 Alternatives for Specifying Time

Suppose a 200-mg oral dose is administered at 6:00 A.M. The model is to be coded with a one-compartment model with first-order oral absorption. Three alternatives for coding a data record describing this dose are provided in Table 4.13.

Note the value of time in each of these examples. Time can be clock TIME as shown in the first line of code. TIME can be a real number expression, not necessarily starting at time equal to 0, or TIME can represent elapsed time that does start at time equal to 0 with the first dose the patient received.

4.5.2 Infusions and Zero-Order Input

Suppose a 500-mg infusion is to be administered over a period of 10 minutes, beginning at 1:00 P.M. If only IV drug administration is included in the dataset, then two alternatives for coding this infusion record in the dataset are shown in Table 4.14.

In the first alternative, PREDPP uses the value of AMT and RATE to administer 500 mg at the rate of 3000 mg/hour. At this rate, the drug runs out after 10 minutes, resulting in a 10-minute duration. With the second alternative, RATE = -2 instructs NONMEM to construct the infusion as an amount given over a particular duration. Here, the duration is defined in the DUR column in the dataset. The $INPUT line would include an arbitrary variable name for this column, for example, DUR, and the parameter $D1$ must be set equal to that variable name in the control stream: $D1 = DUR$.

TABLE 4.13   Example records demonstrating alternative expressions for specifying the value of time

ID	TIME	AMT	DV	EVID	MDV	CMT
1	6:00	200	.	1	1	1

ID	Time	AMT	DV	EVID	MDV	CMT
1	6:0	200	.	1	1	1

ID	Time	AMT	DV	EVID	MDV	CMT
1	0	200	.	1	1	1

TABLE 4.14   Example records demonstrating alternative methods to define a zero-order input dosing record

ID	TIME	AMT	RATE	DUR	DV	EVID	MDV	CMT
1	0	500	3000	.	.	1	1	1

ID	TIME	AMT	RATE	DUR	DV	EVID	MDV	CMT
1	13:00	500	-2	0.167	.	1	1	1

TABLE 4.15 Example of dosing and observation records in a NONMEM dataset

ID	TIME	AMT	ADDL	II	DV	EVID	MDV	CMT	TAD
1	0	250	19	12	.	1	1	1	0
1	1.0	.	.	.	10.6	0	0	2	1.0
1	220	.	.	.	12.3	0	0	2	4.0

Another alternative to this last example is to estimate the duration of the infusion, if there are sufficient data present to inform the fitting of the infusion process. To do so, the duration data need not be present, and $D1$ would be modeled using at least a fixed-effect parameter, for example, $D1 = THETA(n)$. This latter example might be a useful approach to estimate drug input as a zero-order process when the duration of input (i.e., the length of time that the drug is absorbed) is not precisely known, for example, following administration of a membrane-controlled transdermal product, since a reservoir of drug in the skin might contribute to continued absorption after the patch is removed from the skin.

4.5.3 Using ADDL

Fitting data with NONMEM using PREDPP requires interweaving the records of doses and observations in a time-oriented series of events within each individual's records. Suppose an oral 250-mg dose of an antibiotic is administered twice daily for 10 days and that plasma samples are collected on days 1 and 10. These doses and observations might be coded as shown in Table 4.15.

In Table 4.15, TAD is computed as the *time since last (or most recent) dose*. Including this variable value for each observation can aid in presenting plots of the data, where the concentration profile is assembled from data across two or more dosing intervals. The values of CMT given earlier assume that the dose is administered into compartment 1, the absorption compartment for this orally administered drug, and that the observations are made in compartment 2, the central compartment.

Another important behavior of NONMEM that is important to understand, especially when using ADDL, has to do with the order of records. If when using ADDL to specify a series of doses, an observation record occurs at the exact time of an implied dose, NONMEM assumes that the implied dose enters the system first, followed by the concentration. If this situation arises because the study design mandates that samples are collected immediately prior to dosing on certain visits, we need to find another way to code such records. One way to use ADDL and still ensure that the dosing and observation events occur in the correct order is to add an extremely small amount of time (say, seconds) to the time on the dosing record. For example, if the initiating dosing record for the series of once-daily doses administered is recorded at TIME = 8.0 (hours), instead, set the dose time to 8.001 hours. In this way, all doses in the series will be administered a number of seconds after the clock time at which they were recorded, which will prevent samples collected at the same time (8.0 hours) from being predicted after the dose event.

4.5.4 Steady-State Approach

An example that demonstrates the advantage of the SS approach to coding a dataset is given here. Assume an oral dose of 25 mg is administered to patient 12 twice daily for 6 months. Assume also that the elimination half-life is short and SS conditions are achieved after 36 hours, and suppose that samples are collected at 1 and 3 hours after the dose on the morning of day 48. One method that could be considered to record the doses in the dataset is to insert 95 individual dose records, two a day from day 1 to day 47 plus one dose on the morning of day 48. This approach would not be the most efficient manner to specify the dosing history. Another alternative is to use the ADDL item to insert one dose record with TIME=0, ADDL=94, and II=12. The simplest method, however, is to use the SS option to specify that the dose immediately prior to the first observation was given under SS conditions. Oftentimes, case report forms are designed to capture the exact dosing information (date, time, amount, etc.) of the dose administered immediately prior to a sample. In this case, the information needed for this dose record is easily obtained. Considering the dose time in hours following the first dose at an assumed time=0 [$(48 - 1) \times 24 = 1128$], this situation might be coded as shown in Table 4.16.

The use of SS=1 with II=12 instructs NONMEM that enough doses have been administered 12 hours apart to bring the system up to SS conditions some time prior to 1128 hours.

4.5.5 Samples Before and After Achieving Steady State

In many PK studies, some samples are collected before SS conditions are reached as well as after a dose at SS. For example, suppose 50-mg oral doses are administered three times a day for 5 days and that SS is reached after about 48 hours. If samples are collected after the second dose and another sample is collected on day 5, the SS data item could be used to simplify coding of the dosing history as shown in Table 4.17.

TABLE 4.16 Example of an SS dosing scenario

ID	TIME	AMT	SS	II	DV	EVID	MDV	CMT	TAD
12	1128	25	1	12	.	1	1	1	0.0
12	1129	.	.	.	12.7	0	0	2	1.0
12	1131	.	.	.	24.3	0	0	2	3.0

TABLE 4.17 Example of an SS dosing scenario with observations made before and after achieving SS conditions

ID	DAY	TIME	AMT	SS	II	DV	EVID	MDV	CMT	TAD
1	1	0	50	0	.	.	1	1	1	0.0
1	1	8	50	0	.	.	1	1	1	0.0
1	1	12	.	.	.	16.3	0	0	2	4.0
1	5	8	50	1	8	.	1	1	1	0.0
1	5	9.5	.	.	.	2.0	0	0	2	1.5

TABLE 4.18   Example of an SS dosing scenario with an additional dose

ID	DATE	TIME	AMT	SS	II	DV	EVID	MDV	CMT	TAD
1	11/20/10	18:00	250	0	.	.	1	1	1	0
1	11/22/10	7:00	250	2	24	.	1	1	1	0
1	11/22/10	10:30	.	.	.	23.4	0	0	2	3.5

4.5.6   Unscheduled Doses in a Steady-State Regimen

Another situation arises when a patient takes an unscheduled dose in the midst of the regularly scheduled SS dosing scenario. Suppose a patient takes a 250-mg dose of a chronically administered medication once daily at 7:00 A.M. for several months. The half-life of the drug is around 24 hours, so SS can be assumed to have been achieved after 5 days. Through careful questioning, it is confirmed that the patient has followed their morning dosing schedule precisely for at least the last week, but the patient also states he took an extra dose at 6:00 P.M. 2 days prior to the present office visit, at which time a blood sample was collected at 10:30 A.M. for assay of drug concentration. This extra dose cannot be ignored when constructing the dosing profile since its omission would bias the results of the model.

To code this example, the SS dosing history and the extra dose that occurred 2 days prior should be superimposed. Since chronic dosing began at some unspecified time in the past, the SS option is a logical choice to reflect the pattern of the dosing regimen and our knowledge. A DATE plus TIME approach could be considered to code this example since we know the date of the office visit and the date and time of the extra dose. Example data records are shown in Table 4.18.

The use of SS = 2 for the chronic regimen tells NONMEM that this dose can be assumed to be at SS, but does not reset the prior compartment amounts (so as to not obliterate the impact of the extra dose record). This superimposes the concentrations from the two dose records. If a sample had been collected on 11/21/10, this construction would not be correct, as the doses implied by the SS record would not have entered the system at that point.

There are many correct alternatives for coding this event history. This pattern of events could also be described without the use of DATE. One option would be to arbitrarily impute the time of the extra dose as time zero and adjust the other event times accordingly.

4.5.7   Steady-State Dosing with an Irregular Dosing Interval

Using the SS or ADDL dosing items requires using the II data item to inform NONMEM of the frequency of dosing implied for the past or future doses. II can have only a single value for a record, and thus, the implied dosing interval is constant for the record. Administration of some drug products, however, will commonly have an irregular pattern within a day. For example, a drug might be administered three times a day but only during the waking hours.

TABLE 4.19   Example of SS dosing with an irregular dosing interval

ID	DATE	TIME	AMT	SS	II	DV	EVID	MDV	CMT	TAD
1	13	14:00	10	1	24	.	1	1	1	0
1	13	20:00	10	2	24	.	1	1	1	0
1	14	8:00	10	2	24	.	1	1	1	0
1	14	8:30	.	.	.	1.25	0	0	2	0.0

The following scenario illustrates how to adjust the code to accommodate this situation. Suppose, for example, oral doses of 10 mg are administered three times daily at 8:00 A.M., 2:00 P.M., and 8:00 P.M. for 14 days, with SS conditions achieved after 10 days of dosing. If a sample was collected from the patient at 8:30 A.M. on day 14, the following records, as shown in Table 4.19, would correctly specify the daily dosing intervals as well as the observation record:

The dosing history is given by inserting a separate dosing record for each time of day when doses are administered and giving the individual records a 24-hour dosing interval. The first dosing record has SS = 1, initializing the system at SS on this once-daily dose. SS = 2 is used on the two subsequent dosing records to superimpose the two additional series of once-daily doses onto the first dosing series. The doses are specified in order of occurrence with the last dose being the dose immediately prior to sample collection. If the exact date and time of the last three doses prior to blood sample collection were recorded for a dosing interval that varied in duration over a 24-hour period, this method may be considered to specify SS conditions.

4.5.8   Multiple Routes of Administration

Some studies or clinical situations will have concentration data that is collected following doses from multiple routes of administration. An absolute bioavailability study is an example in which subjects would receive IV and oral administration on alternate study periods. In a clinical setting, concentration data may be available from a patient following both IV and oral administration. When data following oral administration are modeled, an absorption compartment will be included. Absorbed drug will be modeled with one or more compartments, one of which is the central compartment. Intravenously administered drug is entered as a bolus or infusion into the central compartment. Suppose ADVAN2 is used to specify the model for the following data, where the depot or absorption compartment is CMT = 1 and the central compartment is CMT = 2. Both the IV (bolus) dose and the observations will occur in compartment CMT = 2, as shown in Table 4.20.

Subject 1 received an oral dose since CMT = 1 on the dosing record, while subject 2 received an IV bolus dose since CMT = 2. For both subjects, each of the observation records occurs in CMT = 2, the central compartment.

TABLE 4.20 Example of dosing from multiple routes of administration

ID	TIME	AMT	DV	CMT	EVID	MDV
1	0	20	.	1	1	1
1	2.5	.	43.6	2	0	0
1	10	.	12.3	2	0	0
2	0	10	.	2	1	1
2	2.0	.	109.7	2	0	0
2	9	.	29.6	2	0	0

TABLE 4.21 Example of records describing a dose followed by simultaneous PK and PD observations

ID	TIME	AMT	DV	CMT	EVID	MDV
1	0	100	.	1	1	1
1	10	.	635	1	0	0
1	10	.	45	3	0	0

4.5.9 Modeling Multiple Dependent Variable Data Types

In PK/PD models or simultaneous models of parent and metabolite concentrations, multiple types of DV data are modeled. These data must all be included in the column for the DV data item. The CMT data item may be used to specify the type of observation and to which model compartment these data apply.

The following example assumes a two-compartment PK model with IV bolus dosing, and the third compartment is an *effect* compartment in a PK/PD model. The data records are shown in Table 4.21.

Here, a single 100-mg IV bolus dose is given at time zero into the first compartment. Ten hours later, a PK and PD measurement is made simultaneously. The second record is the PK sample, since CMT = 1. The third record is the PD observation, since CMT = 3.

4.5.10 Dataset for $PRED

As a final example, a model could be completely specified within a $PRED block without using the features of the PREDPP routines. In this case, NONMEM is providing nonlinear regression tools, but is not keeping up with doses, time, and compartment amounts, or advancing a PK model for the user. $PRED datasets will have structure more similar to those used with other nonlinear regression programs, where every record is an observation record and all data necessary for the regression are present on every record. The concept of dosing records is not considered in these datasets.

A simple example is a dataset of C_{max} and delta-QT$_c$ data. For these data, a regression model exploring the relationship of C_{max} and QT$_c$ might be applied.

TABLE 4.22   Example data records for a $PRED model

ID	PER	DOSE	C_{max}	DQTC
1	1	300	26	5.4
2	1	300	23	3.2
2	2	400	29	3.1
3	1	300	17	4.9

Other data, such as DOSE in this example, may be included as indicator variables, group assignments, or predictors of submodels, but NONMEM does not recognize these data inherently as a dose of drug into a PK system, as it would if PREDPP were used. Example data records are shown in Table 4.22.

4.6 BEYOND DOSES AND OBSERVATIONS

4.6.1 Other Data Items

Analysis datasets may include many items of data in addition to those described earlier that were related to doses, observations, and housekeeping items that NONMEM may use or require to run. Most commonly, additional data items will be included as potential covariates of model parameters or as descriptors of the study design, such as dose amount or group information. Covariate values or other study information might simply be included for use in subsetting the data or results. Evaluating subsets is a frequent and sometimes essential task for understanding the relationships in the data and the model performance or predictions in certain subgroups. Evaluating goodness of fit by dose groups can sometimes reveal nonlinearity, which may not be easily observed in goodness-of-fit plots with all data combined.

As mentioned previously, all data in NONMEM datasets are required to be numerical or to be dropped in the $INPUT line, with the exceptions of TIME, which may include the ":" character, and DATE, which may include the "/" or "-" characters and not be dropped. Frequently, character format data in the source data must be converted to a numerical descriptor for use in the analysis dataset. Coding these descriptors and creating meaningful names can perhaps reduce the occurrence of errors in the interpretation and communication of results. For example, we frequently code the value of sex using a logical variable named SEXF that has a value of 1 for female and 0 for male. With a clear variable name, such SEXF, it is easy to read the data and know the correct interpretation of values.

In addition, variable names can be made to clearly identify units. DOSEMG, WTKG, and HTCM each clearly communicate their meaning and units as dose in milligrams, weight in kilograms, and height in centimeters, respectively. Such practices help reduce errors in dataset construction.

Clinical data such as race, age, weight, organ-function status, lab-test values, concomitant disease, times and amounts of doses, and time of blood collection for PK measurements are typically found in different panels or data files from the clinical trial database. The task of accessing and properly merging these data to create an accurate dataset for PK or PK/PD analysis can require significant effort and programming skill. An essential piece of putting together the data needed for analysis is the presence of a unique merge key between datasets. Study number, clinical trial subject ID number, time and date, and treatment code are examples of data that might be used to merge records from different panels of the clinical trial databases. Careful attention must be given when assembling the data to know that merge keys are unique and that there are not missing values for a merge key in any dataset in which that key is used.

What does one do when one of the essential merge keys is missing from a record or when multiple records have the same merge key values? The data manager has substantial responsibility to find mismatched or incomplete merge records, missing values, or other problems of *missingness* in the data. Values of other variables might also be missing, and the approach to addressing this situation requires careful thought and sometimes regulatory agreement. Decisions regarding imputation of missing values and the assumptions necessary to support these imputations will need to be made. A *best practice* is to define how missing data will be treated in the data analysis plan, which should be developed prior to the release of the data or the start of the analysis, at the latest.

Some considerations in the approach to imputing data include questions such as the following: What fraction of the data is missing? Are these missing data primarily in one group or another? Are missing values occurring at a specific time in the concentration–time profile? The answers to these questions may help to select the most appropriate method to deal with such data.

4.6.2 Covariate Changes over Time

In some circumstances, it will be important to include changes in covariate values over time. For instance, if a long-term study is conducted in which drug treatment affects body weight and body weight is to be explored as a covariate of PK parameters, it will be important to collect repeated measurements of body weight over the duration of the study. The current value of body weight can then be included on dosing or observation records, if the measurement coincides with these events, or body weight can be updated on an *other*-type event record, with EVID=2.

One caution to consider is the default behavior that NONMEM uses when implied doses are used to express a series of dosing events (e.g., ADDL). The values of *other user-supplied data items* on an implied record come from the following record, rather than the prior record. This may not be the behavior one would expect. Consider the records shown in Table 4.23 as an example.

TABLE 4.23   Example records demonstrating a changing covariate over time

ID	TIME	DV	AMT	ADDL	II	WTKG
100	0		100	8	12	84
100	2	56.5	.	.	.	84
100	26	61.3	.	.	.	84
100	98	60.4	.	.	.	86.5

Subject 100 receives the first dose at time equal to 0 followed by 8 additional doses given every 12 hours. This is 9 total doses, given on day 1 until the morning of day 5. Dosing events thus occur at 0, 12, 24, 36, 48, 60, 72, 84, and 96 hours. A baseline body weight of 84 kg is recorded prior to the first dose. This value is carried over onto subsequent records until an update in the data occurs. A body weight of 86.5 kg is measured on the morning of day 5. Blood samples for drug assay are collected at two hours after the morning doses on days 1, 2, and 5, and concentrations are recorded. The default behavior of NONMEM is that the weight of 86.5 kg is used on the implied dosing records between the 26-hour and 98-hour physical records. Thus, if a parameter in the model is computed based on WTKG, its value will be updated as of the 36-hour implied dose to 86.5 kg. One might expect that the update occurs when the WTKG is physically updated starting at 96 hours. This behavior can be controlled using the $BIND statement. The reader may want to refer to the NONMEM user's guides for additional information on use of $BIND (Beal et al. 1989–2011).

4.6.3   Inclusion of a Header Row

NM-TRAN reads the dataset specified in the $DATA statement of the control file and formats this into the very specific format required by the NONMEM program. If included, a header row defining names for the data items in the dataset is not used by NM-TRAN. Instead, NMTRAN gets the names and order of the data items from the $INPUT statement in the control file. Inclusion of a header row is most useful to the human reader of a dataset but must be *skipped* when importing the data file via the control stream or with graphing or other postprocessing software, though that may differ on a program-by-program basis. One might easily write software that strips off the header row and uses those items for variable names.

For some earlier versions of NONMEM, one needed to make sure there was a carriage return after the last row of data in a dataset. This is no longer the case with more recent versions.

REFERENCES

Beal SL, Sheiner LB, Boeckmann AJ, Bauer RJ, editors. *NONMEM 7.2.0 Users Guides*. Hanover: Icon Development Solutions; 1989–2011.

R Development Core Team (2013). *R: A Language and Environment for Statistical Computing*. Vienna: R Foundation for Statistical Computing. Available at http://www.R-project.org/. Accessed December 16, 2013.

SAS Institute Inc. *SAS and all other SAS Institute Inc. product or service names are registered trademarks or trademarks of SAS Institute Inc*. Cary: SAS Institute Inc; 2002–2010.

CHAPTER 5

MODEL BUILDING: TYPICAL PROCESS

5.1 INTRODUCTION

Owing to the hierarchical nature of population pharmacokinetic/pharmacodynamic (PK/PD) nonlinear mixed effect models as well as the typical complexity of such model development efforts, a general framework is proposed. This framework consists of the basic steps of the process for the development of such models (in the context of their application in a drug development endeavor). A high-level description of the proposed process is illustrated in Figure 5.1; each of the steps outlined in the figure will be discussed in this or subsequent chapters of this text.

A framework consisting of the modeling-related steps (i.e., basic model, addition of structural features, addition of statistical features, model refinement, and model testing) was first proposed by Sheiner and Beal in the *Introductory Workshops* they offered in the early nineties, and became fairly standard practice amongst many pharmacometricians (Beal and Sheiner 1992). Ette and colleagues extended this process beyond modeling to address steps that should be taken in advance of modeling and steps that may be taken after a final model is selected to address the application of the model to the problem at hand (Ette et al. 2004). Today, however, many modelers have adopted their own unique variations on this framework in terms of the extent to which process steps are completed and the order in which some steps are undertaken.

5.2 ANALYSIS PLANNING

Analysis planning is perhaps the most important step in any data analysis and modeling effort but particularly so in pharmacometric model development and analysis. Whether the analysis planning process entails the development of a formal, controlled, and approved document or simply a bullet-point list describing the main components of the plan, it is critical to take the time to complete this step prior to initiating data analysis.

Introduction to Population Pharmacokinetic / Pharmacodynamic Analysis with Nonlinear Mixed Effects Models, First Edition. Joel S. Owen and Jill Fiedler-Kelly.
© 2014 John Wiley & Sons, Inc. Published 2014 by John Wiley & Sons, Inc.

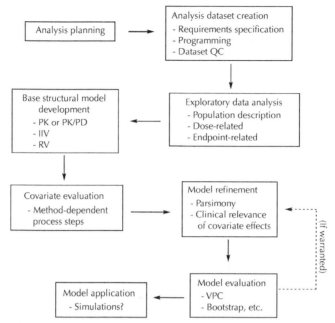

FIGURE 5.1   Typical pharmacometric model building process.

Statistical analysis plans (SAPs) have long been used by statisticians in various fields of study to promote the ethical treatment of data and to ensure the consistency and repeatability of analyses. Development of an analysis plan prior to locking the study databases, unblinding the treatment codes, and/or analysis commencement is perceived to be good statistical practice to minimize potential bias and lend credibility to analysis findings. A well-written SAP should contain enough detail to enable two independent analysts following the plan to come to essentially the same conclusions. International Conference on Harmonization (ICH) guidelines on *Statistical Principles for Clinical Trials* (European Medicines Agency (EMA) 1998) recommend finalization of the SAP before the study blind is broken, in addition to documentation of such activities. The two most relevant regulatory guidance documents for population PK/PD modelers (*FDA Guidance for Industry, Population Pharmacokinetics* (Food and Drug Administration 1999) and EMEA CHMP *Guideline on Reporting the Results of Population Pharmacokinetic Analyses* (EMA 2007)) both refer to the importance of analysis planning by stressing the need to specify analysis assumptions and decision-making rules, as well as deviations from the planned analyses.

The mere act of prespecifying, in detail, the major analysis steps and contingencies often results in a discovery of some sort: a feature of the data requiring further processing for analysis, an exploratory plot that might provide additional insight prior to modeling, a modeling assumption not likely to be met, a data editing rule requiring refinement, or an additional model worthy of consideration. Besides the improvement in analysis quality that derives from such careful a priori planning, obtaining input and/or approval of a pharmacometric analysis plan from team members representing other disciplines will likely result in greater buy-in and support for analysis results. The benefit of project team alignment prior to analysis and agreement with the planned approach to support eventual claims based on modeling efforts will only serve to further ingrain and instantiate the use of modeling and simulation techniques as an essential critical path activity.

Team members representing various functional areas can provide differing types of input and derive different kinds of benefits from involvement in the analysis planning process. Data management personnel responsible for preparing the data for analysis will derive insight from an understanding of the objectives for modeling and simulation efforts, appreciation for the types of data that are most critical to meeting analysis assumptions, and in addition, can provide insight and refinement of data editing rules. Consistent involvement of data management personnel in analysis planning and dataset creation can also provide an opportunity for standardization of code and processes. Involvement of clinicians in the selection and specification of covariates to be considered may prevent wasted time and effort in evaluating factors not likely to be clinically relevant or physiologically plausible even with statistically significant results. The input of a clinician or clinical disease specialist is perhaps most important in the planning of clinical trial simulation efforts where knowledge of factors that might influence response and an understanding of patient population characteristics, especially those that might impact expectations about compliance or drop-out behavior, is essential to the eventual usefulness and applicability of the results.

Other benefits of careful analysis planning performed with team input include greater transparency for life cycle and resource management, the ability to include modeling results and milestones in development program timelines, and the ability to devote time and resources to the consideration of explanations for possible findings prior to the availability of final results, when the timelines for delivery of knowledge are compressed. The proposed team-oriented analysis planning process can result in immediate reductions in time to complete modeling and simulation efforts and prepare the subsequent summary reports if the analysis planning effort is directly translated into the development of code (and even report text) based on the plan. Critical stopping and decision points, when a team-based review of results may be helpful for further planning, may also be elucidated based on the plan.

Appendix 5.1 contains recommendations for pharmacometric analysis plan content.

5.3 ANALYSIS DATASET CREATION

As discussed in Chapter 4, while NONMEM requires a specific structure and format for the dataset in order for it to be properly understood and interpreted by the software, one of its greatest strengths is its tremendous flexibility in accommodating different types of dosing regimens and patterns as well as variations in particular individual dosing histories. This capability, in conjunction with the statistical advantages of mixed effect modeling with sparse data, makes the NONMEM system an ideal platform for model development efforts utilizing the often-messy real-world (Phase 2/3) clinical trial data where protocol violations, data coding errors, dosing and sampling anomalies, and missing data abound. In addition, datasets consisting of pooled data from various trials or phases of development often require significant standardization efforts to normalize the data fields and values for appropriate model interpretation.

As the complexity of the trial design(s) and the messiness of the constituent datasets increase, so does the complexity of the analysis dataset creation task. While an analysis dataset for a standard Phase 1 single ascending dose or age-gender effect crossover study may be achievable using data import and manipulation techniques in a spreadsheet program such as Microsoft Excel®, a dataset for even a single Phase 3 trial or a pooled dataset consisting of several trials requires many complex data merging and manipulation tasks to create the appropriate dosing and sampling event records for the variety of scenarios that are frequently encountered. Such tasks therefore require the use of a programmatic approach and a fair amount of programming expertise, as it would otherwise be almost completely untenable using a more manual approach.

The creation of an analysis-ready dataset involves processing and cleaning the source data based on requirements developed to support the analysis plan. Anomalies in dosing history or sampling frequency will need to be coded so as to be understood accurately by the program, inconsistencies in units or coding of variables must be standardized, and new variables, required by NONMEM or the objectives of the analysis, may need to be created based on the data fields collected during the trial(s). Codification of the steps involved in creating accurate dosing and sampling records for each individual, while required, comes with its own numerous opportunities for the introduction of errors into the dataset. As such, a detailed plan for dataset review and checking should be implemented with each major dataset version or modification.

5.4 DATASET QUALITY CONTROL

Especially important when analysis datasets are created by someone other than the modeler, quality control review of an analysis dataset should consist of at least two major steps: (i) data checking of individual fields and relational data checking and (ii) dataset structure checking. When different individuals are responsible for the tasks of dataset creation and model development, written documentation of the analysis dataset requirements is generally prepared. The quality control process is then utilized as an opportunity to check not only the data and the dataset but importantly the understanding and interpretation of the requirements. Two different interpretations of the same written requirements may result in two different datasets—one, both, or neither of which may be *correct* (meaning as intended by the individual generating the requirements).

Quality checking of individual data fields may consist of a review of frequency tables for categorical or discrete variables and summary statistics (minimum, maximum, mean, standard deviation (SD), median, etc.) of continuous variables based on expectations of the values. Relational data checks may consist of programmatic calculations, such as the amount of time between a given PK sample and the previous dose or a count of the number of samples of various types collected from each subject. These relational checks depend, in part, upon a comparison of the information collected in more than one field of the source datasets. Knowledge of the protocol(s) and/or trial design(s) is typically required to adequately interpret such edit checks.

For NONMEM analysis datasets, quality checking of the dataset structure requires an understanding of both the analysis plan and the intended modeling approach (if not detailed in the plan) as well as the rules and requirements for NONMEM datasets as described in Chapter 4. Quality control review of the NONMEM dataset structure may involve individual field and relational edit checks of NONMEM-required variables in addition to a pass through NM-TRAN and a careful check of NONMEM's FDATA file. The topic of quality control will be discussed in more detail in Chapter 12.

5.5 EXPLORATORY DATA ANALYSIS

Beyond these quality checks, a thorough exploratory review of the data performed by creating graphical and tabular summaries should be conducted prior to running the first model (Tukey 1977). The overarching goal of a careful and deliberate exploratory data analysis (EDA), conducted prior to modeling, is to explore the informational content of the analysis dataset relative to the models to be evaluated. In essence, EDA is a structured assessment of whether the data collected will support the intended analysis plan. A simple and common example illustrating the benefit of EDA lies in the value of the simple concentration versus time (since previous dose) scatterplot. When the protocol allows for subjects to come to the clinic on PK sampling visits at any time following the previous dose in an effort to obtain a random distribution of sampling times relative to dosing, it is critical to understand the reality of this distribution prior to model fitting. If the actual distribution of sampling times relative to dosing is essentially bimodal with the vast majority of sample times clumped at either 1–2 hours postdosing or 10–12 hours postdosing, the PK structural models that may be considered are therefore limited. In this case, attempting to fit two-compartment distribution models to such a dataset may well prove fruitless without consideration of fixing key parameters of the model. If the informational content of the dataset relative to the intended or expected model is significantly lacking, the model development strategy to be employed may require modification.

When the sampling strategy and resulting data are more informative, EDA can serve to set up some expectations for models that are likely to be worthy of testing or not testing. Importantly, if informative plots are constructed, EDA can also serve to highlight important trends in the data, which may warrant consideration of other specific plots that can be constructed to further investigate trends or provide some insight into likely covariate effects. Graphical and tabular summaries of the data created during EDA may also help to identify outliers requiring exclusion and extreme data values worthy of further investigation.

The typical objectives of EDA are therefore, at least threefold: (i) to understand the realities of the opportunities for variability based on study design or execution (i.e., explore the study execution and compliance issues present in the dataset, understand the analysis population, and explore the characteristics of any missing data), (ii) to search for large, obvious trends in the data that will facilitate modeling efforts, and

(iii) to identify potential outliers or high-influence points that may be important to understand for the modeling.

5.5.1 EDA: Population Description

One important component of a thorough EDA entails a description of the population to be analyzed. Summary statistics should be computed describing the number of subjects to be modeled and patient characteristics in the overall dataset as well as separately by study, if data from various studies are to be pooled for analysis. If different dose levels will be evaluated, such summary statistics may also be computed by dose or treatment group in order to evaluate the distribution of subjects and patient features across the anticipated distribution of drug exposure. Table 5.1 and Table 5.2 provide examples of such summary tables generated to describe the population. Frequency distributions of patient characteristics (age, weight, race, gender, etc.) as illustrated in Figure 5.2, boxplots of continuous characteristics plotted versus categorical characteristics (e.g., age or weight versus ethnicity or gender) as in Figure 5.3, and scatterplots of the relationships between continuous patient characteristics should be generated, as in Figure 5.4, and evaluated for a thorough understanding of the patient population to be modeled.

TABLE 5.1 Summary statistics of patient characteristics by study

	Study 1	Study 2	Study 3	Pooled dataset
Weight (kg)				
Mean (SD)	74.0 (13.1)	76.3 (15.1)	81.7 (16.8)	79.2 (17.3)
Median	70.1	75.4	79.9	78.5
Min, max	44.3, 109.1	51.9, 107.9	48.3, 131.4	44.3, 131.4
n	50	50	200	300
Age (years)				
Mean (SD)	24.6 (4.7)	27.2 (6.8)	44.7 (11.2)	41.9 (12.1)
Median	23.0	25.6	45.2	40.7
Min, max	18. 39	19, 45	26, 61	18.61
n	50	50	200	300
Gender				
Female *n* (%)	28 (56.0)	26 (52.0)	113 (56.5)	167 (55.7)
Male *n* (%)	22 (44.0)	24 (48.0)	87 (43.5)	133 (44.3)
Race				
Caucasian *n* (%)	24 (48.0)	19 (38)	123 (61.5)	166 (55.3)
Black *n* (%)	12 (24.0)	11 (22.0)	29 (14.5)	52 (17.3)
Other *n* (%)	14 (28.0)	11 (22.0)	31 (15.5)	56 (18.7)
Asian *n* (%)	0 (0.0)	9 (18.0)	17 (8.5)	26 (8.7)
Renal function				
Normal *n* (%)	39 (78.0)	37 (74.0)	133 (66.5)	209 (69.7)
Mild impairment *n* (%)	10 (20.0)	9 (18.0)	45 (22.5)	64 (21.3)
Moderate impairment *n* (%)	1 (2.0)	4 (8.0)	19 (9.5)	24 (8.0)
Severe impairment *n* (%)	0 (0.0)	0 (0.0)	3 (1.5)	3 (1.0)

TABLE 5.2 Summary statistics of patient characteristics by dose group

	100-mg dose	200-mg dose
Weight (kg)		
Mean (SD)	78.7 (16.1)	79.9 (17.1)
Median	76.5	79.5
Min, max	44.3, 120.6	52.7, 131.4
n	120	180
Age (years)		
Mean (SD)	36.9 (9.6)	42.5 (11.6)
Median	34.7	42.7
Min, max	18, 39	28, 61
n	120	180
Gender		
Female *n* (%)	77 (64.2)	90 (50.0)
Male *n* (%)	43 (35.8)	90 (50.0)
Race		
Caucasian *n* (%)	24 (48.0)	19 (38)
Black *n* (%)	12 (24.0)	11 (22.0)
Other *n* (%)	14 (28.0)	11 (22.0)
Asian *n* (%)	0 (0.0)	9 (18.0)
Renal function		
Normal *n* (%)	39 (78.0)	37 (74.0)
Mild impairment *n* (%)	10 (20.0)	9 (18.0)
Moderate impairment *n* (%)	1 (2.0)	4 (8.0)
Severe impairment *n* (%)	0 (0.0)	0 (0.0)

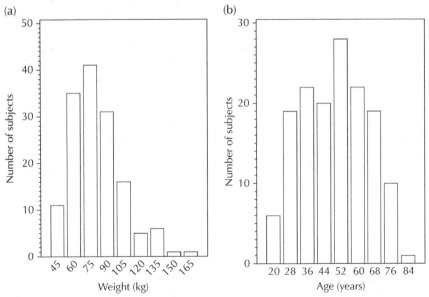

FIGURE 5.2 Frequency distributions of patient characteristics. Panel (a) illustrates the distribution of weight and Panel (b) provides the distribution of age in the population; the number below each bar represents the midpoint of the values in that bar.

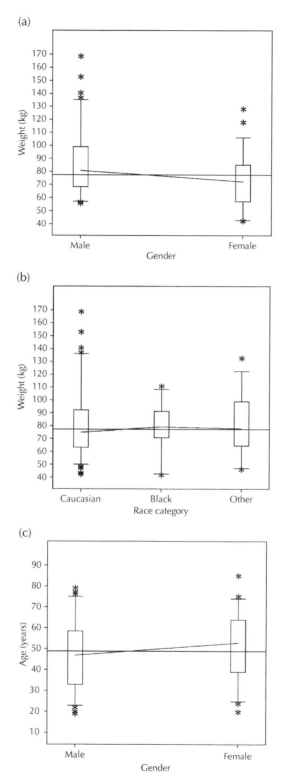

FIGURE 5.3 Boxplots of continuous patient characteristics versus categorical characteristics. Panel (a) illustrates the distribution of weight by gender. Panel (b) provides the distribution of weight by race group. Panel (c) illustrates the distribution of age by gender.

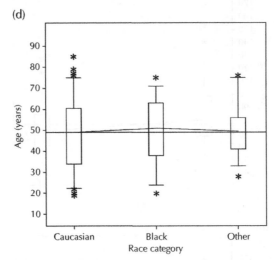

FIGURE 5.3 (*Continued*) Panel (d) provides the distribution of age by race group in the population; the box spans the interquartile range for the values in the subpopulation, the whiskers extend to the 5th and 95th percentiles of the distributions, with the asterisks representing values outside this range, and the boxes are joined at the median values.

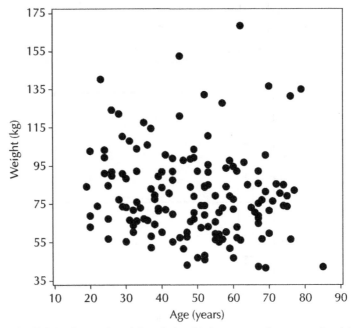

FIGURE 5.4 Scatterplot of the relationship between patient age and weight.

5.5.2   EDA: Dose-Related Data

In all population datasets, but in particular, those that include subjects studied at a variety of different dose levels, it is important to understand various aspects of the dose distribution to appropriately interpret and understand the resulting exposure distribution. Variables to be explored include the dose amount, the frequency of dosing, the length of drug infusions, the number of infusions received if this could vary between subjects, and if relevant, the overall length of drug treatment. Figure 5.5 illustrates an example frequency distribution of dose amount. In addition, derived dose-related data items required by NONMEM to describe dosing histories should also be described and explored (e.g., ADDL, II, and SS) via graphical or tabular frequency distributions. Table 5.3 illustrates a summary of dose-related data items; variables such as SS can be checked for the presence of only allowable values, and other variables, such as II, can be checked for unusual values, which may indicate an outlier or data error. Review of the distribution of such variables may help to identify possible anomalies in data collection or dosing histories as well as debug potential coding errors and/or improve code development to adequately capture the various typical as well as unusual patient behaviors with respect to dosing.

5.5.3   EDA: Concentration-Related Data

For population PK modeling efforts, a thorough understanding of the concentration and sample collection related data is critical as the drug concentration is the dependent variable (DV) to be modeled. As previously discussed, frequency distributions of the

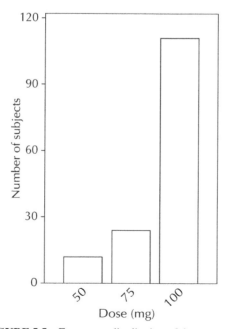

FIGURE 5.5   Frequency distribution of dose amount.

TABLE 5.3 Summary of select NONMEM dose-related data items

ADDL	n,%
0	100, 33.3%
41	7, 2.3%
42	192, 64.0%
43	1, 0.3%
SS	n,%
0	100, 33.3%
1	199, 66.3%
2	1, 0.3%
II	n,%
0	100, 33.3%
24	200, 66.7%

times of sample collection relative to dosing and of the number of samples collected per subject enable a thorough understanding of the informational content of the PK samples in the dataset. Figure 5.6 illustrates an example frequency distribution of the time of sampling relative to the previous dose administration. With respect to the drug and/or metabolite concentrations, summary statistics characterizing the concentrations and the number of samples measured to be below the limit of quantification (BLQ) of the assay, overall and stratified by the applicable dose level, in addition to the timing of such samples relative to dosing, may be informative in selecting an appropriate method of handling such samples in the modeling. Table 5.4 provides an example summary table illustrating the extent of samples determined to be BLQ of the assay. A variety of methods to treat such samples have been proposed (Beal 2001; Ahn et al. 2008; Byon et al. 2008), and the intended method or the means to determine the handling of such samples should be described in the analysis plan.

Perhaps the single most important and informative plot of PK data is the scatterplot of drug concentration level plotted against time of sampling. Because the Phase 2 and 3 data typically collected for population analysis are generated from sparse sampling strategies, where interpretation of the appropriateness and assessment of a given level are difficult at best, this simple scatterplot of concentration versus time since last dose (TSLD) for the population as a whole provides, in one picture, the basis for the population model to be developed. Figure 5.7 illustrates an example of a concentration versus TSLD scatterplot, using a semi-log scale for the y axis.

Even for this simple plot, however, a variety of plotting techniques can be employed to make the interpretation more useful. First, the sample time plotted on the x axis may be the time of the sample either relative to the last dose of study medication or relative to the first dose. Normalizing all of the samples relative to the last dose allows for a gross assessment of the shape of the PK profile, while consideration of the samples relative to the first dose may allow for an assessment as to whether the subjects are at steady state or when they come to steady-state conditions, as well as whether the PK of the study drug is stationary over time during the course of treatment. If a sufficient subset of the data consists of trough levels, this subset may be plotted against time since

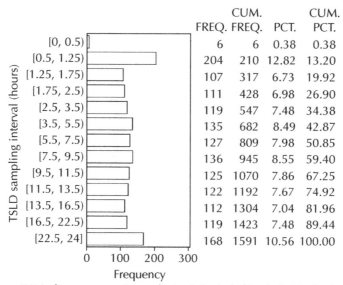

		CUM. FREQ.	FREQ.	PCT.	CUM. PCT.
[0, 0.5)		6	6	0.38	0.38
[0.5, 1.25)		204	210	12.82	13.20
[1.25, 1.75)		107	317	6.73	19.92
[1.75, 2.5)		111	428	6.98	26.90
[2.5, 3.5)		119	547	7.48	34.38
[3.5, 5.5)		135	682	8.49	42.87
[5.5, 7.5)		127	809	7.98	50.85
[7.5, 9.5)		136	945	8.55	59.40
[9.5, 11.5)		125	1070	7.86	67.25
[11.5, 13.5)		122	1192	7.67	74.92
[13.5, 16.5)		112	1304	7.04	81.96
[16.5, 22.5)		119	1423	7.48	89.44
[22.5, 24]		168	1591	10.56	100.00

[]/() indicates respective endpoint is included/excluded in the interval

FIGURE 5.6 Frequency distribution of TSLD (time of sampling relative to the most recent previous dose administered). Summary statistics are also provided to quantify the frequency of sampling in various time bins or ranges of TSLD.

TABLE 5.4 Summary of BLQ data by dose and sampling timepoint

Sampling timepoint (hours since last dose)	100-mg dose group ($n = 120$)	200-mg dose group ($n = 180$)
0.5	0.5% BLQ	0.1% BLQ
	99.5% > BLQ	99.9% > BLQ
1.0	0% BLQ	0% BLQ
	100% > BLQ	100% > BLQ
2.0	0% BLQ	0% BLQ
	100% > BLQ	100% > BLQ
4.0	0% BLQ	0% BLQ
	100% > BLQ	100% > BLQ
8.0	1.5% BLQ	0% BLQ
	98.5% > BLQ	100% > BLQ
12.0	4.7% BLQ	0.6% BLQ
	95.3% > BLQ	99.4% > BLQ
24.0	11.2% BLQ	3.7% BLQ
	88.8% > BLQ	96.3% > BLQ

first dose (TSFD) for a more refined evaluation of stationarity over the treatment and collection period. Figure 5.8 and Figure 5.9 illustrate trough concentrations plotted against the time since the start of treatment. In Figure 5.9, a smooth line is added to highlight the mean tendency of the data over time.

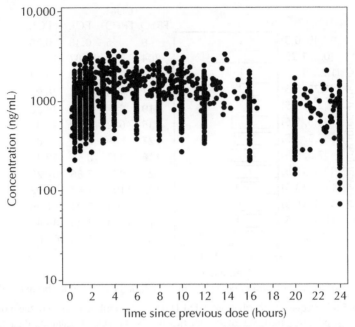

FIGURE 5.7 Scatterplot of drug concentration versus TSLD. A semi-log scale is used for the *y* axis and time of sampling is normalized to time relative to the most recent dose administration.

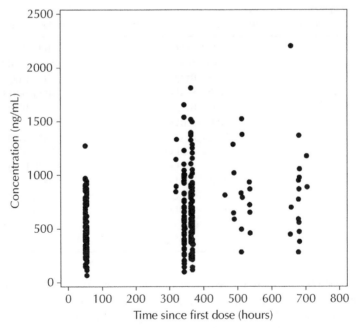

FIGURE 5.8 Scatterplot of trough concentrations versus time since the start of treatment.

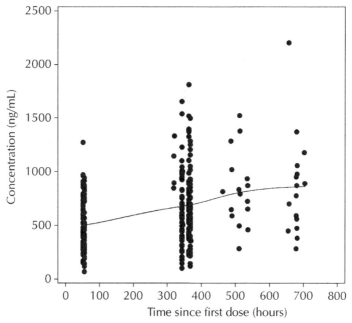

FIGURE 5.9 Scatterplot of trough concentrations versus time since the start of treatment with a smoothing spline through the data. A smoothing spline is added to the scatterplot to illustrate the central tendency of the trough concentrations over time.

Perhaps the more important consideration in the interpretation of this plot is the treatment of the dose level. When dose is properly accounted for, an assessment may be made as to whether a given level may be considered unusual relative to others or within the typical range of variability observed for the particular compound. Without accounting for dose, overinterpretation of a particularly high or low concentration level is possible. For example, if the most extreme (highest) concentration level observed was known to be from a subject receiving the highest dose, it would not be considered as likely to be an outlier as if it were known to be from a subject receiving the lowest dose level. Importantly, any assessment of potential outliers from this plot is minimally a three-pronged evaluation with consideration given to whether the given concentration level is: (i) unusually high or low in the overall sample of concentrations or within the profile of concentration values from the individual (if available), (ii) unusually high or low in comparison to other samples collected following the same or similar dose levels, and (iii) unusually high or low in comparison to other samples collected at a similar time relative to dosing. Concentrations that test positive for each of these considerations may warrant further investigation as potential outliers. Appropriate consideration of factors such as the dose level and the timing of the sample relative to dosing (as in the model), may allow the analyst to hone in on the legitimately unusual samples and avoid spending unnecessary time investigating concentrations that are simply near the tails of the distribution and not necessarily unusual.

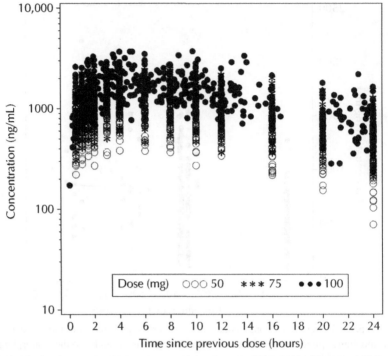

FIGURE 5.10 Scatterplot of drug concentrations versus TSLD with different symbols used to represent the different dose groups.

The treatment of dose level in the scatterplot of concentration versus time can be handled in several different ways, each of which may provide a slightly different picture of the informational content of the dataset. The single scatterplot of concentration versus time in the entire population of interest can be drawn using different symbols and/or symbol colors for the concentrations measured following different dose levels; this technique is illustrated in Figure 5.10. Alternatively, separate scatterplots can be generated for the data following different dose levels. If this technique is used, it may be useful to maintain similar axis ranges across all plots in order to subsequently compare the plots across the range of doses studied; this is illustrated in Figure 5.11. Either of these options for the treatment of dose level allows for a simplistic evaluation regarding dose proportionality across the studied dose range. Yet another option for this type of assessment is to dose-normalize the concentration values by dividing each concentration by the relevant dose amount prior to plotting versus time. If differing symbols or colors are used for the various dose groups in a dose-normalized plot, confirmation that the different dose groups cannot be easily differentiated because of substantial overlap may provide adequate confirmation of dose proportionality in a given dataset. Figure 5.12 and Figure 5.13 illustrate dose-normalized concentrations plotted versus time since the previous dose, with different symbols used to represent the different dose groups; in Figure 5.13, a smoothing spline is added for each dose

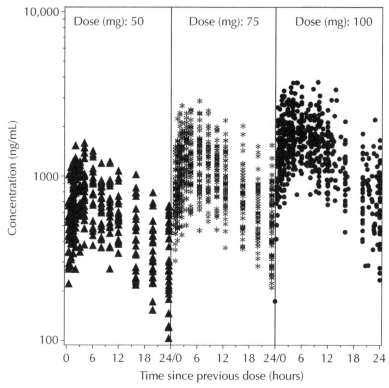

FIGURE 5.11   Scatterplot of drug concentrations versus TSLD with different panels used to compare the data following different dose levels. Solid triangles represent data following the administration of the 50-mg dose, asterisks represent data following the administration of the 75-mg dose, and solid dots represent data following the administration of the 100-mg dose.

group. The addition of the smoothing splines to the dose-normalized plot in Figure 5.13 serves to further illustrate (in this case) the similarity between the disposition following each of the dose levels.

   If full- or relatively full-profile sampling strategies (four to six or more samples following a given dose) were implemented in the various studies to be analyzed, plotting this subset of the analysis dataset, joining the points collected from a given individual may be illustrative in understanding the shape of the PK profile and highlighting potential differences across patients. If sampling strategies are sparse (three or fewer samples following a given dose), joining such points within an individual's data can be a misleading illustration of the PK profile when considered on a patient-by-patient basis. Figure 5.14 illustrates this type of plot for a sample of patients with full-profile sampling. When multiple troughs are collected from each individual, joining such levels across time in the study or time since first dose can provide an assessment of PK stationarity as discussed earlier. Figure 5.15 illustrates such a plot for a small number of subjects with two trough samples collected, and with a larger sample and/or more samples per subject, the overall trends across the data would be clear from a plot of this type.

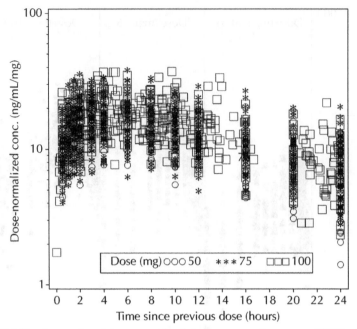

FIGURE 5.12 Scatterplot of dose-normalized drug concentrations versus TSLD with different symbols used to represent the different dose groups.

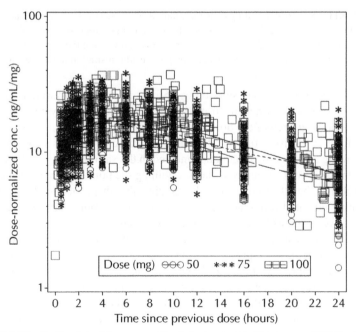

FIGURE 5.13 Scatterplot of dose-normalized drug concentrations versus TSLD with different symbols used to represent the different dose groups and smoothing splines added for each dose group.

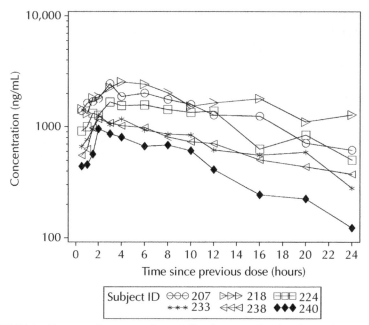

FIGURE 5.14   Concentration versus time profiles for a sample of patients with full-profile sampling. A semi-log scale is used for the y axis.

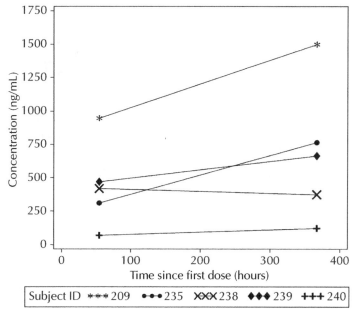

FIGURE 5.15   Scatterplot of trough concentrations versus time since the start of treatment, joined by subject.

The concentration or *y* axis may be plotted on either a semi-logarithmic or a linear scale, and probably should be plotted on each, since different information in the data is emphasized by the different plot formats. The linear scale for concentration allows for a straightforward means to interpret the exact value of a given concentration level, which may be useful in facilitating comparisons to known levels or summary statistics such as the mean or median concentration value. On a linear scale, the higher end of the concentration profile is emphasized in comparison to the log-scale version of the same plot, allowing for a perhaps closer examination of the peak, the absorption profile, and early distributional portion of the PK profile. When plotted on a semi-logarithmic scale, the lower end of the concentration profile is stretched in comparison to the linear scale version, thereby allowing for a closer examination of the later (elimination) phase of the PK profile. Figure 5.16 and Figure 5.17 illustrate linear scale *y*-axis versions of Figure 5.11 and Figure 5.14 for comparison. Furthermore, when plotted on a semi-log scale, the concentration versus time profile can be assessed for concordance with first-order (FO) processes, and the appropriate compartmental PK model for the data can be

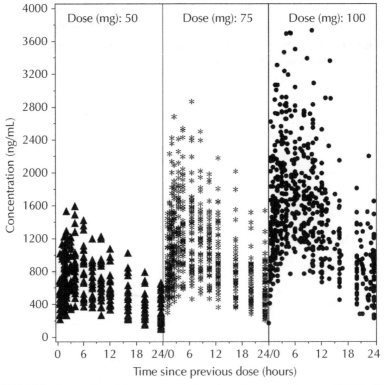

FIGURE 5.16   Scatterplot of drug concentrations (on a linear scale) versus TSLD with different panels used to compare the data following different dose levels. Solid triangles represent data following the administration of the 50-mg dose, asterisks represent data following the administration of the 75-mg dose, and solid dots represent data following the administration of the 100-mg dose.

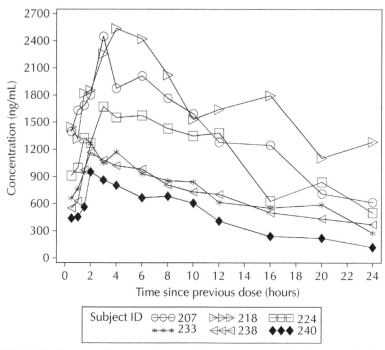

FIGURE 5.17 Concentration (on a linear scale) versus time profiles for a sample of patients with full-profile sampling.

considered. If the concentration data following the peak exhibit a single linear slope, a one-compartment disposition model may be a reasonable characterization of the data. However, if the concentration data following the peak exhibit bi- or triphasic elimination, characterized by multiple linear segments, each with different and progressively shallower slopes over time, then a two- or three-compartment disposition model may be an appropriate characterization of the data. Furthermore, a distinctly concave shape to the concentration data following the peak level may indicate the presence of Michaelis–Menten (nonlinear) elimination. These types of assessments of the shape of the PK profile are not possible when concentration versus time data are plotted on a linear y-axis scale for concentration. Figure 5.18 illustrates the shape of some of these profiles for comparison.

A final plotting technique, which may be considered with concentration versus time data, is the use of a third stratification variable (other than or in addition to dose). For example, if the drug under study is known to be renally cleared, an interesting plot to consider for confirmation of this effect in a particular dataset is concentration versus time for a given dose, with different symbols and/or colors used for different categories of renal function. Obvious separation of the renal impairment groups in a concentration versus time scatterplot would provide empiric evidence to support the influence of renal function on the PK of the compound. Figure 5.19 and Figure 5.20 illustrate this plot, before and after smooth lines are added to further illustrate the differences between the renal function groups. Trellis-style graphics, as

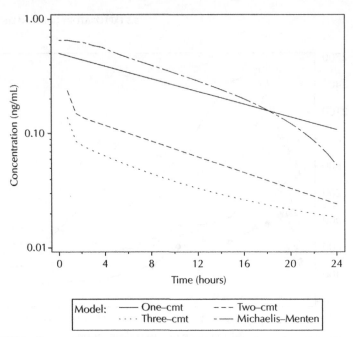

FIGURE 5.18 Representative concentration versus time profiles for various disposition patterns.

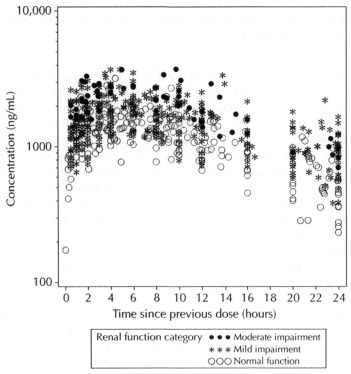

FIGURE 5.19 Scatterplot of drug concentrations versus TSLD with different symbols used to represent the different renal function categories.

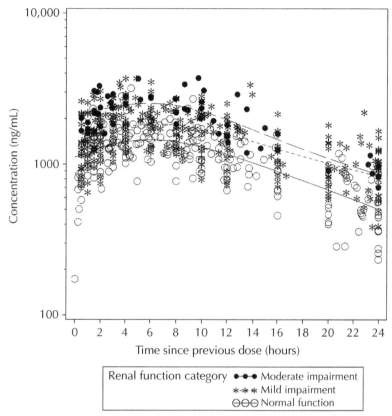

FIGURE 5.20   Scatterplot of drug concentrations versus TSLD with different symbols used to represent the different renal function categories and smoothing splines added for each renal function category.

implemented in R, offer an alternative method for illustrating the potential effect of a third variable (R Core Team 2013). Such graphs provide a matrix of plots, each representing a different subset of the population based on the distribution of the third variable. Stratification of the concentration versus time scatterplot with different covariates under consideration allows for a quick and simple assessment of the likelihood of influence of such potential factors. Highly statistically significant covariate effects are often easily detected from such plots. Figure 5.21 illustrates the concentration versus time data, plotted in a trellis style with different panels for the different renal function categories.

5.5.4   EDA: Considerations with Large Datasets

Special consideration of alternative plotting techniques may be warranted when datasets for analysis are extremely large. In this situation, scatterplots of the sort discussed in Section 5.5.3, especially those utilizing the entire dataset, may be largely uninterpretable as many points will plot very near each other resulting in a large

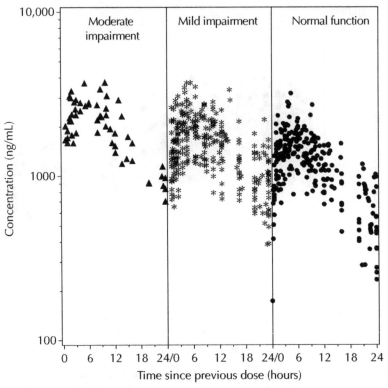

FIGURE 5.21   Scatterplot of drug concentrations versus TSLD with different panels used to compare the data from the different renal function categories. Solid triangles represent data from subjects with moderate renal impairment, asterisks represent data from subjects with mild renal impairment, and solid dots represent data from subjects with normal renal function.

inkblot from which no apparent trend can be deciphered. In this situation, the choice of plotting symbol can make a large difference and an open symbol (which uses less ink) may be preferable to a filled symbol. Figure 5.22 illustrates a scatterplot of a very large dataset using open symbols. The overlay of a smoothing line (spline) on such dense data is one technique that may help the analyst detect a trend or pattern where one cannot be easily seen by eye; Figure 5.23 shows the same data with a smoothing spline added. Stratification and subsetting techniques as described in the previous section also offer a method of breaking down a large dataset into more manageable subsets from which patterns may be observable. Figure 5.24 illustrates the large dataset plotted in different panels, stratified by study, revealing different underlying patterns in the different studies. A final technique, which may be considered when even the subsets of data are quite dense, is random thinning. With a random thinning procedure, points to be plotted are randomly selected for display in a given subset plot. For EDA purposes, it may be appropriate to apply this technique to the entire dataset, generating numerous subset plots such that each point is plotted exactly once, and ensuring that no point goes unobserved or unplotted. For illustration of very large datasets as in a publication, a single random subset plot that preserves

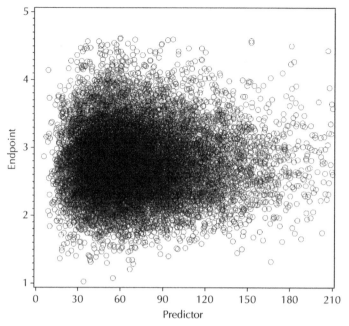

FIGURE 5.22   Scatterplot of an endpoint versus a predictor variable for a large dataset using open symbols.

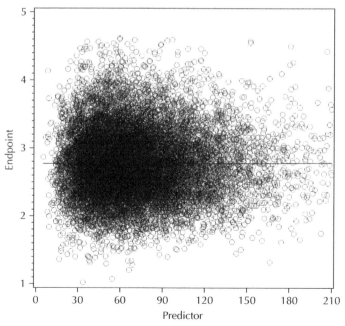

FIGURE 5.23   Scatterplot of an endpoint versus a predictor variable for a large dataset using open symbols and a smoothing spline added.

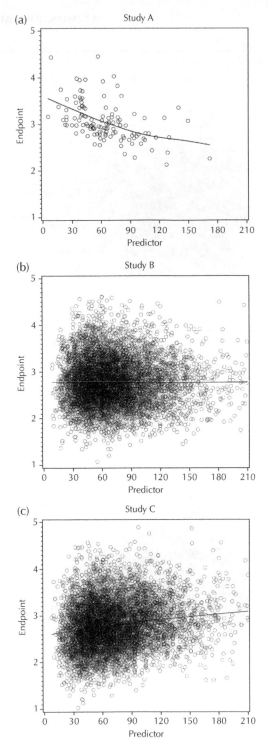

FIGURE 5.24 Scatterplot of an endpoint versus a predictor variable, plotted separately by study with smoothing splines. Panel (a) represents the endpoint versus predictor data for the subjects from Study A. Panel (b) is for Study B. Panel (c) is the data from Study C.

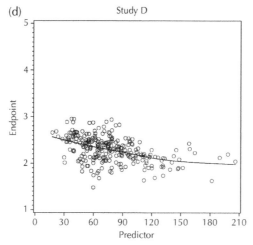

FIGURE 5.24   (*Continued*) Panel (d) is the data from Study D.

at least most of the features of the overall dataset may be more appropriate. Software tools with interactive plotting features may also be useful in evaluating large datasets by implementing graph building or stripping features.

5.5.5 EDA: Summary

Exploratory data analysis is a critical, though sometimes overlooked, step in a comprehensive and deliberate model building strategy. Analysts with the discipline to thoroughly explore and understand the nuances of a dataset prior to attempting model fitting will reap the rewards of efficiency in subsequent steps. A sure strategy for repeating analysis steps, starting and restarting model development efforts, and spending more time and effort than necessary includes initiating model fitting without fully appreciating the intricacies of the analysis dataset through EDA.

With an understanding of the studies to be included, the population to be studied, and some expectations regarding the PK characteristics of the drug, EDA can be effectively planned and scripted at the time of drafting the analysis plan (i.e., well before trial databases are locked and data are even available for processing). Importantly, EDA plots and tables should be recreated following any significant change to the analysis population, such as the exclusion of a particular study from the analysis dataset. Neglecting to do so may result in the same potential misunderstandings and inefficiencies that result from not performing EDA in the first place.

Data summaries, EDA plots, and tables should be included in presentations, reports, and publications of population modeling efforts. Such displays are the most effective way to demonstrate the features of a large complicated dataset, especially one consisting of several studies pooled together, and to facilitate understanding of the informational content of the data to be modeled.

5.6   BASE MODEL DEVELOPMENT

With a solid understanding of the informational content of the analysis dataset relative to the models to be considered for evaluation, initial model fitting may be attempted. The approach proposed herein (and adopted by the authors) involves starting with a parsimonious simplistic model sufficient only to characterize the overall nature of the data and subsequently building in layers of complexity as more knowledge is gained and more variability is explained with model additions and improvements. Thus, the base structural model initially attempted may be defined as a model that may be considered to be appropriate to describe the general and typical PK characteristics of the drug (i.e., one-compartment model with first-order absorption and linear elimination), including the estimation of interindividual variability (IIV) on only a limited number of PK parameters and including the estimation of residual variability using a simplistic error model. During the process of establishing an adequate base structural model, additional PK parameters may be estimated (e.g., absorption lag time and relative bioavailability fraction) as needed, and based on the model fit and diagnostics, IIV may be estimated on additional (or all) parameters, and the residual variability model (i.e., weighting scheme for the model fit) may be further refined.

Considering these features part of a sufficient base structural model, when an adequate fit is obtained (see Section 5.6.1) following the evaluation of such model components, the model may be designated as the base structural model. Generally, a base structural population PK model will not include the effect of any individual-specific patient factors or covariates on the parameters of the model. However, in some circumstances, the inclusion of a patient covariate effect, especially one with a large and highly statistically significant effect on drug PK, is a necessary component to obtaining an adequate base structural model. Other possible exceptions to this precept might include estimating the effect of weight or body size in a pediatric population as an allometric scaling factor on relevant PK parameters. (See Section 5.7.4.3.2 for a description of the functional model form typically used for allometric scaling of PK parameters.)

5.6.1   Standard Model Diagnostic Plots and Interpretation

The table file output from NONMEM contains several statistics useful in interpreting the results of a given model fit. In addition to the requested values (i.e., those specified in the $TABLE record), NONMEM appends the following values at the end of each record of the table file: DV, PRED, RES, and WRES. The first value, DV, is the value of the dependent variable column of the dataset. The second value, PRED, is the population-level model-predicted value corresponding to the measured value in DV. The final two values, RES and WRES, are the residual and weighted residual corresponding to the given measured value and its prediction. The residual, RES, is simply the difference between the measured and predicted values, or DV-PRED.

Positive values of RES indicate points where the population model-predicted value is lower than the measured value (underpredicted), and negative values for RES indicate an overprediction of the point (PRED > DV). The units for RES are the units of the DV, for instance, ng/mL, if the DV is a drug concentration. The weighted residual, WRES, is calculated by taking into account the weighting scheme, or residual variability model, in effect for this particular model fit. Because the weighting scheme effectively normalizes the residuals, the units for WRES can be thought of as an indication of SDs around an accurate prediction with WRES = 0. In fact, the WRES should be normally distributed about a mean of 0 with a variance of 1. Therefore, WRES values between −3 and +3 (i.e., within 3 SDs of the measurement or true value) are to be expected, and WRES values greater in absolute value than 3 are an indication of values that are relatively less well-fit, with a larger WRES indicating a worse fitting point.

5.6.1.1   *PRED versus DV*
Perhaps the most common model diagnostic plot used today is a scatterplot of the measured values versus the corresponding predicted values. This plot portrays the overall goodness-of-fit of the model in an easily interpretable display. In the perfect model fit, predictions are identical to measured values and all points would fall on a line with unit slope indicating this perfect correspondence. For this reason, scatterplots of predicted versus observed are typically plotted with such a unit slope or identity line overlaid on the points themselves. For the nonperfect model (i.e., all models), this plot is viewed with an eye toward symmetry in the density of points on either side of such a unit slope line across the entire range of measured values and the relative tightness with which points cluster around the line of identity across the range of measured values. Figure 5.25 illustrates a representative measured versus population-predicted scatterplot with a unit slope line. With regard to symmetry about the unit slope line, the fit of this particular model seems reasonably good; there are no obvious biases with a heavier distribution of points on one or the other side of the line. However, when the axes are changed to be identical (i.e., the plot is made square with respect to the axes) as in Figure 5.26, a slightly different perspective on the fit is obtained. It becomes much more clear that the predicted range falls far short of the observed data range.

5.6.1.2   *WRES versus PRED*
Another plot illustrative of the overall goodness-of-fit of the model is a scatterplot of the weighted residuals versus the predicted values. The magnitude of the weighted residuals (in absolute value) is an indication of which points are relatively well-fit and which are less well-fit by the model. A handful of points with weighted residuals greater than |10| (absolute value of 10) in the context of the remainder of the population with values less than |4| indicate the *strangeness* of these points relative to the others in the dataset and the difficulty with which they were fit with the given model. Closer investigation may reveal a coding error of some sort, perhaps even related to the dose apparently administered prior to such sampling, rather than an error in the concentrations themselves. In addition to the identification of poorly fit values, the plot of WRES versus PRED also illustrates potential patterns of misfit across the range of predicted values. A good model fit will be indicated in this plot by a symmetric distribution of points around WRES = 0

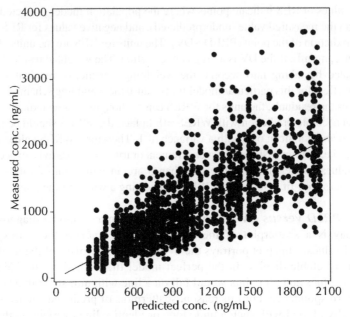

FIGURE 5.25 Scatterplot of observed concentrations versus population predicted values illustrating a reasonably good fit. Note that the axes are scaled to the range of the data.

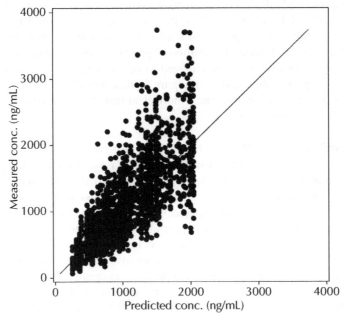

FIGURE 5.26 Scatterplot of observed concentrations versus population predicted values with equal axes.

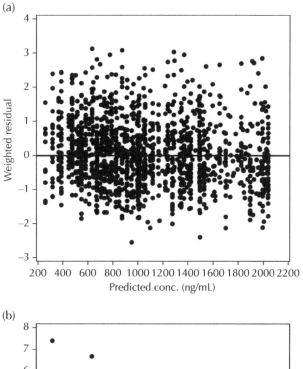

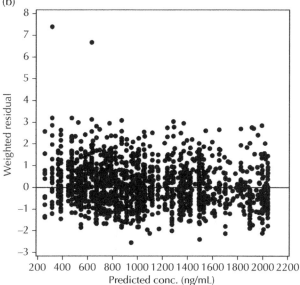

FIGURE 5.27   Scatterplot of weighted residuals versus population predicted illustrating a good fit. Panel (a) includes no apparent outlier points, while Panel (b) includes two apparent outliers associated with high weighted residuals.

across the entire range of predicted values. Figure 5.27 illustrates a good-fitting model in panel (a) and a similarly good-fitting model in panel (b) with two outlier points associated with large weighted residuals. Obvious trends or patterns in this type of plot, such as a majority of points being associated with exclusively positive or negative WRES (thus indicating systematic under- or overprediction, respectively) in a certain range of predicted values may indicate a particular bias or misfit of the model. The plot in Figure 5.28 illustrates clear trends, associated with certain misfit. A classic pattern in this plot with a specific interpretation is the so-called U-shaped trend shown in Figure 5.29, whereby a majority of WRES are positive for low values of the predicted values, become negative for intermediate values of PRED, and finally, are mostly positive again for the highest predicted values. Generally speaking, for PK models, this pattern is an indication that an additional compartment should be added to the model. For other models, it would be an indication that the shape of the model requires more curvature across the range of predictions.

Another pattern sometimes observed in WRES versus PRED plots is an apparent bias in the distribution of WRES values, evident as a lack of symmetry about WRES=0, often with a higher density of points slightly less than 0 and individual values extending to higher positive values than negative ones. Figure 5.30 illustrates this pattern, which may or may not be consistent across the entire range of PRED values. This pattern is often an indication that a log-transformation of the DV values in the dataset and the use of a log-transformed additive residual variability model may be appropriate. The log-transformation of the data will often result in a more balanced and less biased display of WRES versus PRED. When the log-transformed additive error model is used, both the DV and PRED values displayed in diagnostic plots may be either plotted as is (in the transformed realm) or back-transformed (via exp(DV) and exp(PRED)) to be presented in the untransformed realm.

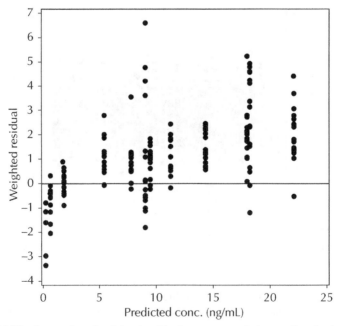

FIGURE 5.28   Scatterplot of weighted residuals versus population predicted values illustrating a poorly fitting model.

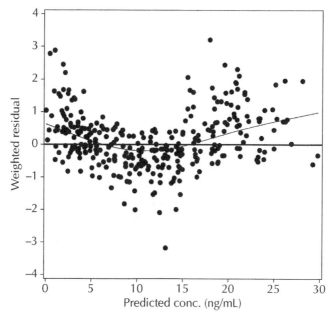

FIGURE 5.29   Scatterplot of weighted residuals versus population predictions illustrating a U-shaped pattern, indicative of the need for an additional compartment in the model.

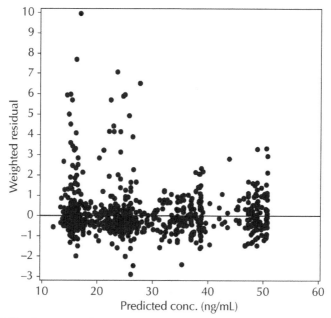

FIGURE 5.30   Scatterplot of weighted residuals versus population predictions illustrating the need for log-transformation.

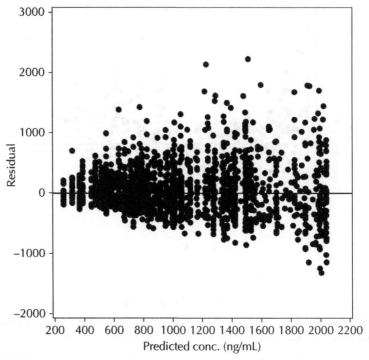

FIGURE 5.31 Scatterplot of residuals versus population predictions illustrating the fan-shaped pattern indicative of the proportional residual variability model.

5.6.1.3 RES versus PRED In contrast to the WRES versus PRED plot, where a consistent spread in WRES is desired across the PRED range, the RES versus PRED plot may indicate vast disparity in the dispersion about RES=0 and still portray a good fit. While symmetry about RES=0 is still considered ideal, a narrower spread at the lower predictions which gradually increases to a much wider dispersion at the higher end of the predicted range is a reflection of the weighting scheme selected via the residual variability model. The commonly used proportional residual variability model which weights predictions proportionally to the square of the predicted value, thereby allows for greater variability (i.e., more spread) in the higher concentrations as compared to the lower concentrations. Figure 5.31 is a scatterplot of residuals versus population predictions illustrating this pattern. Since RES are simply the nonweighted difference between the measured value and the corresponding prediction, these values can be interpreted directly as the amount of misfit in a given prediction in the units of the DV. Figure 5.32 illustrates a representative residuals versus population predictions plot indicative of a good fit when an additive error model is used.

5.6.1.4 WRES versus TIME Since PK models rely heavily on time, another illustrative plot of model goodness-of-fit is WRES versus TIME. This plot may sometimes be an easier-to-interpret version of the WRES versus PRED plot described above. Initially considering time as the TSLD of study drug, the plot of WRES versus

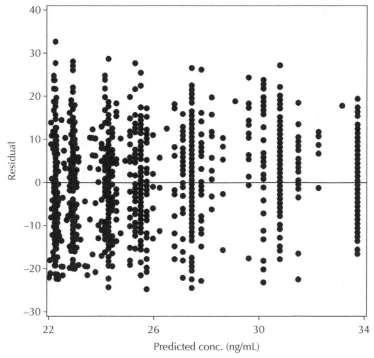

FIGURE 5.32   Scatterplot of residuals versus population predictions illustrating a constant spread across the range of predictions indicative of an additive error model.

TSLD allows one to see where model misfit may be present relative to an expectation of where the peak concentration may be occurring (usually smaller values of TSLD) or where troughs are most certainly observed (the highest TSLD values). Figure 5.33 provides an example of such a plot for a model that is fit well, where there are no obvious patterns of misfit over the time range. Considering time as the TSFD of study drug, again this plot allows one to consider misfit relative to time in the study and perhaps more easily identify possible problems with nonstationarity of PK or differences in the time required to achieve steady-state conditions. Figure 5.34 demonstrates some obvious patterns of bias in the plot of weighted residuals versus TSFD, indicating that the model is not predicting well over the entire time course.

5.6.1.5 *Conditional Weighted Residuals (CWRES)*   Andrew Hooker and colleagues illustrated in their 2007 publication that the WRES values obtained from NONMEM and commonly examined to illustrate model fit are calculated in NONMEM using the FO approximation, regardless of the estimation method used for fitting the model (Hooker et al. 2007). In other words, even when the FOCE or FOCEI methods are used for estimation purposes, the WRES values produced by the same NONMEM fit are calculated based on the FO approximation. Hooker et al. derived the more appropriate conditional weighted residual (CWRES) calculation (based on the FOCE objective function) and demonstrated that the expected

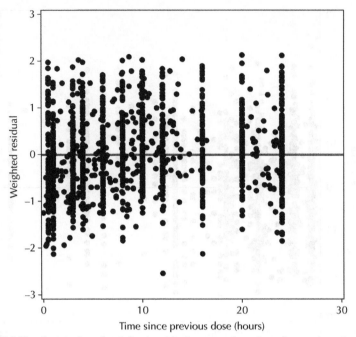

FIGURE 5.33 Scatterplot of weighted residuals versus time since the previous dose illustrating a good fit.

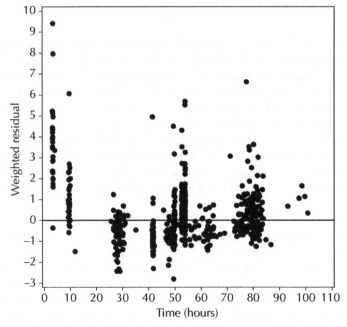

FIGURE 5.34 Scatterplot of weighted residuals versus TSFD illustrating patterns indicative of a biased fit over the time course of treatment.

properties of standard WRES (i.e., normal distribution with mean 0 and variance 1) quickly deteriorate, especially with highly nonlinear models and are a poor and sometimes misleading indicator of the model fit. The CWRES, however, obtained using the alternative calculation, maintain the appropriate distributional characteristics even with highly nonlinear models and are therefore, a more appropriate indicator of model performance. The authors conclude that the use of the standard WRES from NONMEM should be reserved for use with only the FO method.

Hooker et al. (2007) also showed that CWRES, calculated based on the FOCE approximation, can be computed using the FO method in combination with a POSTHOC step. Thus, in those rare cases where conditional estimation is not possible due to model instability or excessively long run times, this feature allows one to understand the possible improvement in model fit that may be obtained with a conditional estimation method by comparing the WRES obtained to the CWRES. An important caveat to the use of CWRES, however, is that with NONMEM versions 6 or lower, the calculation of the CWRES is not trivial. To facilitate the use of this diagnostic, Hooker et al. (2007) have implemented the CWRES calculation in the software program, Perl Speaks NONMEM, along with the generation of appropriate diagnostic plots in the Xpose software (Jonsson and Karlsson 1999; Lindbom et al. 2005). NONMEM versions 7 and above include the functionality to calculate CWRES directly from NONMEM and request the output of these diagnostics in tables and scatterplots.

Based on Hooker et al.'s (2007) important work, and in order to avoid the selection of inappropriate models during the model development process based on potentially misleading indicators from WRES, the previously described goodness-of-fit plots utilizing weighted residuals should always be produced using CWRES in place of WRES when conditional estimation methods are employed. These plots include WRES versus PRED and WRES versus TIME, as well as examination of the distribution of WRES. Figure 5.35 and Figure 5.36 provide plots of conditional weighted residuals versus population predictions and time since first dose, in both cases indicating a good-fitting model.

5.6.1.6 *Typical Value Overlay Plot* Another diagnostic plot supportive of the appropriateness of the selected structural model is a representation of the predicted concentration versus time profile for a typical individual overlaid on the (relevant) raw data points, as in Figure 5.37. Such a plot illustrates whether the so-called typical model fit captures the most basic characteristics of the dataset. To obtain the typical predictions for such a plot, a dummy dataset is first prepared containing hypothetical records for one or more *typical* subjects. For example, if the analysis dataset contains data collected following three different dose levels, the dummy dataset may be prepared with three hypothetical subjects, one receiving each of the three possible doses. The analyst will need to consider whether a predicted profile following a single dose (say, the first dose) is of interest or if a more relevant characterization of the fit would be for a predicted profile at steady state (say, following multiple doses) and create the appropriate dosing history for each subject in the dummy dataset. In order to obtain a very smooth profile of predicted values for each hypothetical subject, multiple sample records are included for each of the three subjects, at very

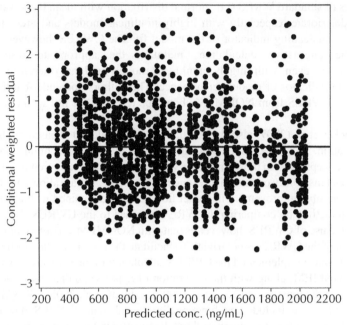

FIGURE 5.35 Scatterplot of conditional weighted residuals versus population predictions illustrating a good fit.

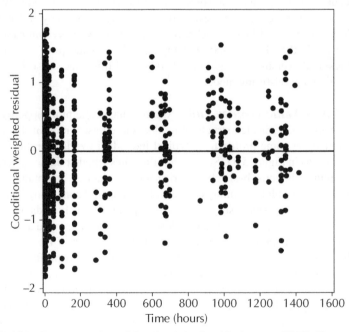

FIGURE 5.36 Scatterplot of conditional weighted residuals versus TSFD illustrating a good fit.

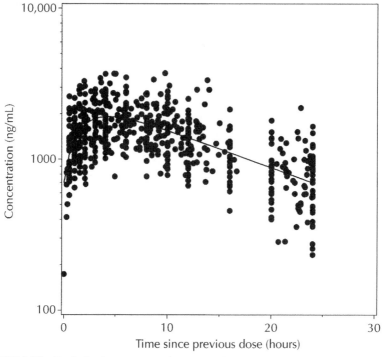

FIGURE 5.37 Typical value concentration versus time profile overlaid on the raw concentration versus time since previous dose data.

frequent intervals following dosing for one complete interval. Sample records are created with AMT=".", MDV=0, and DV="." in order to obtain a prediction at the time of each dummy sample collection. If the fit of a base model is to be illustrated with this method, the dataset need contain only those columns (variables) essential to describe dosing and sampling to NONMEM (i.e., the required data elements only).

A control stream is then crafted for prediction purposes which reads in the dummy dataset, adjusting the $DATA and $INPUT records as needed to correspond to the dummy dataset. If an MSF file was output from the model run of interest, it may be read in using a $MSFI record and the $THETA, $OMEGA, and $SIGMA records eliminated. However, if an MSF file does not exist, the final parameter estimates from the fit of the model to be used may be copied into the $THETA, $OMEGA, and $SIGMA records as fixed values. For the purposes of this deterministic simulation, the values in $OMEGA and $SIGMA are, in fact, not used and so these values may also be input with 0s. The $ESTIMATION record may either be eliminated or be specified with the MAXEVAL option set equal to 0 function evaluations. Either method prevents the minimization search from proceeding and essentially uses the estimates specified in $THETA, without a minimization search, to generate predictions for the hypothetical subjects in the dummy dataset. In the absence of the estimation step, the $COV record should either be commented out or not be included.

The resulting table file may then be used to plot the predicted profile for each hypothetical subject in one or multiple displays in order to compare the predictions resulting from various doses, dosing regimens, or over a time scale of interest. This

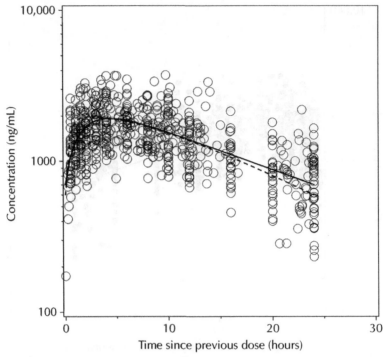

FIGURE 5.38 Typical value concentration versus time profiles for a one- and two-compartment model fit overlaid on the raw concentration versus time since previous dose data. The solid line indicates the typical profile associated with the one-compartment model and the dashed line indicates the typical profile associated with the two-compartment model.

technique can also be applied to plot predicted profiles for specified values of a relevant covariate, as described below, in detail. Based upon the intended purpose of the display, it may be of interest to overlay such predicted profiles on the original raw data or an appropriate subset of the raw data (say, the data following a particular dose). This technique can be particularly useful in illustrating the differences between the profiles resulting from two different nonhierarchical models. For instance, if one wishes to compare the predicted profiles resulting from a particular one- and a two-compartment model in relation to the population data, two such control streams would be created and run, as described above, and the table files set together with each other and the raw data in order to overlay the two predicted profiles on the raw dataset. Figure 5.38 illustrates the typical value profiles for two competing models overlaid on the raw data; in this case, it is apparent that there is not much difference between the predicted typical profiles for these otherwise very different structural models (except at the earliest times).

5.6.1.7 Typical Value Overlay Plot for Models with Covariate Effects   If the influence of significant covariate effects on the predicted concentration versus time profile is to be illustrated with this technique, consideration should also be given to the specified characteristics of the subjects to be included in the dummy dataset. For example, if the model includes the effects of two demographic covariates, such as weight and race

with three levels each, nine subjects might be included in the dummy dataset, for all combinations of the different levels of the weight distribution and the different race groups ($3 \times 3 = 9$). For a continuous covariate like weight, an arbitrary weight value from the lower end of the weight distribution, the population median weight, and an arbitrary weight value from the upper end of the weight distribution might be selected (e.g., the 5th percentile, 50th percentile, and 95th percentile, so as not to select values at the very extremes of the studied population, assuming the interest is in a typical subject's profile).

The control stream would be created and run as described above for the standard typical value overlay plot description, using the model that includes the covariate effects of interest to illustrate. The resulting table file may then be used to plot the predicted profile for each hypothetical subject in one or multiple displays in order to compare the predictions resulting from the covariates of interest in the model or from particular values of a continuous covariate. For example, if creatinine clearance is a statistically significant and clinically relevant factor in explaining intersubject variability in drug clearance, and predictions were generated for subjects with five different levels of creatinine clearance using the method described above, a single plot may be created with the five predicted profiles overlaid on the original raw dataset, where the symbols for the data points differ for various ranges of creatinine clearance, to roughly correspond with the five selected levels of interest. Figure 5.39 illustrates the overlay of

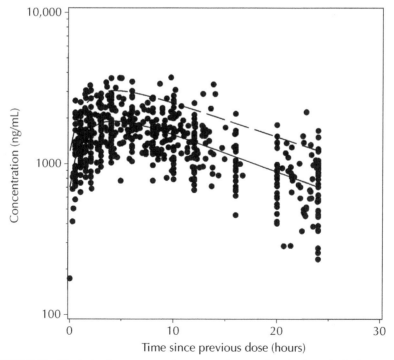

FIGURE 5.39 Typical value concentration versus time profiles for hypothetical subjects representing two different patient types overlaid on the raw concentration versus time since previous dose data.

the predicted profiles associated with two different patient types on the raw data; if desired, different symbols could also be used for the raw data to correspond with these patient types and further illustrate the correspondence of the model fits with the observed data. If the dataset is sufficiently large and/or fewer levels of the covariate of interest are to be displayed, such a plot might be stratified by each range of the covariate. For example, this could result in three separate plots, each illustrating a subset of the original dataset that corresponds to the subjects with creatinine clearance values in the lowest third of the distribution, the middle third, and the upper third, each with the relevant predicted profile overlaid. When separate plots like these are presented side-by-side, care should be taken to maintain the same axis ranges across each plot in order to best illustrate differences across the subsets; if the axis ranges are allowed to adjust to the data represented in each plot, it becomes more difficult to illustrate differences and the reader has to work a bit harder to draw the appropriate conclusions. Most software packages will, by default, allow the axis ranges to adjust to the data to be presented in the plot, and the resulting plots may be inappropriately interpreted if not carefully examined.

5.6.2 Estimation of Random Effects

With respect to the estimation of parameters describing IIV in PK parameters (i.e., ETAs), one should carefully consider the informational content of the dataset when postulating how many interindividual random-effect terms to include in a given model in addition to which ones (on which parameters) to estimate. If the informational content of a dataset is richer around the trough than it is around the peak or during absorption, it may be possible to obtain a good (precise) estimate of IIV on drug clearance only. However, if most subjects also had at least one blood sample drawn within the early time period after dosing, with some subjects having more than one sample in this time window, the estimation of IIV on either central volume, absorption rate, or both, in addition to clearance, may well be possible. A recommendation for strategy with respect to the estimation of IIV terms is to begin with the smallest number of IIV terms the dataset would be expected to support based on the EDA. Then, with successful estimation of this subset of possible ETAs, a systematic evaluation of the estimation of additional ETAs, one at a time, can be considered until the maximum number supported by the data is determined.

In the early stages of model development, when much variability remains to be characterized or explained, it is not uncommon to encounter difficulty in obtaining successful minimization for a particular model due to one or more ETA terms being inestimable. In addition to the minimization errors or warnings, an inestimable ETA will often be returned with an estimate close to 0. One should be careful not to interpret this as an indication of the lack of IIV in a particular parameter, or even the extent of such IIV being small. On the contrary, this is more often an indication of the particular dataset's inability to support the estimation of independent variability terms (random effects) given the rest of the terms of the model. However, the inability to estimate a particular IIV term at an early stage of model development is not necessarily an indication that this characterization will forevermore be impossible with this dataset. Sometimes, an inappropriate characterization of the residual variability model, resulting in interplay between the interindividual random-effect terms and the residual error random-effect terms can result in an inestimable ETA. Once the residual variability model is more appropriately characterized, however, a particular ETA term may become estimable.

5.6.2.1   *Diagnostic Plots for Random-Effect Models*   The standard diagnostic plots discussed in Section 5.6.1 describe various ways to view the typical value or population-level predictions (i.e., PRED) and residuals based on these (i.e., RES, WRES, and CWRES) from the model. These predictions for the concentration at a given time following a given dose can be obtained by plugging in the typical values of the PK parameters (THETA terms), along with the dose and time, into the equation for the PK model. Therefore, these predictions represent the expected value for a typical subject. It is also important to understand that these predictions, by definition, often give rise to a limited number of unique predicted values, especially when the study to be analyzed includes a limited number of doses and a fixed sampling strategy. A *striped* pattern evident in a plot of DV versus PRED is often observed in this situation and is merely an indication of the underlying design, the stage of model development, and the type of typical value predictions that are being plotted. Figure 5.40 provides an example of this type of pattern in a plot of the observed value versus the population predictions. As model development continues, and subject-specific covariate values

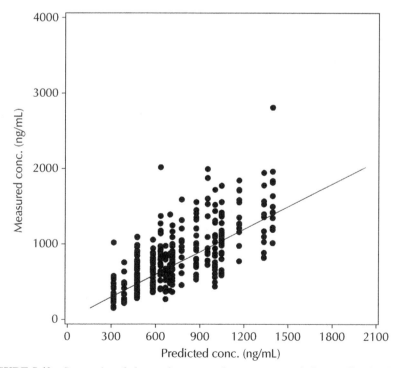

FIGURE 5.40   Scatterplot of observed concentrations versus population predicted values illustrating a limited number of predicted values based on the design and the model.

are included in the model, the striped pattern will tend to fall away, as predictions become more subject specific. However, the fact remains that the population predictions (PRED) for a given concentration measured at a particular time after a particular dose for a subject with the same covariate values relevant to the model (say, the same weight and CrCL) would be identical.

However, with only a few lines of code, one can also obtain individual-specific predictions and residuals to plot and consider in evaluating the model fit and appropriateness. NONMEM's F used in coding the residual variability model is, by definition, the individual predicted concentration value. It is individual-specific in that it includes all of the subject-specific ETA terms included in the model, thus giving rise to different predictions for each individual in the dataset. Since this F value may not be output directly from NONMEM (in the table file output from $TABLE or in a scatterplot from $SCAT), it must be renamed in order to be output (Beal et al. 1989–2011). One typical method to generate these individual predictions along with individual residuals and individual weighted residuals is shown below in code that can be used in NM-TRAN.

```
$ERROR
IPRED = F
W=F
IRES = DV-IPRED
IWRES = IRES/W
Y = IPRED + W*EPS(1)
```

The code above culminates with the expression of residual variability using a constant coefficient of variation error model. With the typical code specified above, one can easily change to an additive, log-transformed, or additive plus constant coefficient of variation model by changing the definition of W (the weighting term).

For additive error, use $W=1$; for log-transformed additive error (exponential error in the un-transformed domain), use IPRED=LOG(F) and $W=1$ (but note other caveats about the use of the LOG() function in Section 3.5.3.1); for proportional or constant coefficient of variation (CCV) error, use $W=F$ as shown above in the example; and for additive plus CCV, use either (i) $W={\tt SQRT}\,(1+{\tt THETA}\,(n)\,**2\,*F**2)$ or (ii) $W={\tt SQRT}\,(F**2+{\tt THETA}\,(n)\,**2)$, where THETA($n$) is defined as the ratio of the additive to proportional components of residual variability (RV) in (i) or the proportional to the additive components of RV in (ii). THETA(n) should be initialized in $THETA with a lower bound of 0 for either parameterization. Note also that for each of these residual variability models implemented with this coding structure, the IWRES value calculated as shown above (i.e., IRES/W) needs to be divided by the estimate of EPS(1) (σ_1^2) in order to maintain the appropriate scaling.

An alternative framework for coding the residual variability structure is provided below. Similar to the previous structure, to use this alternative method only the definition of W would change with the implementation of differing models. This structure fixes the value of EPSILON(1) on $SIGMA to a variance of 1 for σ^2. In contrast to the previous coding method, one advantage to this coding is that the IWRES values are scaled by this weighting and, therefore, are provided on an appropriate and similar scale to the population WRES, which facilitates interpretation.

```
$ERROR
IPRED = F
W = THETA(X)                       ; for additive RV
W = THETA(Y)*IPRED                 ; for proportional or CCV RV
W = SQRT(THETA(X)**2
    + (THETA(Y)*IPRED)**2)         ; for additive plus CCV RV
W = SQRT(THETA(Y)**2
    + (THETA(X)/IPRED)**2)         ; for additive plus CCV RV
                                     on a log-scale (to use
                                     this model and coding,
                                     the data must be log-
                                     transformed and IPRED must
                                     be defined as LOG(F))
IWRES = (DV - IPRED) / W
Y = IPRED + W*EPS(1)

$SIGMA 1 FIX
```

By fixing the estimate of EPS(1) to 1, the theta parameters estimated above represent the SDs of the corresponding variability components.

As the reader will certainly appreciate by now, there are often several ways to accomplish similar tasks in NONMEM. Yet, another alternative to the residual variability coding provided above is the following:

```
$ERROR
IPRED = F
W = SQRT(IPRED**2*SIGMA(1,1)
    + SIGMA(2,2))                  ; for additive plus CCV RV
IWRES = (DV - IPRED) / W
Y = IPRED + IPRED*EPS(1) + EPS(2)

$SIGMA 0.04 10
```

With this variation, the IWRES does not need to be scaled and no thetas are required to code the residual variability elements. In addition, the interpretation of the two epsilon terms is facilitated and alternative structures can easily be evaluated by simply fixing one or the other epsilon term to 0.

With any of the variations for residual variability coding described earlier, in addition to the IPRED value that can be output to a table file or included in diagnostic plots, the IRES and IWRES values are also calculated and defined as expected based on the IPRED definition. The IRES values are the individual-specific residuals or the difference between the measured value and the individual-specific prediction based on the model (including ETA terms). IRES values (similar to RES) are, therefore, calculated in units of the measured dependent value. The individual weighted residual (IWRES) is the individual-specific weighted residual based on the model (THETAs and ETAs) and considering the weighting scheme implemented in the residual variability model; it is the individual residual scaled by the defined weighting factor, W.

5.6.2.2 IPRED versus DV Although PRED versus DV is the most common model diagnostic plot used today, the IPRED versus DV plot is likely the most commonly reported and published model diagnostic plot. A scatterplot of IPRED versus DV compares the measured values with the corresponding individual-specific predicted values. This plot portrays the goodness-of-fit of the model after accounting for the influence of the subject-specific random-effect terms. Because much of the unexplained variability in PK models lies in the between-subject realm, once these differences are accounted for, the DV versus IPRED plot often demonstrates a large improvement over the similar DV versus PRED version. In the perfect model fit, individual predictions are identical to measured values and all points would fall on a line with unit slope indicating this perfect correspondence. Scatterplots of individual predicted versus observed values are typically plotted with such a unit slope or identity line overlaid on the points themselves. For the nonperfect model (i.e., all models), this plot is viewed with an eye toward symmetry in the density of points on either side of such a unit slope line across the entire range of measured values and the relative tightness with which points cluster around the line of identity across the range of values. Systematic under- or overprediction of points in this plot indicate an issue with the model fit that cannot be corrected with the flexibility introduced through interindividual random-effect terms. Figure 5.41 illustrates a representative scatterplot of observed concentrations versus individual predicted values.

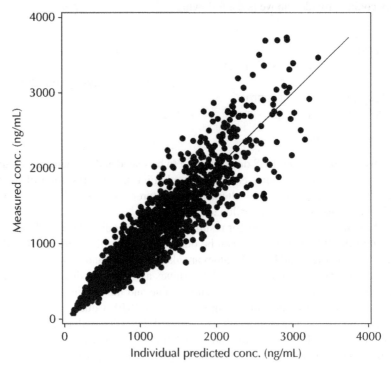

FIGURE 5.41 Scatterplot of observed concentrations versus individual predicted values illustrating a good fit.

5.6.2.3 *IWRES versus IPRED and |IWRES| versus IPRED* Two plots illustrative

of the appropriateness of the selected residual variability model are variations of the
scatterplot of the individual weighted residuals versus the individual predicted values.
As with the population weighted residuals (WRES), the magnitude of the IWRES (in
absolute value) is an indication of which points are relatively well fit and which are
less well fit by the model. A model fit with appropriately characterized residual
variability will be indicated in these plots by a symmetric distribution of points around
IWRES = 0 across the entire range of individual predicted values and a flat and level
smooth line in the |IWRES| versus IPRED version. Figure 5.42 illustrates a model
with no apparent misfit in the specification of residual variability. Obvious trends or
patterns in either of these plots, such as a gradually increasing spread of IWRES with
increasing IPRED values, indicate greater variability in higher predictions as compared
to lower ones and the possible inappropriate use of an additive RV model when a CCV
model may be warranted; this is illustrated in Figure 5.43. Conversely, decreasing
spread in IWRES with increasing IPRED may indicate that an additive model would
be a more appropriate characterization of the data than a CCV model; this pattern is
illustrated in Figure 5.44.

Note that a number of different variations on the predictions, residuals, and
weighted residuals may now be requested directly from NONMEM, with version 7.
In addition to the (standard) conditional weighted residuals, conditional predictions
(CPRED) and conditional residuals (CRES) may be requested. In addition,

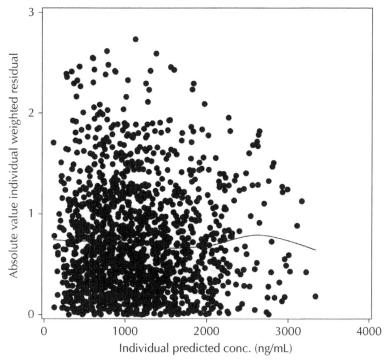

FIGURE 5.42 Scatterplot of the absolute value of the individual weighted residuals versus
the individual predictions, indicating no lack of fit.

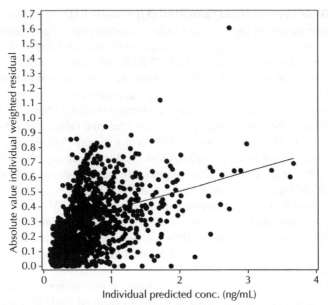

FIGURE 5.43 Scatterplot of the absolute value of the individual weighted residuals versus the individual predictions, indicating an increasing spread with increasing individual predictions. This pattern may result from the inappropriate use of an additive RV model when a CCV model may be warranted.

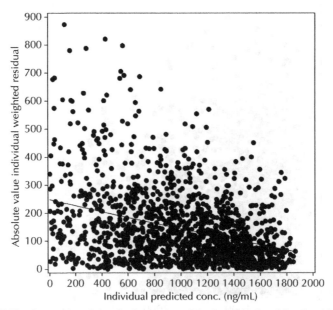

FIGURE 5.44 Scatterplot of the absolute value of the individual weighted residuals versus the individual predictions, indicating a decreasing spread with increasing individual predictions. This pattern may result from the use of a proportional or CCV RV model when an additive model would be more appropriate.

conditional weighted residuals with interaction (assuming that the INTERACTION option was specified on $EST) named CWRESI, along with the corresponding CPREDI and CRESI, the conditional predictions and residuals accounting for eta–epsilon interaction, may be requested for output in $TABLE or for use in plotting with $SCAT (Beal et al. 1989–2011). Refer to Chapter 3 for additional detail on the $TABLE and $SCATTERPLOT records.

5.6.3   Precision of Parameter Estimates (Based on $COV Step)

While the significance of a successful $COVARIANCE step has been a point of contention and disagreement among pharmacometricians, when successfully completed, the output from this step can be used as an indication of the precision of the NONMEM parameter estimates. When the $COV step has been requested along with a particular model estimation and it completes successfully, standard errors are obtained for each element of THETA, OMEGA, and SIGMA which was estimated. Considering each of these standard errors in relation to the corresponding parameter estimate (i.e., as a percentage: standard error of the estimate divided by the final parameter estimate times 100 or $SE(\theta_n)/FPE(\theta_n) \times 100$) allows one to compare the relative precision by which each of the fixed- and random-effect parameter estimates were obtained; for random-effect terms, we can similarly calculate the %RSE (or percent relative standard error) as $SE(\omega_n^2)/FPE(\omega_n^2) \times 100$ for the parameter, ETA(n). This statistic is sometimes referred to as a percent standard error of the mean (%SEM) and sometimes as a percent relative standard error (%RSE). Generally speaking, fixed-effect estimates with relative precisions below 30% are regarded as precisely estimated. Random-effect estimates are often obtained with less precision and values below 40–50% are generally regarded as reasonably precisely estimated.

An alternative calculation for the precision of random-effect terms is sometimes used. The calculation above for the %RSE of an element of OMEGA was performed on the variance (squared) scale. If one wishes to calculate the relative standard error of the random-effect terms on the SD scale (since we often think of these estimates in %CV terms anyway), one could take advantage of the delta method that uses the FO approximation of the variance, and the corresponding estimate of %RSE for an element of OMEGA or SIGMA would be calculated as follows:

$$\%RSE\left(\omega_{1,1}^2\right) = \frac{SE\left(\omega_{1,1}^2\right)}{2 \times FPE\left(\omega_{1,1}^2\right)} \times 100$$

The $COV step output also includes the correlation matrix of the estimates. Elements of this correlation matrix indicate how independently estimates of the various parameters were obtained. For example, a pair of estimates associated with a high absolute value in the correlation matrix (say, with absolute value>0.9) may be considered highly correlated. Highly correlated parameters are not considered to reflect independent estimates, and based upon the sign of the correlation matrix element indicate the direction of the correlation. A positive and high value (e.g., 0.92) for the correlation between two parameters indicates that, in the minimization step, as different values were tried for these two parameters, increasing one estimate has the effect of increasing the other in order to obtain a successful minimization. Conversely, a high negative value (e.g., –0.95) indicates that as one estimate increases, the other must decrease to obtain as good a model fit. Both cases illustrate the extent to which such highly correlated parameter estimates rely on each other (based on the size of the value in absolute terms) and, therefore, indicate a detriment in the overall goodness of fit of such a model. Ideally, none of the elements of the correlation matrix will be greater in absolute value than 0.9, thus indicating that all estimates are reasonably independent of all others.

A model with high correlations amongst many or all structural parameters would typically be rejected as a candidate model and would not generally be considered an acceptable model to describe the given dataset. At times, however, a singular pair of correlated estimates cannot be avoided for a given dataset and model, such as when highly correlated estimates of E_{max} and EC_{50} parameters are obtained and are an indication of a lack of informational content of the dataset to describe this relationship. Oftentimes, this situation arises when the range of administered doses is too narrow and/or most of the range of doses provides a response at or near the maximal effect. If such an E_{max}-type model is considered to be the most appropriate description of the data and a simpler, more empirical model is not desired, then along with the results and description of such a model, a listing of the highly correlated parameters and the degree of correlation should be provided. When requesting and successfully obtaining the $COV step, it is good practice to always review the output of the correlation matrix in assessing the fit of a particular model.

5.7   COVARIATE EVALUATION

There are many methods and philosophies surrounding the process for evaluating the influence of covariates on PK model parameters. Regardless of the selected method, the intention of such evaluations is usually to describe and explain inter- and intra-subject variability in PK parameters with patient factors that are typically known or can be collected in the population of interest. Many covariate evaluations are performed to address a regulatory authority's interest in understanding the PK of the compound in what are considered special populations (e.g., the elderly, children, and various racial or ethnicity groups). Covariate models also enrich the opportunity for individualization in dosing regimen. For many applications, the influences of so-called demographic or intrinsic factors on the PK of a drug are of interest. These factors may be those patient characteristics that are recorded for each subject at a baseline study visit and describe patient-specific factors such as the subject's gender, race, ethnicity, age, weight, and height, for instance. Depending upon the population, covariates that describe something about the current disease status and/or medical history for each patient may also be collected. For the purposes of covariate evaluations, these factors can often be considered to be time invariant or stationary for the duration of study (i.e., the length of the clinical trial treatment period). The inclusion of a stationary or time-invariant covariate effect in a population PK model would be expected to explain and, therefore, reduce the unexplained intersubject variability in the parameter that is most directly affected by the covariate. Obviously, some of these factors, such as ethnicity and gender, will not change within the study period, while others may be changing slightly over the time period of study, such as weight and age, but typically, not to an extent that would be considered important to capture. On the other hand, if the compound of interest is indicated for weight loss and the PK of the drug were known to be related to weight, changes in a subject weight during the course of treatment may be large enough to represent an important source of PK variability. In the end, the choice of whether to consider a particular covariate as stationary or time varying rests on the data collected during the study and an understanding of the population to be studied, the trial design, and the goals of the analysis.

In longer term studies (i.e., those of a year or more in duration), the extent to which a covariate, such as renal function, measured by creatinine clearance, may be changing could be particularly important to capture, especially if the drug elimination is largely renal. Other covariates that are sometimes studied as time-varying factors include laboratory measures of hepatic function, such as total bilirubin or alanine aminotransferase (ALT), which may be measured at multiple study visits, as well as indicator variables for food intake or concomitant medications of interest with the potential to induce a drug–drug interaction. Generally speaking, if a particular covariate of interest has been collected on multiple occasions during the treatment period, it may be considered for evaluation as a time-varying covariate effect. In addition to the between-patient differences in time-varying covariate data, because such factors are changing (potentially) with each observation record in the dataset, these covariates would be expected to reduce not only some of the unexplained intersubject variability in the related PK parameter but also some of the unexplained residual variability.

Concomitant medication use represents a common extrinsic factor that might be explored as a time-varying covariate. Concomitant medication data are typically captured on case report forms using the start and stop dates of each medication. One simplistic method for capturing such concomitant medication information in a NONMEM dataset is to set an indicator or flag variable to a value of 1 on each dosing or sampling record when the concomitant medication was coadministered with the study drug and a value of 0 on each dosing or sampling record when the drug was not coadministered. To do so, the date (and time) of each event record in the NONMEM dataset would be compared to the start and stop dates (and times, if available) of the concomitant medication history data. Since the concomitant medication history is not typically collected with as much rigor and care as other study data, this task can be fraught with challenges and necessitate several assumptions. For example, if the month and day for a start date of a particular concomitant medication is missing (as is quite often the case), one must decide what values to impute in order to set the indicator flag. Similarly, if the year of the start date of a concomitant medication is missing, one may wish to assume that the year is at least 1 year before the first visit date. If a particular medication or several medications are of most interest to study and there is opportunity to provide prospective input during study protocol development, case report form pages can be designed to capture more complete and better information regarding the usage of the particular concomitant medications (e.g., the inclusion of check boxes regarding coadministration with each study drug dose or sample) at little additional cost.

With regard to the evaluation of concomitant medication effects, another useful treatment of the data involves grouping of concomitant medications into classes based on their enzymatic activity (e.g., CYP 3A4 inhibitors versus inducers) for PK models or their mechanism of action for PD models. The end result is then a quantification of the influence of various medications of a particular type on the PK of the study drug (e.g., study drug clearance is increased by 31.6% in the presence of CYP 3A4 inducers). This method may be particularly advantageous when the frequency of use of individual medications is low or the overall number of concomitant medications is quite large. Input from clinical pharmacists on the team in the determination of the particular classifications of medications to be studied as well as the assignment of particular medications to classes represent a prime opportunity for collaboration that may result in greater understanding and acceptance of modeling results at the conclusion of the effort.

Perhaps another of the more important considerations in covariate evaluation has to do with the process for selecting which covariates to study and on which parameters to evaluate each covariate. If appropriate care is taken at the time of drafting the analysis plan, one can avoid unnecessary difficulty in imagining a rationale for an unanticipated and seemingly unexplainable relationship. After all, using an α value of 0.05 for the determination of the statistical significance of covariate effects in the model, if we undertook to consider the effects of 100 covariate-parameter pairs or possible relationships in a given model, we would expect 5 relationships to be detected purely by chance. While 100 effects may be quite high, even half of this would leave approximately 2–3 effects to be detected by chance alone, and therefore, most likely quite difficult to explain. Therefore, a logical and strategic policy in selecting covariate effects to be evaluated is careful consideration of the following: the pharmacology of the compound and patient factors that may be expected to alter the drug ADME, the patient population of interest and their likely medical history and concomitant medication profile, typical and common demographic factors, including those special populations of interest from a regulatory perspective, and, so as not to completely prevent the possibility of a serendipitous finding, any other data collected during the trial which might be reasonably thought to explain interpatient variability in PK and/or PD.

5.7.1   Covariate Evaluation Methodologies

Given the importance of covariate evaluations to population modeling, several different methodologies have been proposed over the last two decades to systematically approach the addition of explanatory factors to population PK and PK/PD models. In deciding which to approach to pursue, the analyst desires to achieve a balance between the time required to test possible models including such potentially explanatory factors, the explanatory *power* of the additional parameters describing these relationships, and the usefulness of the resulting model including such effects. If time (and computing resources) available for modeling were unlimited, after selecting the appropriate list of covariates to be evaluated, one might consider testing every possible model for each covariate-parameter combination that could be constructed. However, since the real world imposes many limitations on our ability to consider a given problem for as long as we might like, systematic approaches are necessary to maximize the yield from our efforts.

5.7.2 Statistical Basis for Covariate Selection

There are many ways to measure the improvement in a model resulting from the addition of a covariate effect. First and foremost, a statistical measure of model improvement is desirable for use in decision making (i.e., the yes/no selection of one model over another) such that we can quantitate the differences between models. Theoretically, the addition of effects (parameters) to a model must decrease the minimum value of the objective function (MVOF) in comparison to a model with fewer estimated parameters. The question then becomes how much of a change in the MVOF is meaningful to indicate an important model addition?

Before considering the statistical basis for model improvement through covariate additions, we must understand the concept of hierarchical (or nested) models. Two models are considered hierarchical, or nested, when setting one (or more) parameter(s) in the larger model (i.e., the one with more parameters) to the null hypothesis value(s) makes the models identical. For example, consider a simple model including the effect of gender on drug clearance, where:

$$CL_i = \theta_1 + \theta_2 \times SEXF_i$$

This model is considered hierarchical in comparison to the simple base model:

$$CL_i = \theta_1$$

This is because, in the larger model including the gender effect, when θ_2 is set to its null hypothesis value of 0, indicating no effect of gender on clearance, the larger model resolves to the smaller one, as shown below:

$$CL_i = \theta_1 + \theta_2 \times SEXF_i = \theta_1 + 0 \times SEXF_i = \theta_1$$

An example of two models (one including a covariate effect) that would not be considered hierarchical might be:

$$CL_i = \theta_1 \times WTKG_i \quad \text{and} \quad CL_i = \theta_1$$

since there is no single fixed value for θ_1 which allows the two models to be identical. However, the following two models could be considered hierarchical because when θ_2 is fixed to 0, the models resolve to the same equation:

$$CL_i = \theta_1 \times WTKG_i \quad \text{and} \quad CL_i = \theta_2 + \theta_1 \times WTKG_i$$

The discussion that follows regarding the statistical basis for comparisons between models assumes that the models to be compared are hierarchical in nature.

Recalling that the MVOF for a particular model is proportional to minus twice the log-likelihood of the data, a likelihood ratio test allows for comparison between the MVOFs of two hierarchical models. The likelihood ratio test further defines the difference between the two MVOF values to be chi-square distributed with v degrees of freedom, where v = the number of additional parameters (either fixed- or random-effect terms) in the larger of the two hierarchical models (Freund 1992). This then allows for comparison of this calculated difference to a test statistic, in order to determine the probability (p value) associated with observing the given difference between models. In comparison to the appropriate test statistic based on the prespecified α value for testing, if the difference between the two MVOFs is larger than the statistic, the addition of the covariate effect is considered statistically significant. If the difference is equal to or smaller than the test statistic value, then the covariate effect is not considered a statistically significant addition to the model.

As an example, let us suppose that the MVOF obtained from the estimation of the base model, including no covariate effects, was 1000. Now, in order to consider the influence of various covariate effects, suppose an α value of 0.05 was prespecified in the analysis plan as the significance level associated with covariate additions to the model. Therefore, covariate effects associated with $v = 1$ degree of freedom would require a decrease in the MVOF of at least 3.84 to achieve statistical significance ($X^2_{\alpha = 0.05, v = 1} = 3.84$). Furthermore, suppose that two covariate effects (gender and weight) were considered separately, each by adding one covariate to the base model. If the model including the effect of gender resulted in a MVOF of 997.500 and the model including the effect of weight resulted in a MVOF of 981.326, we would calculate the two differences between the hierarchical models: base—(base + gender effect) = 1000 – 997.5 = 2.5 and base—(base + weight effect) = 1000 – 981.326 = 18.674. The comparison of these differences to the test statistic associated with the prespecified level of significance indicates that the gender effect would not be considered statistically significant, since the difference of 2.5 < 3.84. However, the addition of the weight covariate would be considered a statistically significant addition to the model since the difference in MVOF associated with this addition, 18.674, is greater than 3.84. For reporting purposes, various statistical packages, such as SAS® or R, may be used to compute the approximate p value associated with a particular MVOF difference and number of degrees of freedom, based on a X^2 distribution function.

It is important to note here that several authors have studied the properties of these likelihood ratio test comparisons under different conditions in order to evaluate the appropriateness of this procedure in the selection of covariate effects via an assessment of how closely the resulting p values correspond with the nominal level of significance of these tests (Wahlby et al. 2001; Beal 2002; Gobburu and Lawrence 2002). A consistent finding among these evaluations is that use of NONMEM's FOCE method, in particular, with the INTERACTION option specified, results in much better agreement with nominal significance levels for covariate evaluation than does the default FO method. Since the vast majority of modeling work being done with NONMEM today utilizes the FOCE method, and when possible, the INTERACTION option as well, these publications serve to reinforce the appropriateness of this methodology in this circumstance but also to warn against likely bias in the reported p value for covariate assessments if the FO method is used.

It is also important to note that comparisons of MVOF values between models are not valid if any changes are made to the dataset. A difference in even one concentration value in a dataset of thousands of samples will affect the MVOF and render a comparison of models based on the MVOF inappropriate. Thus, if a dataset error is detected during the covariate evaluation process, the tentative model at the point of the error detection should be re-estimated with the corrected dataset and the resulting MVOF used as the new value for comparison of subsequent models based on the hierarchical model framework discussed previously.

5.7.3 Diagnostic Plots to Illustrate Parameter-Covariate Relationships

Given a list of covariates to be considered and the parameters upon which the potential influence of a covariate(s) are to be tested, a first step in the covariate evaluation process involves plotting the data to assess the extent and nature of relationships evident in the data. Using the table file output from the base model, scatterplots of the empirical Bayesian estimates (EBEs) of the PK or PD parameters versus the covariates of interest can be generated. Examples of such plots for clearance and volume versus weight, age, and creatinine clearance are provided in Figure 5.45 and Figure 5.46. For discrete covariates, boxplots of the EBEs for the various levels of each categorical covariate can be generated. If desired, smoothing splines can be added to the scatterplots and the medians of the boxplots can be joined across categories to assist in identifying possible relationships. Figure 5.47 and Figure 5.48 illustrate plots of the EBEs of clearance and volume versus gender and race.

These plots may be used in several different ways. First, these plots facilitate the selection of relationships between parameters and covariates to be modeled. Second, selection of potential functional forms to describe these possible relationships is made easier. And finally, possible high influence covariate values, which may cause difficulties in subsequent covariate models, may be identified.

The plots in Figure 5.45, Figure 5.46, Figure 5.47, and Figure 5.48 provide examples of the patterns that may be observed in such plots. A pattern or trend in any of these plots may be considered an indication that a possible relationship may be detected or that a portion of the unexplained IIV in that parameter may be explained by the corresponding covariate. With respect to the testing of specific models including covariate effects, the analysis plan should specify how this assessment is to be made. Sometimes analysis plans are written to include an (albeit subjective) assessment as to whether a trend is evident in this plot of the relationship between the

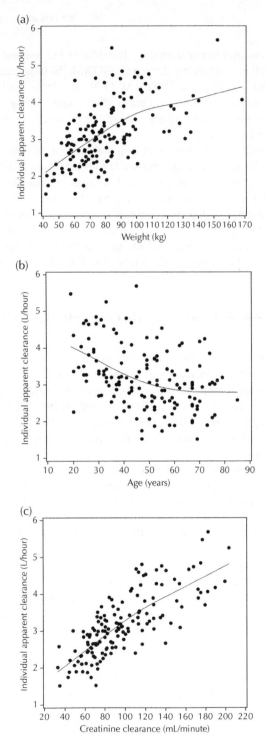

FIGURE 5.45 Scatterplots of the EBEs of clearance versus continuous covariates. Panel (a) shows the plot of clearance versus weight, Panel (b) shows the plot of clearance versus age, and Panel (c) shows the plot of clearance versus creatinine clearance.

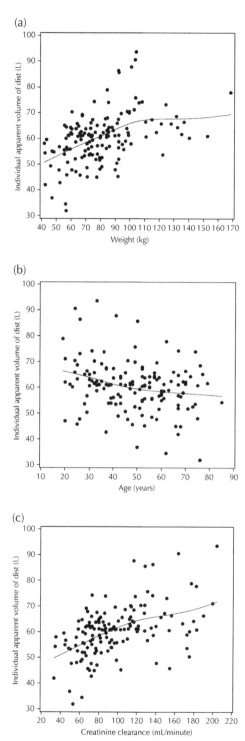

FIGURE 5.46 Scatterplots of the EBEs of volume versus continuous covariates. Panel (a) shows the plot of volume versus weight, Panel (b) shows the plot of volume versus age, and Panel (c) shows the plot of volume versus creatinine clearance.

145

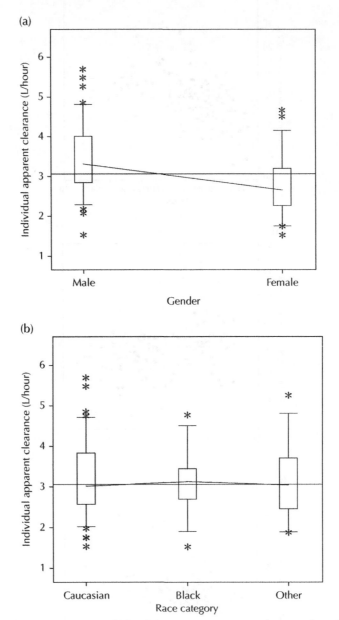

FIGURE 5.47 Boxplots of the EBEs of clearance versus categorical covariates. Panel (a) shows the plot of clearance versus gender and Panel (b) shows the plot of clearance versus race. The box represents the 25th to 75th percentiles of the data, with the whiskers extending to the 5th and 95th percentiles of the data and the asterisks representing values outside this range; the boxes are joined at the median values.

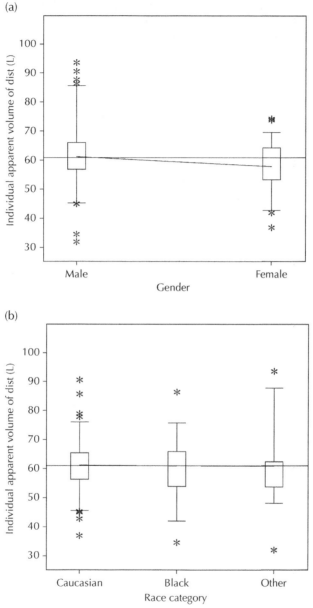

FIGURE 5.48   Boxplots of the EBEs of volume versus categorical covariates. Panel (a) shows the plot of volume versus gender and Panel (b) shows the plot of volume versus race. The box represents the 25th to 75th percentiles of the data, with the whiskers extending to the 5th and 95th percentiles of the data and the asterisks representing values outside this range; the boxes are joined at the median values.

parameter and the covariate. If (and only if) a trend is noted, then a model(s) will be tested to estimate the effect of the covariate on the parameter. Alternatively, the plan may indicate that all prespecified relationships between parameters and covariates will be estimated in NONMEM. In this case, the plots may be used to select which functional forms are worthy of consideration.

The former method described above (testing only those parameter-covariate models where a relationship is evident from the plots) may seem a logical and efficient choice to avoid fitting a potentially large number of models where no effect is likely to be detected; however, care should be taken to avoid potentially misleading findings as a result of a phenomenon called Bayesian shrinkage (to be described in more detail in Chapter 7) (Savic and Karlsson 2009). In their publication, Savic and Karlsson warned against over-reliance on such plots, especially in situations where there may be significant shrinkage in the distributions of the EBEs. In this case, Savic and Karlsson suggested the estimation of all tentative models in NONMEM (the latter method described earlier).

5.7.4   Typical Functional Forms for Covariate-Parameter Relationships

Now that we have an understanding of how to statistically compare models, we can move our attention to methods for the mathematical parameterization of models to include the effects of covariates in a meaningful and readily interpretable way. Various functional forms, or model structures, are commonly used to relate the effects of covariates to PK or PD parameters. Some of these typical forms for the parameter-covariate submodel include additive shifts, proportional shifts, linear, power, exponential, and piece-wise linear forms. Each of these will be explored in the following sections, in turn, as each has different properties and is associated with different assumptions about its parameters.

5.7.4.1 Dichotomous Predictors   Covariates with only two possible levels, such as gender, are the easiest type to both model and interpret. Dichotomous covariate effects can be coded in a few different ways, as described below:
Additive shift model:

$$CL_i = \theta_1 + \theta_2 \times SEXF_i$$

Proportional shift model:

$$CL_i = \theta_1 \times (1 + \theta_2 \times SEXF_i)$$

Alternatively, using an IF–THEN coding structure:

```
IF (SEXF.GT.0.5) THEN
TVCL = THETA(1)
ELSE
```

```
TVCL = THETA(2)
ENDIF
CL = TVCL*EXP(ETA(1))
```

Each of these parameterizations requires two parameters to estimate the drug clearance for males and females. In the first case above, the additive shift model estimates the clearance for males (where SEXF=0) using θ_1 and the increment or decrement in clearance associated with female gender (where SEXF=1) as the positive or negative θ_2 that is added to the male clearance value. In the second case with the proportional shift model, again θ_1 represents the male clearance value, but with this model θ_2 represents the proportional increase or decrease over the male clearance value, associated with female gender. It is important when using either the additive or proportional shift models described earlier that neither lower nor upper bounds be set on the fixed-effect estimate for θ_2. While a lower bound of 0 may be perfectly appropriate for θ_1 to prevent a negative clearance value, a lower bound of 0 on θ_2 would restrict the search space to allow for only solutions whereby the clearance for females is greater than that of males. In the third and final option presented above, the drug clearance is coded as θ_1 for males and θ_2 for females. With this variation, it would be appropriate to set lower bounds of 0 on both θ_1 and θ_2.

Note that in the IF–THEN coding of the third example, the conditional IF statement uses a SEXF value of 0.5 to differentiate between males and females, when the data include only values of 0 for males and 1 for females. This is an intentional selection in order to avoid possible problems that sometimes occur when an exact value is utilized in an IF statement. Due to rounding and numerical representation issues with electronic data, it has been shown that certain numbers may be problematic to use based on rounding of repeating decimals, and IF statements utilizing these numbers may fail to recognize and categorize them appropriately. Therefore, this technique of selecting a value not exactly represented in the data may be safer way to ensure that the subjects are categorized correctly and dealt with accordingly.

5.7.4.2 *Categorical Predictors*   When covariates are discrete variables, but can take on more than two (i.e., n) possible levels, $n-1$ indicator variables are commonly created for use in covariate modeling. Each of these n indicator variables can take on two possible values, typically 0 or 1, for ease of implementation as described in the following text.

For example, perhaps a RACE variable was collected with values of 1=Caucasian, 2=Black/African American, 3=Asian, and 4=Other. Based on this variable, three indicator variables would be created: one for Black/African American race (RACB), one for Asian race (RACA), and one for "Other" races (RACO). Refer to Section 3.5.2.4 for an example of the creation of such indicator variables. In each case, a value of 1 for the indicator would denote a positive identification for that group with 0 indicating that the subject is not a member of the corresponding group. In this way, when looking across all of the newly created indicator variables for a particular covariate, each subject has at most a single positive value. If all of the values are 0, the subject belongs to the reference population, which in this case, is Caucasian race.

Using these indicator variables in place of the original race variable, one could then code the effect of race on drug clearance using an additive shift model as shown below:

$$CL_i = \theta_1 + \theta_2 \times RACB_i + \theta_3 \times RACA_i + \theta_4 \times RACO_i$$

Note that no indicator variable is required for the population considered to be the reference group (in this case, Caucasian race). The estimate for θ_1 in this example is the typical drug clearance for the Caucasian population, and θ_2, θ_3, and θ_4 are the positive or negative shifts from this estimate for Black subjects, Asian subjects, and subjects coded as race Other, respectively. As in the previous additive shift model example, neither lower nor upper bounds would be set for θ_2, θ_3, or θ_4. Sometimes, the reference group might have been selected because it is the group with the highest representation in the dataset; however, in order to avoid possible situations where PK parameters, such as clearance, become negative, one may consider selecting the population with the lowest mean clearance as the reference population. In this way, the estimates for the typical shifts for the other populations will be positive, thus avoiding negative clearance values.

5.7.4.3   Continuous Predictors   The variety of possible functional forms for parameter-covariate submodels with continuous predictor variables is considerably greater than for discrete covariates. Some of the typically encountered forms used to describe the relationship between continuous covariates and PK or PD parameters include linear, power, exponential, and piece-wise linear.

5.7.4.3.1   Linear Models   A linear form for the parameter-covariate submodel implies that over the range of observed covariate values, the PK or PD parameter either increases or decreases (monotonically) with increasing values of the covariate at a rate estimated by the positive or negative slope parameter (θ_2), as in Figure 5.49. If the linear function has an estimated intercept term (θ_1), then, depending on the parameterization (i.e., if not centered—see Section 5.7.5), a portion of the parameter may be considered independent of the covariate and is estimated to be present even when the covariate is not measured or has a value of 0.

Linear models for covariates generally take on the following form:

$$CL_i = \theta_1 + \theta_2 \times WTKG_i$$

where θ_1 is the clearance (intercept) when weight$=0$, θ_2 is the (positive or negative) slope estimate reflecting the change in clearance per unit change in weight, and $WTKG_i$ is the body weight of the ith subject.

Examination of a plot of individual estimates of clearance (y axis) versus subject weight (x axis) may be useful in the determination of appropriate initial estimates for linear model parameters. The graphing program may also be used to add a line of best fit to the plot or the analyst may choose to simply *eyeball* the relationship. For a simple linear model, selection of two points on the line of best

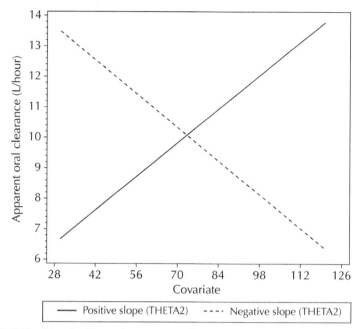

FIGURE 5.49 Lineplot illustrating representative linear models for the relationship between apparent oral clearance and a covariate.

fit would allow for the simple calculation of an approximate slope (as the change in y values divided by the corresponding change in the x values for the two selected points) and the determination of the y intercept where the line appears to cross the y axis.

5.7.4.3.2 Power Models A power model form allows for much greater flexibility in the relationship between the parameter and the covariate, as shown in Figure 5.50. Its typical parameterization is as follows:

$$CL_i = \theta_1 \times WTKG_i^{\theta_2}$$

where θ_1 is the clearance (coefficient) when weight $= 1$; θ_2 is the (positive or negative) exponent estimate reflecting the change in the natural log of clearance per unit change in the natural log of weight; and $WTKG_i$ is the body weight of the ith subject. The specific value of the exponent term and its sign, in conjunction with the sign of the coefficient term (θ_1), allows for the relationship to take on a variety of different shapes as shown in Figure 5.50. Although most of these shapes appear nonlinear over the weight range, this model form is an inherently linear form in that it is considered linear in the parameters. To illustrate this point, taking the natural logarithm of both sides of the equation results in a linear model, for example:

$$\ln(CL_i) = \ln(\theta_1) + \theta_2 \times \ln(WTKG_i)$$

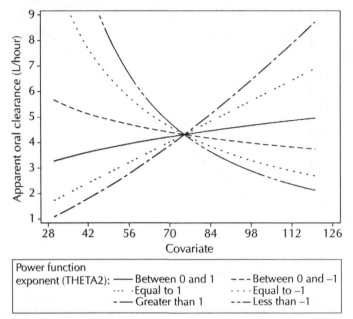

FIGURE 5.50 Lineplots illustrating representative power models with varying exponents for the relationship between apparent oral clearance and a covariate.

thus allowing for the interpretation of the model parameters (as above) in linear model equivalents. Figure 5.51 presents the representative power model curves shown in Figure 5.50 after natural log transformation to illustrate their linear counterparts. Due to its flexibility and the use of only two parameters (as with a linear model), the power model functional form is found to be an appropriate characterization of many relationships and is often associated with lower objective function values than other model forms. Based on this transformation, examination of a plot of individual estimates of ln-transformed clearance (y axis) versus ln-transformed subject weight or other covariate (x axis) may be useful in the determination of appropriate initial estimates for power model parameters as described previously for the linear model.

The classic parameterization associated with the introduction of an allometric relationship between PK parameters and weight generally invokes the power model with a fixed value for the exponent (θ_2) as shown below:

$$CL_i = \theta_1 \times WTKG_i^{0.75}$$

$$V_i = \theta_2 \times WTKG_i^{1.0}$$

For clearance parameters, an exponent of 0.75 is typically used and for volume parameters, an exponent of 1.0 is used based on a well-described scientific framework that can be related to basic physiologic functions (Anderson and Holford 2009).

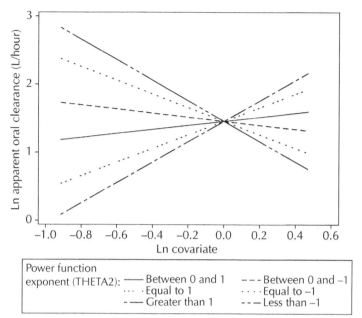

FIGURE 5.51 Lineplots illustrating the natural log transformation of representative power models for the relationship between apparent oral clearance and a covariate.

5.7.4.3.3 Exponential Models The exponential functional form, as shown in Figure 5.52, appropriately describes relationships between parameters and covariates that take on a different shape than those illustrated in Figure 5.49, Figure 5.50, and Figure 5.51. The assumptions of the exponential model are also different than those relevant for the other forms. The typical parameterization of the exponential model is as follows:

$$CL_i = \theta_1 \times e^{\theta_2 \times WTKG_i}$$

where θ_1 is the clearance (coefficient) when weight=0; θ_2 is the (positive or negative) exponent estimate reflecting the change in the natural log of clearance per unit change in weight; and $WTKG_i$ is the body weight of the ith subject. As for the power model discussed earlier, although the shape of the relationship between clearance and body weight is not linear with an exponential relationship, this model form is also an inherently linear form in that it is linear in the parameters. As above, taking the natural logarithm of both sides of this equation results in the following linear model, for example:

$$\ln(CL_i) = \ln(\theta_1) + \theta_2 \times WTKG_i$$

thus allowing for the interpretation of the model parameters (as above) in linear model equivalents. Figure 5.53 presents the representative exponential model curves shown in Figure 5.52 after natural log transformation to illustrate their linear counterparts.

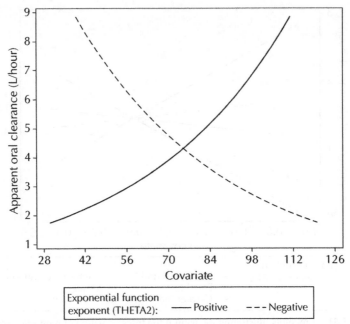

FIGURE 5.52 Lineplots illustrating representative exponential models for the relationship between apparent oral clearance and a covariate.

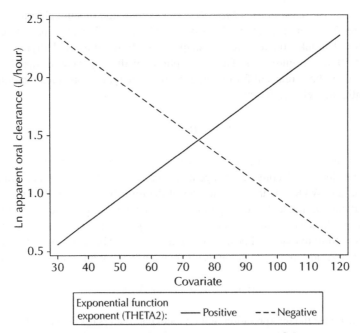

FIGURE 5.53 Lineplots illustrating the natural log transformation of representative exponential models for the relationship between apparent oral clearance and a covariate.

As described previously for the linear and power models, examination of a plot of individual estimates of ln-transformed clearance (*y* axis) versus (untransformed) subject weight (*x* axis) may be useful in the determination of appropriate initial estimates for exponential model parameters.

   5.7.4.3.4   Piece-wise Linear Models   At times, the relationship between a parameter and covariate takes on a unique shape, sometimes referred to by its *hockey-stick* appearance, whereby the parameter appears to be constant over a range of covariate values and linearly increasing or decreasing over another range of values. This type of relationship is often fit quite nicely with a piece-wise linear model form. Figure 5.54 illustrates two examples of a piece-wise linear relationship. This model form is flexible allowing for the linearly increasing (or decreasing) portion to occur with either low or high values of the covariate, such that the hockey stick can be oriented in either direction and pointing either upward or downward. With this type of functional form, two different methods can be attempted: (i) one in which the inflection point (the bend in the hockey stick) is selected and fixed based on the data or (ii) one in which the inflection point is an estimated parameter. While the second method has the added benefit of allowing for the best estimate of the change point to be selected based on the data (i.e., slightly less subjective), it also requires one additional parameter to be fit.

   The typical forms for a piece-wise linear model, in the case where (1) the constant portion of clearance is associated with values of weight less than or equal to

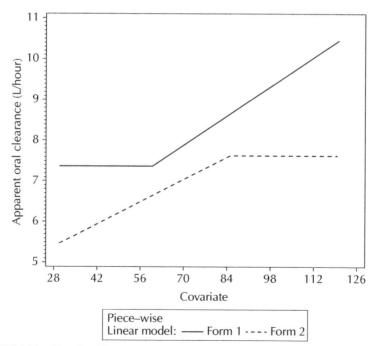

FIGURE 5.54   Lineplots illustrating representative piece-wise linear models for the relationship between apparent oral clearance and a covariate.

70 kg and (2) where the constant portion of clearance is associated with values greater than or equal to 70 kg, are as follows:

$$(1) \quad CL_i = \theta_1 + \theta_2 \times 70 \times (1 - WTindic_i) + \theta_2 \times WTKG_i \times WTindic_i$$

where θ_1 is a portion of the clearance when weight = 70 or less; θ_2 is the (positive or negative) slope estimate reflecting the change in clearance per unit change in weight (for weight values >70 kg); WTindic_i is an indicator variable for the ith subject defined as 1 when body weight is greater than or equal to 70 kg and 0 when body weight is less than 70 kg; and $WTKG_i$ is the body weight of the ith subject and

$$(2) \quad CL_i = \theta_1 + \theta_2 \times 70 \times WTindic_i + \theta_2 \times WTKG_i \times (1 - WTindic_i)$$

where θ_1 is the clearance (intercept) when weight = 0; θ_2 is the (positive or negative) slope estimate reflecting the change in clearance per unit change in weight (for weight values <70 kg); WTindic_i is an indicator variable for the ith subject defined as 1 when body weight is greater than or equal to 70 kg and 0 when body weight is less than 70 kg; and $WTKG_i$ is the body weight of the ith subject.

Building on the piece-wise linear parameterization, in order to allow even greater flexibility with this form, the model can be coded in such a way as to estimate the covariate value at which the estimation of clearance changes from a linear function to a constant value or from a constant to a linear function. This, of course, requires the estimation of one additional parameter over the standard piece-wise linear described above with the hard-coded inflection point. The equations used to code the situation where the constant portion of clearance is associated with values greater than or equal to the estimated inflection point are as follows:

```
CRCINF = THETA(1)     ; CRCINF is used to denote the
estimated inflection point in CRCL

CRIND = 0             ; CRIND is an indicator value
IF (CRCL>=CRCINF) CRIND = 1

TVCL = THETA(2) + THETA(3)*CRCINF*CRIND +
THETA(3)*CRCL*(1-CRIND)

CL = TVCL*EXP(ETA(1))
```

So, using the code above, drug clearance is estimated to be linearly related to creatinine clearance at values of creatinine clearance less than CRCINF (with slope = θ_3) and constant at values greater than or equal to CRCINF.

5.7.5   Centering Covariate Effects

Another important consideration in constructing models including the influence of covariate factors on PK or PD parameters is the practice of centering covariate effects (Draper and Smith 1981a). Centered models for covariate effects prevent the estimation of parameters defined by data completely outside the observed range and provide improved precision of parameter estimates over uncentered models. The models presented in Section 5.7.4 are all uncentered models for ease of exposition in describing the relevant mathematical functions and associated properties. A careful review of this section, however, reveals that for each functional form presented for continuous covariates, the intercept or coefficient parameter in every case was defined as the drug clearance when the covariate was equal to a value of either 0 or 1. For most common continuous covariates considered, values of either 0 or 1 are either extremely unlikely or impossible. Generally speaking, typical continuous covariates include demographic factors like age, weight, body mass index (BMI), and body surface area (BSA), in addition to measures of renal or hepatic function such as creatinine clearance, ALT, or aspartate transaminase (AST). Considering the simple linear model presented in Section 5.7.4.3.1, an estimate of drug clearance when weight is equal to 0 is not only useless information but also implausible in that little or no data are available to support the estimation of such a parameter. With the data collected in a typical clinical trial conducted in an adult population, how could we know what the drug clearance would be when weight is equal to 0? This is exactly the point supporting the need for centering.

Centering is a reparameterization of the parameter-covariate submodel allowing for the intercept or coefficient parameter to be defined within the range of the observed data, thus improving the precision of the estimate. In order to derive the centered equations, we begin with the uncentered simple linear model presented in Section 5.7.4.3.1:

$$CL_i = \theta_1 + \theta_2 \times WTKG_i$$

with parameters defined as presented earlier. Without changing the equation, if the term $\theta_2 \times medWTKG$, where medWTKG is the median body weight in the population, is both added to and subtracted from the linear model, we obtain:

$$CL_i = (\theta_1 + \theta_2 \times medWTKG) + \theta_2 \times WTKG_i - \theta_2 \times medWTKG$$

Then, rearranging terms, we could write:

$$CL_i = \theta_1' + \theta_2 \times (WTKG_i - medWTKG)$$

where θ_1' is the drug clearance when body weight is equal to the median body weight of the population. Clearly, an estimate of drug clearance obtained for body weight near the middle of the distribution (e.g., at the mean or median value of the population) of observed body weights is more meaningful and more easily interpreted than the value of clearance associated with an unobservable weight (i.e., weight=0). Examining the equation above, it is as if we are applying a simple linear model to the relationship between drug clearance and the difference between body weight and the median body weight, or a body weight normalized by subtracting off the median value of the distribution. In practice, either the mean or median value may be used for centering, as for most typical populations either value will be near the *center* of the range of values. Figure 5.55 illustrates the relationship between individual estimates of drug clearance and creatinine clearance, before and after the creatinine clearance values are centered, in this case, by subtracting the mean value in the population.

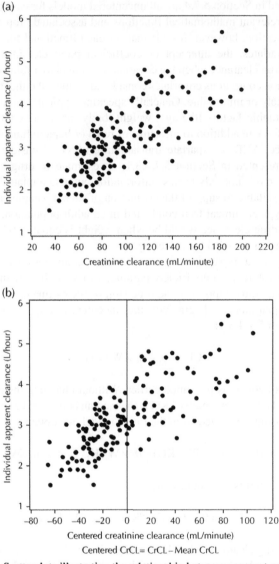

FIGURE 5.55 Scatterplots illustrating the relationship between apparent oral clearance and creatinine clearance. Panel (a) shows the plot of drug clearance versus (raw) creatinine clearance and Panel (b) shows the plot of drug clearance versus centered creatinine clearance.

This reparameterization also provides beneficial statistical properties for our model. Based on the confidence band about a regression line (see Fig. 5.56), we can see that the most precise parameter estimates will be obtained near the center of the distribution (closest to the mean) of the covariate (independent variable) while the least precise estimates would be obtained near the extremes of the distribution, or worse yet, outside the observed range of the data (Draper and Smith

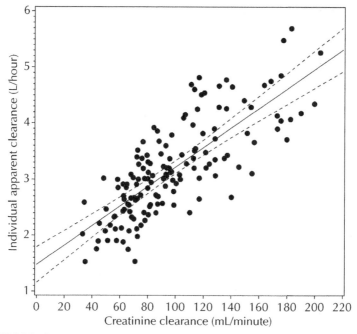

FIGURE 5.56 Scatterplot illustrating the relationship between apparent oral clearance and creatinine clearance with the fitted line and the confidence band about the fitted line.

1981b). This is the basis for the improvement in the precision of the intercept or coefficient parameter estimate that is obtained with a centered model as compared to an uncentered model.

Applying the same reparameterization technique to the power and exponential models, we can derive the following centered versions of these functional forms for the parameter-covariate submodel:

$$CL_i = \theta_1 \times \left(\frac{WTKG_i}{medWTKG} \right)^{\theta_2}$$

and

$$CL_i = \theta_1 \times e^{\theta_2 \times (WTKG_i - medWTKG)}$$

Similarly, the centered piece-wise linear model, based on a specified inflection point, with constant clearance for low values of weight and increasing clearance with higher values of weight would take the form:

$$CL_i = \theta_1 + \theta_2 \times (70 - medWTKG) \times (1 - WTindic_i) + \theta_2 \times (WTKG_i - medWTKG) \\ \times WTindic_i$$

5.7.6 Forward Selection Process

One methodology for the systematic evaluation and selection of covariates is a stepwise forward selection followed by backward elimination procedure. With a forward selection process, covariates are considered for inclusion in the model in various steps or rounds, with a single covariate added at the conclusion of each step. For the first step of the process, the effect of each covariate to be tested would be estimated on a single parameter in a single model separately. For example, consider the parameter-covariate combinations described in Table 5.5 to be evaluated based on the analysis plan.

Thus, round #1 of forward selection would entail the estimation of at least six models, four evaluating covariate effects on drug clearance and two evaluating covariate effects on volume of distribution. More than six models may be required if multiple functional forms are examined for a given parameter-covariate relationship. Looking across the results of each of the six (or more) models, the differences between the MVOF obtained for each model and the MVOF for the reference (base) model are calculated. Based on the prespecified α value for the inclusion of covariates into the model (say, $\alpha = 0.05$), differences of greater than 3.84 (based on $X^2_{a=0.05, \upsilon=1}$) are considered statistically significant additions to the model. A table may be constructed, as shown in Table 5.6, based on the results of each round to facilitate comparison of model results and selection of an appropriate model from each round.

Based on the information in Table 5.6, if the prespecified (analysis plan) criteria for model selection were based solely on the change in the MVOF, the obvious choice of covariate to be added following round #1 would be the effect of creatinine clearance on drug clearance using the power model functional form. However, if the prespecified criteria additionally included a reduction in the magnitude of IIV (in the parameter of interest), the choice is not so clear-cut. While a reduction in IIV on clearance is observed with the addition of the creatinine clearance effect on clearance, a much larger reduction in IIV (on volume of distribution) is obtained with the addition of the effect of weight on volume of distribution. Furthermore, this effect is also statistically significant with $p < 0.05$. So the modeler is faced with a choice: include the covariate associated with the largest reduction in the MVOF and a small

TABLE 5.5 Planned covariates to be evaluated during covariate assessment, and on which parameter each is to be evaluated

Parameter	Covariate
CL	Weight
CL	Age
CL	Race
CL	Creatinine clearance
V	Weight
V	Gender

TABLE 5.6   Summary of a given round of the forward selection process

Parameter	Covariate	Functional form	Decrease in MVOF	Degrees of freedom	p value	Decrease in IIV
CL	Weight	Power	44.927	1	2.05E−11	6.81
CL	Age	Linear	9.532	1	0.002029	1.58
CL	Race	Additive shift	0.551	3	0.759192	0.07
CL	Creatinine clearance	Power	75.987	1	0	10.84
CL	Creatinine clearance	Linear	75.362	1	0	10.72
V	Weight	Power	22.970	1	1.645E−6	13.06
V	Weight	Linear	22.589	1	2.006E−6	12.97
V	Gender	Additive shift	9.741	1	0.001802	9.48

reduction in IIV or the covariate associated with a slightly smaller reduction in MVOF but a much larger reduction in IIV. This example illustrates, in a simple way, some of the nuance and subjectivity involved in model development exercises, even in the presence of a carefully worded analysis plan. Of course, one could choose to follow the prespecified analysis plan *to the letter* which would result in choosing the effect of creatinine clearance on clearance at this round since this effect is statistically significant at $\alpha=0.05$, achieves the largest change in the MVOF, and reduces IIV in the parameter of interest. On the other hand, one could easily justify the selection of the effect of weight on volume at this round, based on the arguably more meaningful impact it has on reducing unexplained IIV, which is, after all, one of the main objectives of covariate evaluations.

In an effort to strip away as much subjectivity as possible from our model development efforts, the example above provides fodder for the specification of additional rule-based criteria in our analysis plans. For example, if we further added to the prespecified criteria for forward selection that the IIV should be reduced by at least 5% CV from the reference model, we move one step closer to this goal. Of course, we will always encounter situations where insight and experience cannot be ignored in an effort to abide by an analysis plan, no matter how carefully considered and worded. For this reason, it is common practice to include a section entitled *Changes to the Planned Analyses* in the technical report summarizing pharmacometric modeling and simulation efforts to describe any deviations that may have occurred from the prespecified planned analysis.

After the selection of the single covariate effect for inclusion in the model following round #1 of forward selection, the diagnostic plots illustrating the remaining relationships between parameters and covariates (based on this model including the effect of one covariate) are produced and examined again to facilitate round #2 of forward selection. In Section 5.7.3, diagnostic plots for illustrating the relationships between parameters and covariates were introduced. A variation on these plots will be presented here, as an option to be considered once one or more covariate effects have been included in the model.

Once a particular covariate effect has been included in the model, we wish to understand whether (i) the addition of the covariate effect to the model was effective in characterizing the trend originally observed in the plot of the EBE of the parameter versus the covariate and (ii) whether any of the remaining covariates may be useful in explaining the remaining unexplained variability (i.e., trends are evident in other plots) after accounting for the first covariate effect. In order to address these issues, we need to examine the suite of scatterplots and boxplots of EBEs versus covariates (as described in Section 5.7.3), specifically looking for the expected relationship between the EBE and the covariate included in the model after round #1 and any other trends between EBEs and other covariates. One can imagine that after several rounds of covariate additions, it can be quite a challenge to keep track of the expected relationships based on factors in the model and the undiscovered relationships based on factors not yet included.

A solution to this problem is to create an alternative version of these diagnostic plots, sometimes referred to as a *delta-plot* or *delta-parameter plot*. Examples of delta-plots for clearance and volume versus continuous and categorical predictors are shown in Figure 5.57, Figure 5.58, Figure 5.59, and Figure 5.60. Instead of plotting the EBE of the parameter(s) on the y axes of these plots, we plot the difference between the EBE and the typical value of the parameter instead. This difference quantifies the remaining unexplained variability in the parameter or the variability not yet accounted for by the covariates included in the model. In fact, this difference is exactly equivalent to the IIV random effect, or η, if an additive model is used for IIV. If an exponential or other model form is used to describe the IIV, this difference is merely a transformation of the η random-effect term.

The major advantage to the delta-parameter versus covariate plots over the EBE versus covariate plots is that, regardless of the round of selection or the particular covariates included or excluded from the model at a particular stage, all plots are examined with a single objective: to identify possible trends, indicating further model improvement is required. One does not need to keep track of which covariates are in or out of the model, with differing expectations of what to find in these plots. If a trend is identified in a given scatterplot or boxplot based on a delta-parameter, a model to estimate a covariate addition or improvement would be considered. Once a covariate is included in the model, if a delta-parameter versus covariate plot for that relationship reveals a remaining trend, this is an indication that the functional form utilized to describe the relationship might be in need of additional refinement. When no trends are apparent in any of the delta-parameter versus covariate plots, we would conclude that the remaining unexplained variability in these parameters is not likely to be related to the covariates under consideration and no further additions of covariate effects may be warranted. Some modelers prefer to examine plots of the η terms themselves versus covariates with a similar objective in mind.

The process of evaluating diagnostic plots to guide the consideration of models to be tested in each round of forward selection, followed by the estimation of appropriate models testing specific parameter-covariate relationships is repeated after each addition of a new statistically significant covariate effect to the model. Forward selection is concluded when no further covariate effects reach statistical significance based on the prespecified criteria in the analysis plan.

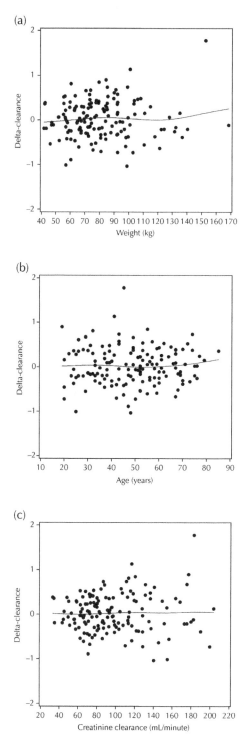

FIGURE 5.57 Scatterplots of delta-clearance versus continuous covariates. Panel (a) shows the plot of delta-clearance versus weight, Panel (b) shows the plot of delta-clearance versus age, and Panel (c) shows the plot of delta-clearance versus creatinine clearance.

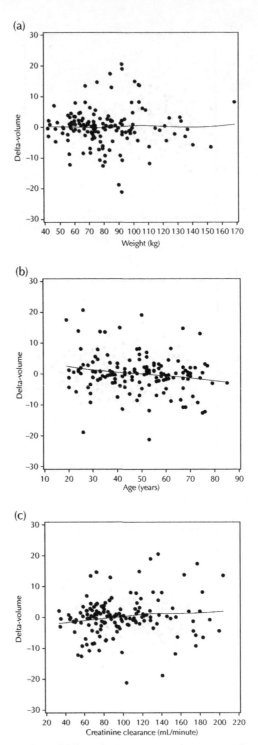

FIGURE 5.58 Scatterplots of delta-volume versus continuous covariates. Panel (a) shows the plot of delta-volume versus weight, Panel (b) shows the plot of delta-volume versus age, and Panel (c) shows the plot of delta-volume versus creatinine clearance.

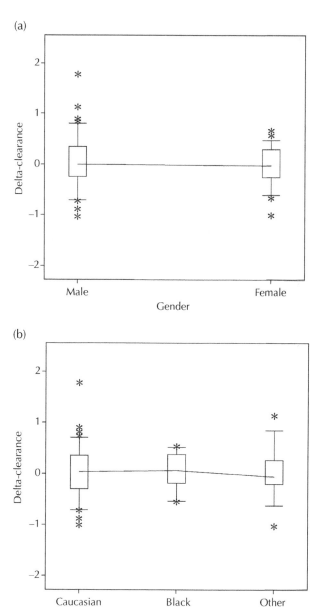

FIGURE 5.59 Boxplots of delta-clearance versus categorical covariates. Panel (a) shows the plot of delta-clearance versus gender and Panel (b) shows the plot of delta-clearance versus race. The box represents the 25th to 75th percentiles of the data, with the whiskers extending to the 5th and 95th percentiles of the data and the asterisks representing values outside this range; the boxes are joined at the median values.

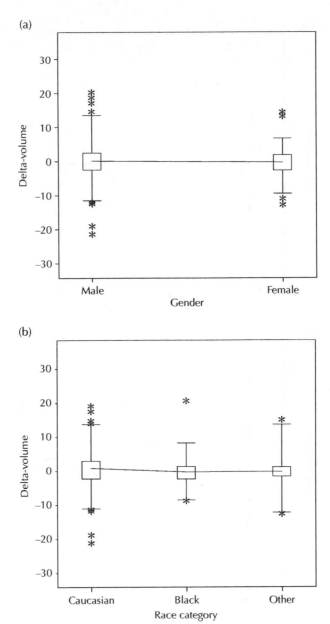

FIGURE 5.60 Boxplots of delta-volume versus categorical covariates. Panel (a) shows the plot of delta-volume versus gender and Panel (b) shows the plot of delta-volume versus race. The box represents the 25th to 75th percentiles of the data, with the whiskers extending to the 5th and 95th percentiles of the data and the asterisks representing values outside this range; the boxes are joined at the median values.

5.7.7   Evaluation of the Full Multivariable Model

The stage of model development that follows the completion of forward selection is referred to as the full multivariable model evaluation stage. It is at this stage of development that the random-effect models are refined. If there are PK or PD parameters on which IIV was not estimable with the base structural model, an attempt may be made at this stage to estimate such terms. Sometimes the inclusion of important covariate effects in the model, and the accompanying reduction in unexplained variability, allows for the estimation of IIV terms that were not estimable prior to the evaluation of covariates.

Once all IIV terms have been added to the model, consideration may be given to whether the default assumption of no covariance between IIV terms is appropriate. Pair-wise scatterplots of η terms can be generated to assist with this assessment. Such plots (sometimes referred to as η biplots) and the corresponding statistics such as the r^2, or correlation coefficient, of this relationship provide information regarding whether or not a relationship between these terms is evident. Example eta biplots are provided in Figure 5.61. Other plotting features, such as horizontal and vertical reference lines at $\eta = 0$ (cross-hairs), are also helpful in detecting trends in these plots. If trends are detected, the covariance between the IIV random-effect terms (i.e., the off-diagonal elements of the Ω matrix) may be estimated. The NM-TRAN coding for estimation of off-diagonal elements of Ω and Σ is provided in Section 3.6.

Sometimes the decision of whether to estimate an off-diagonal element of Ω in the model is not so straightforward. Clearly, if all indicators of an improved model fit were present—a reduction in the MVOF, reasonable parameter estimates with good precision, improvement (or at least a lack of detriment) in goodness-of-fit plots, etc.—then the decision to include the estimated random effect would be easy. In the following case, the decision is not as simple and clear-cut. Suppose in comparison to the appropriate reference model, in this case the full multivariable model following forward selection, the estimation of the covariance term between the IIV on clearance and the IIV on volume of distribution results in a reduction in the MVOF of 52 points. However, the standard error associated with this parameter estimate is 92% of the estimate and the precision of the estimate of IIV on clearance also worsened (from 34% of the estimate prior to the estimation of the covariance term to 61% of the estimate after including the covariance), while the IIV on volume was relatively unchanged. One might further consider the precisions of other parameter estimates as well as diagnostic plots of goodness-of-fit, but for the purpose of this example, we will suppose these indicators were all similar between models. In this situation, the modeler has the choice of accepting the additional term in the model (which presumably is a more appropriate characterization of the IIV since the η biplot indicated a trend and the MVOF is considerably reduced), along with the detriment in the precision of the parameter estimates, *or* rejecting this addition in favor of more precisely estimated parameters.

One additional piece of evidence that may be useful in making the decision to keep or reject this term is the condition number of the model. The condition number may be determined with the eigenvalues of the variance–covariance matrix. The

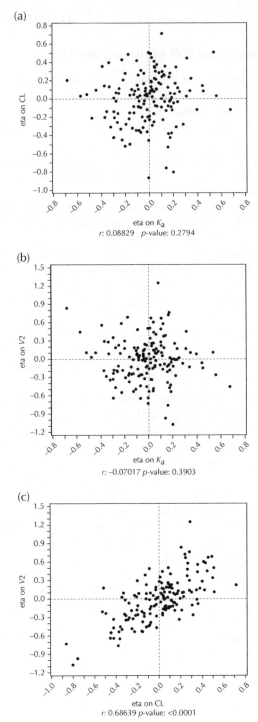

FIGURE 5.61 Bivariate scatterplots of random-effect terms (eta biplots). Panel (a) shows the plot of eta_{CL} versus eta_{K_a}, with no apprent trend, Panel (b) shows the plot of eta_{V2} versus eta_{K_a}, with no apparent trend, and Panel (c) shows the plot of eta_{V2} versus eta_{CL}, with a positive relationship evident.

eigenvalues may be requested using the PRINT=E option on the $COVARIANCE record (see Section 3.8). Taking the ratio of the largest to the smallest eigenvalue ($\lambda_{largest}/\lambda_{smallest}$), one can compute the condition number of the model (Bonate 2006). While the exact value of the condition number is a useful diagnostic in itself, the change in condition number with a change to the model is also informative. If the condition number following the addition of the covariance term to the model indicates that the model has now become ill conditioned when it previously was not, the term should probably not be added. However, if the condition number is relatively similar, with no indication of ill conditioning, one might choose in favor of accepting the term in the model.

The final consideration with respect to the appropriateness of the random-effect terms at this full multivariable model stage is a check on the residual variability model selection. Similar to the considerations when selecting a functional form for the RV model at the base structural model stage, we consider the diagnostic plots of IWRES versus IPRED and |IWRES| versus IPRED as well as the final parameter estimates and standard errors for the estimates of the Σ matrix (and corresponding θs if relevant based on the parameterization selected). If no trends are apparent in the scatterplots and the RV parameter estimates are reasonable and precisely estimated, no changes to the model are likely warranted. However, oftentimes after covariates that explain a portion of the previously unexplained variability have been added to the model, improvements in the RV model are warranted and beneficial to the stability of the model at this stage. It is important to note that the conclusion of forward selection often comes with a fairly unstable and/or overparameterized model. This finding occurs, in part, because the forward selection process may have resulted in the addition of covariates that are now unnecessary or extraneous in the presence of other factors and modifications to the random-effect models. For these reasons, the next step in the covariate evaluation process is to consider each fixed-effect covariate term for possible removal from the model.

5.7.8 Backward Elimination Process

The backward elimination step is typically quicker and easier to perform than the forward selection process. During backward elimination, which is also completed in a series of rounds or steps, each covariate effect is tested for removal from the model one at a time. If the model following the full multivariable model stage contains four covariate effects, three factors on clearance and one on volume of distribution, the first round of backward elimination would consist of four models. In each of the four models, one of the covariate effects is removed from the model, while all of the other parameters are kept in and estimated. A table summarizing the results of each round of backward elimination could be created, as shown in Table 5.7, in a similar manner to the one created during each round of forward selection (see Table 5.6 in Section 5.7.6).

Looking across the results of each of the four models, the differences between the MVOF obtained for each model with one covariate effect removed and the MVOF for the reference model (that following refinement of full multivariable model) are

TABLE 5.7 Summary of the first round of backward elimination

Parameter	Covariate	Functional form	Decrease in MVOF	Degrees of freedom	p value
CL	Weight	Power	2.590	1	0.108
CL	Age	Linear	0.950	1	0.330
CL	Creatinine clearance	Power	78.705	1	0
V	Weight	Power	20.822	1	5.04E–6

calculated. Based on the prespecified α value for the maintenance of covariates into the model (say, $\alpha = 0.001$), differences of greater than 10.83 (based on $X^2_{a=0.001,\upsilon=1}$) are considered statistically significant deletions from the model. Based on Table 5.7, and assuming the prespecified (analysis plan) criteria for keeping a covariate effect in the model were based solely on the change in the MVOF, the only covariates that would be considered for removal from the model during this first round of backward elimination would be the effects of age and weight on drug clearance. Since the MVOF increased by only 0.95 and 2.59 with the removal of the age and weight effects, respectively, no statistically significant detriment in the fit is noted after removing each of these parameters from the model. In an effort to develop a parsimonious model that adequately describes the data, the age effect would be removed from the model first (as it was associated with the smallest change in the MVOF) and the new model with covariate effects of weight and creatinine clearance on drug clearance and weight on volume of distribution would be taken into round #2 of backward elimination. This process would be repeated until the removal of each covariate from the model results in a statistically significant detriment to the fit, as measured by increases in the MVOF greater than 10.83.

On a practical note, there are several ways to code the models to be tested at each round of backward elimination. Of course, one could remove the covariate effect parameter by rewriting the relevant portion of the parameter-covariate submodel in the $PK block without the affected theta, renumbering the subsequent thetas in the vector, and removing the appropriate initial estimate in the $THETA record. Perhaps a simpler method, which has the added benefit of requiring less modification to the code and therefore less risk of inadvertent coding errors, is to leave the model in the $PK or $PRED block untouched and simply change the initial estimate for the appropriate THETA to a fixed value equal to the null hypothesis value for that effect. For example, to remove the linear age effect (slope) from the model for clearance, we can leave the model statements in the $PK block exactly as for the full multivariable model:

```
$PK

TVCL = THETA(1) * ((WTKG/MDWT)**THETA(3)) * ((CRCL/
MDCC)**THETA(4)) + THETA(5)*(AGE-MDAG)

CL = TVCL*EXP(ETA(1))
```

and change the $THETA record from:

```
$THETA
(0, 39.2)        ;typical value of drug clearance
(0, 10.3)        ;typical value of volume of
                 distribution
(0.75)           ;typical value of exponent for weight
                 effect on CL
(0.5)            ;typical value of exponent for CRCL effect
on CL
(-0.1)           ;typical value of slope for age effect on CL
...
```

to:

```
$THETA
(0, 39.2)     ;typical value of drug clearance
(0, 10.3)     ;typical value of volume of distribution
(0.75)        ;typical value of exponent for weight effect
              on CL
(0.5)         ;typical value of exponent for CRCL effect
              on CL
(0 FIXED)     ;typical value of slope for age effect on CL
...
```

By fixing the estimate for θ_5 to 0, the null hypothesis value for this term, the age effect on clearance is effectively removed from the model.

5.7.9   Other Covariate Evaluation Approaches

In addition to the comprehensive forward selection followed by backward elimination procedure described above in Sections 5.7.6–5.7.8, a variety of other methods of covariate evaluation have been proposed. One of the earliest alternative methods, proposed by Mandema et al. in 1992, was the use of generalized additive models (GAM) as part of the covariate selection process (Mandema et al. 1992). GAM is a flexible model fitting technique that may be used to evaluate a variety of possible functional forms for the relationships between PK or PD parameters and covariates. Using this technique, the EBEs are regressed against covariates in a step-wise manner outside of NONMEM, using a separate software package, such as S-PLUS® or R (S-Plus 2005, R Core Team 2013). The resulting relationships then provide a reduction in the dimensionality of the covariate evaluation process, by providing a (typically) smaller number of relationships to test in NONMEM in addition to guidance regarding the appropriate functional forms of these relationships.

   In 2001, Kowalski and Hutmacher proposed the use of the WAM (Wald approximation method) algorithm for covariate selection (Kowalski and Hutmacher 2001). This method takes advantage of the flexibility of the power model functional form by allowing only power relationships between parameters and covariates in a semi-automated process of covariate testing. Interest in automating the covariate selection process also stimulated the work of Jonsson and Karlsson in 1998, whose method attempts to automate the covariate testing process by applying a FO-based linear approximation of the influence of covariates on parameters (Jonsson and Karlsson 1998). More recently, Jonsson and Karlsson, along with other colleagues, have extended their automated searching procedure by applying a first-order conditional estimation (FOCE)-based linear approximation with this method (Khandelwal et al. 2011). Finally, Gastonguay (2004) has recently advocated the use of the full covariate approach. With this approach, covariates are preselected and included in the model on the basis of scientific interest, mechanistic plausibility, and exploratory graphics. As such, no hypothesis testing is conducted and the clinical importance of covariate effects is addressed by means of the parameter estimates and associated bootstrap confidence intervals.

5.8   MODEL REFINEMENT

Following the completion of the evaluation of covariate effects, the model should be carefully considered for potential refinement. Each model component should be considered in turn. With regard to fixed-effect structural model parameters, the precision of each estimate should be evaluated with respect to the informational content in the dataset relating to that parameter. If the informational content is low, relatively poorer precision should be expected. Fixed-effect parameters describing covariate influences should be estimated with sufficient precision to support the claim of a significant covariate effect. Based on analysis plan specifications, differing criteria may be utilized for claims of statistical significance and clinical relevance of a covariate influence. If the $COVARIANCE step output was requested from NONMEM, the standard errors of each parameter estimate can be used to calculate a symmetric 95% confidence interval about each parameter estimate. The equations are provided below:

$$95\% \text{ confidence interval lower bound: } FPE(\theta_1) - 1.96 \times SE(\theta_1)$$

$$95\% \text{ confidence interval upper bound: } FPE(\theta_1) + 1.96 \times SE(\theta_1)$$

Where $FPE(\theta_1)$ is the final parameter estimate for θ_1, $SE(\theta_1)$ is the standard error of the estimate for θ_1, and 1.96 corresponds to the one-sided Z-statistic with $\alpha = 0.025$.

For covariate effects, such confidence intervals may be used to support significance by evaluating whether or not such intervals contain the null hypothesis value for that effect. For linear and power parameterizations, the null hypothesis value would be 0, so intervals containing 0 could be deemed not significant. Refinement of such a model containing a nonsignificant covariate effect might include fixing the covariate effect to the null hypothesis value and re-estimating the model.

In addition to the standard and typical goodness of fit diagnostic plots which should be explored and determined to be free of substantial trends, biases, or obvious misfit, additional plots may be considered to support the adequacy of a final model. To further evaluate the assumptions relating to the random-effect

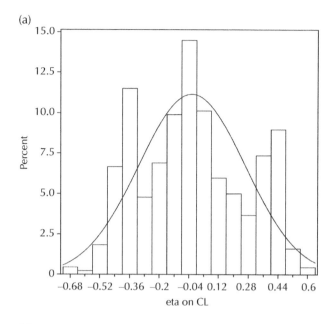

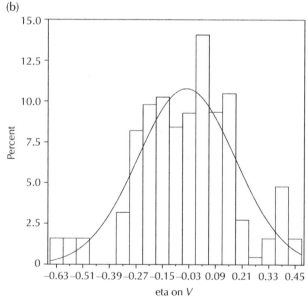

FIGURE 5.62 Histograms of random-effect terms. Panel (a) shows the frequency distribution of eta_{CL} and Panel (b) shows the frequency distribution of eta_V with a normal kernel density estimate overlaid on each plot.

terms in the model, histograms of subject-specific eta estimates may be prepared; these should be examined for symmetry about 0 and a lack of bimodality. Figure 5.62 illustrates example histograms of eta estimates; plots such as these should be examined carefully for an obvious lack of symmetry, extreme outliers, and potential evidence of bimodality. Deficiencies in these displays should be

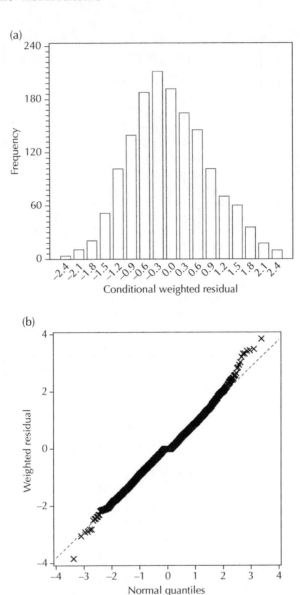

FIGURE 5.63 Distribution of weighted residuals from the proposed final model. Panel (a) shows the histogram of conditional weighted residuals and Panel (b) shows the corresponding Q–Q plot of weighted residuals.

investigated further as they may indicate additional effects or subpopulations that have not been adequately accounted for in the model. In addition to histograms, quantile–quantile (Q–Q) plots exploring the distribution of (conditional) weighted residuals from the final model (in comparison to a normal distribution) should be considered as well. Figure 5.63 illustrates an example histogram of conditional weighted residuals as well as a Q–Q plot of weighted residuals.

APPENDIX 5.1   RECOMMENDED ANALYSIS PLAN CONTENT

REFERENCES

Ahn JE, Karlsson MO, Dunne A, Ludden TM. Likelihood based approaches to handling data below the quantification limit using NONMEM VI. J Pharmacokinet Pharmacodyn 2008;35(4): 401–421. Erratum in: J Pharmacokinet Pharmacodyn 2010 Jun;37(3):305–308.

Anderson BJ, Holford NH. Mechanistic basis of using body size and maturation to predict clearance in humans. Drug Metab Pharmacokinet 2009;24(1):25–36. Review.

Beal SL. Commentary on significance levels for covariate effects in NONMEM. J Pharmacokinet Pharmacodyn 2002;29 (4):403–412.

Beal SL. Ways to fit a PK model with some data below the quantification limit. J Pharmacokinet Pharmacodyn 2001;28(5):481–504. Erratum in J Pharmacokinet Pharmacodyn 2002b;29(3):309.

Beal SL, Sheiner LB. *Course Notes: A Short Course in Population Pharmacokinetic Data Analysis Using the NONMEM System.* San Francisco: University of California at San Francisco; 1992.

Beal SL, Sheiner LB, Boeckmann AJ, Bauer RJ, editors. *NONMEM 7.2.0 Users Guides.* Hanover: Icon Development Solutions; 1989–2011. Available at ftp://nonmem.iconplc.com/Public/nonmem720/guides. Accessed December 14, 2013.

Bonate PL. *Pharmacokinetic-Pharmacodynamic Modeling and Simulation.* New York: Springer Science + Business Media, LLC; 2006. p 65–69.

Byon W, Fletcher CV, Brundage RC. Impact of censoring data below an arbitrary quantification limit on structural model misspecification. J Pharmacokinet Pharmacodyn 2008 Feb;35 (1):101–116.

Draper NR, Smith H. *Applied Regression Analysis.* 2nd ed. New York: John Wiley & Sons, Inc.; 1981a. p 16–17.

Draper NR, Smith H. *Applied Regression Analysis.* 2nd ed. New York: John Wiley & Sons, Inc.; 1981b. p 29–30.

Ette EI, Williams PJ, Lane JR. Population pharmacokinetics III: design, analysis, and application of population pharmacokinetic studies. Ann Pharmacother 2004;38:2136–2144.

European Medicines Agency. Committee for Medicinal Products for Human Use (CHMP). *Guideline on Reporting the Results of Population Pharmacokinetic Analyses.* 2007. Available at www.ema.europa.eu/pdfs/human/ewp/18599006enfin.pdf. Accessed December 14, 2013.

European Medicines Agency. Committee for Proprietary Medicinal Products (CPMP) *ICH E9: Statistical Principles for Clinical Trials.* 1998. Available at www.ema.europa.eu/docs/en_GB/document_library/Scientific_guideline/2009/09/WC500002928.pdf. Accessed December 14, 2013.

Food and Drug Administration, Guidance for Industry, Population Pharmacokinetics. Rockville: Food and Drug Administration; 1999.

Freund JE. *Mathematical Statistics*. 5th ed. Englewood: Prentice-Hall, Inc; 1992. p 442–448.

Gastonguay MR. A full model estimation approach for covariate effects: inference based on clinical importance and estimation precision. AAPS J 2004;6(S1). Available at www.aapsj.org/abstracts/AM_2004/AAPS2004-003431.PDF. Accessed December 14, 2013.

Gobburu JV, Lawrence J. Application of resampling techniques to estimate exact significance levels for covariate selection during nonlinear mixed effects model building: some inferences. Pharm Res 2002; 19 (1):92–98.

Hooker AC, Staatz CE, Karlsson MO. Conditional weighted residuals (CWRES): a model diagnostic for the FOCE method. Pharm Res 2007;24 (12):2187–2197.

Jonsson EN, Karlsson MO. Automated covariate model building within NONMEM. Pharm Res 1998;15:1463–1468.

Jonsson EN, Karlsson MO. Xpose—an S-PLUS based population pharmacokinetic/pharmacodynamic model building aid for NONMEM. Comput Methods Programs Biomed 1999;58 (1):51–64.

Khandelwal A, Harling K, Jonsson EN, Hooker AC, Karlsson MO. A fast method for testing covariates in population PK/PD models. AAPS J 2011;13 (3):464–472.

Kowalski KG, Hutmacher MM. Efficient screening of covariates in population models using Wald's approximation to the likelihood ratio test. J Pharmacokinet Pharmacodyn 2001;28:253–275.

Lindbom L, Pihlgren P, Jonsson EN. PsN-Toolkit—a collection of computer intensive statistical methods for non-linear mixed effect modeling using NONMEM. Comput Methods Programs Biomed 2005; 79 (3):241–257.

Mandema JM, Verotta D, Sheiner LB. Building population pharmacokinetic-pharmacodynamic models I. Models for covariate effects. J Pharmacokinet Biopharm 1992;20:511–528.

R Core Team. *R: A Language and Environment for Statistical Computing*. R Foundation for Statistical Computing, Vienna; 2013. Available at http://www.R-project.org. Accessed December 14, 2013.

Savic RM, Karlsson MO. Importance of shrinkage in empirical Bayes estimates for diagnostics: problems and solutions. AAPS J 2009;11:558–69.

S-Plus [computer program] Version 7. Seattle: Insightful Corporation; 2005.

Tukey JW. *Exploratory Data Analysis*. Reading: Addison-Wesley; 1977.

Wahlby U, Jonsson EN, Karlsson MO. Assessment of actual significance levels for covariate effects in NONMEM. J Pharmacokinet Pharmacodyn 2001;28:231–252.

CHAPTER 6

INTERPRETING THE NONMEM OUTPUT

6.1 INTRODUCTION

The appropriate interpretation of the output from NONMEM may well be considered the art in what is often referred to as the *art and science* of population modeling. The ability to understand the information provided in the various output files and to make appropriate decisions based on this information is one of the more challenging aspects of population modeling.

With enough time and experience comes a knack for zeroing in on the most relevant bits of information from among the plethora of data provided in the output files in order to make appropriate decisions about what steps to take next. Although each modeling exercise is somewhat unique in its particular goals and objectives, the NONMEM output files contain a vast amount of information addressing various aspects of each model. Synthesizing this information to gain a complete and accurate picture of what can be learned from this particular model fit is essential to taking a logical path to a final model. The output described in this chapter will specifically focus on that of the classical estimation methods in NONMEM, though many of the comments are relevant to all of the estimation methods.

6.2 DESCRIPTION OF THE OUTPUT FILES

After running a given typical model with NM-TRAN and NONMEM, several different files are available to the user. These include the *.rpt file, the *.FDATA file, the *.PRDERR file (possibly), the *.FCON file, and any user-requested files, such as the output from the $TABLE step(s) and/or a model specification file, and, with NONMEM version 7, the *.phi file, the *.ext file, the *.coi file, the *.cor file, and the *.cov file (Beal et al. 1989–2011).

While each of these files contains important data and diagnostic information about a particular run, this chapter will focus primarily on reviewing the contents of

Introduction to Population Pharmacokinetic / Pharmacodynamic Analysis with Nonlinear Mixed Effects Models, First Edition. Joel S. Owen and Jill Fiedler-Kelly.
© 2014 John Wiley & Sons, Inc. Published 2014 by John Wiley & Sons, Inc.

the NONMEM report file. This file is the primary repository of results for a given model. Many of the additional files, now produced with version 7, such as the *.phi and the *.ext files, can be very useful to the user interested in programmatically parsing these output files for certain pieces of data to use as an input into another helper program or application.

6.3   THE NONMEM REPORT FILE

The NONMEM report file is a text file consisting of output from the various components of the NONMEM system relevant to a particular model fitting, in addition to error messages and other useful diagnostic data. In Sections 6.3.1–6.3.6 the specific types of output in the NONMEM report file will be reviewed in additional detail.

6.3.1   NONMEM-Related Output

The first section of output in the NONMEM report file consists of information relating to output from the NONMEM portion of the system. Recall that when the NONMEM program is used to run a particular population model, PREDPP may or may not be called, but NONMEM will be called. The output from each of these components of the NONMEM system is provided separately within the NONMEM report file.

After the first few lines of output that detail the licensing information and version of NONMEM being called:

```
License Registered to: XXXX
Expiration Date:    dd MMM yyyy
Current Date:       dd MMM yyyy
Days until program expires :  nn
1NONLINEAR MIXED EFFECTS MODEL PROGRAM (NONMEM) VERSION 7.X.Y
   ORIGINALLY DEVELOPED BY STUART BEAL, LEWIS SHEINER, AND
   ALISON BOECKMANN
   CURRENT DEVELOPERS ARE ROBERT BAUER, ICON DEVELOPMENT
   SOLUTIONS, AND ALISON BOECKMANN. IMPLEMENTATION,
   EFFICIENCY, AND STANDARDIZATION PERFORMED BY NOUS INFO-
   SYSTEMS.
```

the settings of various options are described, along with information regarding how NONMEM has read the data file with respect to the NONMEM-required data items:

```
PROBLEM NO.:   1
'text which follows $PROBLEM goes here'
0DATA CHECKOUT ....

0FORMAT FOR DATA:
(E6.0,E8.0, …
```

Among the items provided in this portion of the output, the total number of data records read from the dataset and the number of data items in the dataset are provided. Verification of these counts is an important step in ensuring that the data file has been read in correctly.

The next portion of the output file provides additional counts which should be verified against checks of the data performed outside of NONMEM in order to ensure that the data have been read in correctly. The number of observation records and number of individuals in the dataset are provided (see the following):

```
TOT. NO. OF OBS RECS:          1109
TOT. NO. OF INDIVIDUALS:         79
```

Since the observation record count is a tally of the records NONMEM considers as observation events (i.e., records where a PK sample or PD endpoint is measured), the difference between the number of data records in the dataset (provided earlier in the report file) and this count of observation records is usually the number of dosing records plus the number of other-type event records (i.e., where EVID=2). The counts of the number of individuals and the number of observation records are perhaps most important to verify when the IGNORE and/or ACCEPT options are specified on the $DATA record. Since the specification of conditions within these options, especially multiple conditions, can be a bit tricky, the counts provided by NONMEM should always be confirmed with independent checks of the expected counts as a verification of the correct specification of the subsetting rules.

Continuing with the NONMEM-related output in the report file, the next section of output reiterates the conditions (size and initial estimates provided) for the THETA vector and the OMEGA and SIGMA matrices. Next, the options requested for estimation and covariance via the $ESTIMATION and $COVARIANCE records are detailed in the output file. Finally, requests for specific output from the $TABLE and $SCAT records are described.

6.3.2 PREDPP-Related Output

The next section of the output file details the requests related to the call to PREDPP, if appropriate. When PREDPP is called (via the $SUBROUTINES record in the control stream), several PREDPP-required variables are needed in the dataset (and $INPUT record), and the coding of the model in the $PK block must correspond with the specification of the model requested through the choice of subroutines. If PREDPP is called, this section of the report file describes the model requested, the compartment attributes of that model and parameterization, the assignment of additional PK parameters, and the location of the PREDPP-required variables in the dataset.

6.3.3 Output from Monitoring of the Search

The next section of the report file is one of the most important sections for the analyst to review in great detail for each model before accepting or further attempting to interpret the results. For the first and last iteration and each interim iteration for which output is requested (via the `PRINT = n` option on the `$ESTIMATION` record), the following information is provided: the value of the objective function at this point in the search, the number of function evaluations used for this iteration, the cumulative number of function evaluations performed up to this point in the search. Also, for each parameter that is estimated, the parameter estimate is given in its original or raw units (with newer versions of NONMEM only), along with the transformed, scaled value of each parameter (called the unconstrained parameters (UCPs), which scale each parameter to an initial estimate of 0.1), and the gradient associated with each parameter at this point in the search (Beal et al. 1989–2011).

The output from the monitoring of the search is provided as a summary of each step, with labeled information at the top of each section for the iteration number, the value of the objective function, and the number of function evaluations. Immediately following this information are specific lines of output for the parameters and the associated gradients for each iteration output. These columns are not labeled with respect to the corresponding parameter but are presented with the elements of the THETA vector first (in numerical sequence), followed by the elements of the OMEGA matrix and, finally, the elements of the SIGMA matrix. If a parameter was fixed (and not estimated) for a particular model, then a column would simply not exist for that parameter. So if THETA(4), the intercompartmental clearance term, was fixed to a value from the literature, the columns in the monitoring of the search section would be ordered as follows: THETA(1), THETA(2), THETA(3), THETA(5), ETA(1), ETA(2), etc., and then EPS(1), followed by any other EPS parameters which might have been used.

In reviewing the detailed output regarding the search, it is important first to ensure that none of the gradients are equal to 0 at the start of the search. A gradient of 0 at the start of the search is an indication that there is a lack of information for NONMEM to use in order to determine the best estimate for that parameter. For example, this situation might arise if the model to be estimated includes an effect of gender on the drug's clearance and the dataset consists entirely of males (the data in the gender column contains the same value for all subjects). In this situation, at the initiation of the search using the user-provided initial estimates, there would be no information to guide the search for an appropriate estimate of the gender effect, and the gradient would start at a value of exactly 0 for this parameter. In this case, no syntax errors would be detected, assuming the model was coded correctly and the variables needed to estimate the effect were found in the dataset. If a thorough EDA had been performed, the analyst would be aware of the gender distribution, and the attempt to fit such a model could have been avoided in the first place. However, assuming the situation may have arisen as an unintended consequence of data subsetting (perhaps via use of the `IGNORE` or `ACCEPT` options on the `$DATA` record), the gradients on the 0th iteration would be the first place to detect such a problem.

One way to think about the value of the gradients is that the gradients provide information about the steepness of the slope of the surface with respect to a particular parameter at a specific point in the search. If you imagine the search process as a stepwise progression from some point on the inside of a bumpy bowl-like surface toward the bottom or lowest point of the bowl, each gradient describes what the surface looks like with respect to that parameter. If the gradient is high (a positive or negative value with a large positive exponent), then the surface is steep with respect to that parameter at that point and the search has not yet reached a sufficient minimum. If the gradient is small, either a value close to the final (*best*) estimate has been found or the model has settled into a local, not global, minimum with respect to that parameter. In addition to checking that the gradients generally get smaller as the search progresses and that no exact 0 values (or values very close to 0) are obtained, the gradients at the final iteration should be checked carefully as well. At the final iteration, all gradients should ideally have exponents equal to or less than +02, and of course, none should be exactly 0.

Generally, the changes in the minimum objective function value from iteration to iteration will be greater at the start of the search than near the end of the search. When the search is nearly complete, the changes to the objective function value typically become very small. After the summary of the final iteration is provided, the happy phrase MINIMIZATION SUCCESSFUL may be found. This declaration is followed by a count of the total number of function evaluations used and the number of significant digits obtained in the final estimates.

When the run fails to minimize for any reason, or minimizes successfully, but is qualified by some other type of warning or an indication of a problem(s) from the COV step, messages to this effect will be found in this general location in the report file. If an error occurs during the search, information about the error will be printed in the output file at the point in the search where it occurred.

Overall, a great deal of information can be learned from a careful review of the output from the monitoring of the search. When errors do occur, the values of the gradients can provide clues about where the problems may lie. When the results are not optimal or do not make sense, the values of the gradients at the point at which the run completed its search may provide insight as to which parameters are causing the difficulty.

When conditional estimation methods are used (e.g., FOCE, FOCE INTER, FOCE LAPLACIAN), additional information is provided following the summary of the monitoring of the search in the output file. Estimates of Bayesian shrinkage are provided for each of the estimated elements of OMEGA and SIGMA. Bayesian shrinkage is discussed in additional detail in Chapter 7. The mean of the distribution of individual eta estimates is also provided (referred to as ETABAR) along with the associated standard error for each estimate and the results of a statistical test of location under the null hypothesis that the mean of each element of OMEGA (i.e., each ETA) is equal to 0. If a p value less than 0.05 is reported, this is an indication that the mean of the distribution for that ETA is statistically significantly not equal to 0, or in other words, a rejection of the null hypothesis.

6.3.4   Minimum Value of the Objective Function and Final Parameter Estimates

Immediately following the monitoring of the search and related summary information about the run, the minimum value of the objective function is provided for the classical methods (FO, FOCE, FOCE with INTERACTION). After the minimum objective function value, the final parameter estimates are provided, first for the theta vector and then for the OMEGA and SIGMA matrices. Parameter estimates that were fixed in the control stream are reported in this section of the output as the fixed value without indication that the value of this parameter was fixed rather than estimated.

6.3.4.1 Interpreting Omega Matrix Variance and Covariance Estimates

Recall that in Chapter 3, a derivation was provided to calculate initial variance estimates for elements of OMEGA and SIGMA when an exponential or proportional error model is implemented, by working backward from an estimate of variability described as a %CV. This same derivation can be applied to the interpretation of the variance estimates obtained from NONMEM for elements of OMEGA and SIGMA. Typically, we wish to describe the magnitude of interindividual and residual variability in terms of a %CV, or at least a standard deviation (SD), which can then be compared in size to another estimate from the data.

Let us begin with a diagonal OMEGA matrix, where each of the PK parameters upon which interindividual variability is estimated is modeled using an exponential error structure. So, a portion of our control stream code might look like the following:

```
TVCL = THETA(1)
CL = TVCL*EXP(ETA(1))
TVV = THETA(2)
V = TVV*EXP(ETA(2))
TVKA = THETA(3)
KA = TVKA*(EXP(ETA(3))
```

If the final parameter estimates obtained from NONMEM are the following:

```
OMEGA - COV MATRIX FOR RANDOM EFFECTS - ETAS *************

            ETA1            ETA2            ETA3
ETA1
+           3.62E-01

ETA2
+           0.00E+00        1.19E-01

ETA3
+           0.00E+00        0.00E+00        5.99E-01
```

we can calculate a corresponding approximate %CV for each variance estimate by taking the square root of the estimate and multiplying it by 100. So, in this case, the %CV of $ETA1 = 60.17\%CV$ ($\sqrt{0.362} \times 100$), of $ETA2 = 34.50\%CV$, and of $ETA3 = 77.40\%CV$.

If the error structures employed were additive instead of exponential or proportional (as may be used with PD parameters where the distribution may be normal as opposed to log normal), then we often describe the magnitude of interindividual variability in these parameters simply in terms of a standard deviation (SD). The SD can be obtained by simply taking the square root of the variance estimate. Assume that the following output was obtained regarding the magnitude of the ETA estimates for two parameters modeled with additive interindividual variability:

```
OMEGA - COV MATRIX FOR RANDOM EFFECTS - ETAS *************

              ETA1                ETA2

    ETA1
    +         1.15E+01

    ETA2
    +         0.00E+00       2.03E+01
```

In this example, we can calculate a corresponding SD for each variance estimate by taking the square root of the estimate. So, in this case, the SD associated with $ETA1 = 3.39 \, (\sqrt{11.5})$ and with $ETA2 = 4.51$. Since these estimates are SDs, they maintain the same units as the parameter with which they are associated.

If a block structure was used to estimate off-diagonal elements of the OMEGA matrix (covariance terms), the interpretation of these estimates is also possible. To describe the magnitude of covariance between two random-effect parameters, a correlation coefficient can be easily calculated. Again, recall the information in Chapter 3 describing a method for obtaining an initial estimate for such a covariance term. We will use this method, working backward again, to derive a correlation coefficient from the covariance estimate.

If the following output is obtained in the report file,

```
OMEGA - COV MATRIX FOR RANDOM EFFECTS - ETAS *************

              ETA1                ETA2

    ETA1
    +         3.61E-01

    ETA2
    +         2.01E-01       1.37E-01
```

we can use the following formula to calculate a correlation coefficient from these estimates to describe the relationship between the two variance estimates (Neter et al. 1985):

$$\rho_{1,2} = \frac{\text{cov}\left(\omega_{1,1}^2, \omega_{2,2}^2\right)}{\left[\sqrt{\omega_{1,1}^2} \times \sqrt{\omega_{2,2}^2}\right]}$$

So, for the estimates in this example, $\rho_{1,2} = 0.201/\left[\sqrt{0.361} \times \sqrt{0.137}\right] = 0.904$, and $\rho_{1,2}^2 = 0.82$, indicating a fairly high degree of correlation.

With NONMEM version 7.2.0, both covariance and correlation matrices to OMEGAs and SIGMAs are provided in the report file. The corresponding correlation matrix output for the estimates of OMEGA provided earlier would be:

```
OMEGA  -  CORR MATRIX FOR RANDOM EFFECTS  -  ETAS  *************

              ETA1                ETA2
ETA1
+             6.01E-01

ETA2
+             9.04E-01      3.70E-01
```

Using this output, the aforementioned calculations are not needed.

6.3.4.2 Interpreting SIGMA Matrix Variance Estimates

The formulas presented in the previous section can also be appropriately applied to estimates of residual variability in the SIGMA matrix when the same error structures are used. Therefore, the formulas provided earlier are applicable when exponential or additive models are used. However, for residual variability, more complex error structures are often used and will be described next.

When a combined additive plus CCV model is implemented using the following parameterization,

```
$ERROR
Y = F + EPS(1) + F*EPS(2)
```

an approximate %CV can be calculated to describe the magnitude of residual variability but will result in a range of values, corresponding to a range of predicted concentration values. The formula is as follows:

$$\%CV = \frac{\sqrt{\left[\sigma_1^2 + F^2 \times \sigma_2^2\right]}}{F} \times 100$$

Clearly, based on this formula, the value of the %CV depends on the value of F, the individual predicted concentration. Furthermore, the %CV estimate will be higher for smaller values of F and lower or smaller for larger values of F.

If the following output is obtained,

```
SIGMA  -  COV MATRIX FOR RANDOM EFFECTS  -  EPSILONS  **********

              EPS1                EPS2
EPS1
+             1.99E-01

EPS2
+             0.00E+00      3.25E-02
```

the calculated %CV would be in a range of 48.1–18.0%CV over a range of individual predicted concentrations of 1–100 ng/mL. An example of one way to present results like these is included in Table 2.3.

Alternatively, the same error model structure could be coded using code like the following:

```
$ERROR
IPRED = F
```

```
W = SQRT(THETA(1)**2 + (THETA(2)*IPRED)**2)
IWRES = (DV - IPRED) / W
Y = IPRED + W*EPS(1)

$SIGMA 1 FIX
```

In this case, notice that the initial estimate of σ_1^2, provided via the $SIGMA record, is fixed at 1. Notice also that two fixed effect parameters, θ_1 and θ_2, are used in the statement defining the weighting factor, W. With this parameterization, θ_1 and θ_2 represent the SD of the additive and proportional components of residual variability, respectively. This coding (as described previously in Section 5.6.2.1 along with other options) has the additional advantage of preserving the appropriate weighting for the individual weighted residuals.

Two additional parameterizations are commonly used to parameterize this model, both using a single EPS and a single THETA, as shown below:

```
$ERROR
IPRED = F
W = SQRT(1 + (THETA(Y)**2*IPRED**2))
IWRES = (DV - IPRED) / W
Y = IPRED + W*EPS(1)

$ERROR
IPRED = F
W = SQRT(THETA(X)**2 + IPRED**2)
IWRES = (DV - IPRED) / W
Y = IPRED + W*EPS(1)
```

Refer to Chapter 5 for a detailed description of the parameters used for these models.

6.3.5 Covariance Step Output

If the covariance step is requested, any output from this step is provided following the final parameter estimates. The first section of output following the parameter estimates contains the standard errors of the estimates. The standard errors of the estimates provide information about how precisely the parameters are estimated. Small standard errors associated with parameters indicate that the parameters are estimated precisely, while large standard errors indicate greater uncertainty in the parameter estimates.

For each element of THETA, OMEGA, and SIGMA for which an estimate was requested (i.e., the parameter was not fixed), a corresponding standard error will be provided if the covariance step completed successfully. Because the standard error estimates are in the same units as the corresponding parameter, but differ from parameter to parameter, comparison of such estimates across parameters is difficult. Simple calculations are often performed to calculate standard errors as relative standard error estimates. This calculation is performed by dividing the standard error of the estimate by the estimate itself, thus expressing each error in terms relative to the estimate. In this way, comparisons of the precision of the estimates, across parameters, are facilitated. More detail regarding calculation of such statistics is provided in Section 5.6.3.

Immediately following the standard errors of the estimates, are the variance–covariance matrix of the estimates, the correlation matrix of the estimates, and the inverse of the variance–covariance matrix of the estimates. While each of these provides useful information, the correlation matrix should be reviewed very carefully with each model. The correlation matrix is a matrix of correlation coefficients describing the correlation between parameter estimates, with values ranging between −1 and +1, where each element describes the extent of correlation between pairs of estimated parameters. Ideally of course, all parameter estimates would be independent of all other parameter estimates. In this case, all off-diagonal elements of the correlation matrix would have relatively low values, say, values between −0.8 and +0.8. Correlations greater than |0.9| or |0.95| indicate that as one estimate moves, so does the other with equally good fit to the data. Correlation estimates that are large and negative indicate that the two parameters are negatively correlated, while large positive estimates indicate positive correlation between the parameters. If large correlations (in magnitude, based on the absolute value) are observed with a particular model fit, this information should be reported along with the parameter estimates and final objective function value to appropriately convey important information about the quality of the fit. A model associated with no large correlations is preferable to one with highly correlated parameters.

With NONMEM versions prior to 7.2.0, the diagonal elements of the correlation matrix of the parameter estimates were presented with values of 1.00 (an indication of the degree of correlation between the parameter and itself). With version 7.2.0, however, diagonal elements are presented as values equal to the square root of the corresponding diagonal element of covariance matrix (or in other words, the standard error) (Beal et al. 1989–2011). Therefore, when searching for high values in the correlation matrix of the parameter estimates output, be careful to consider only the off-diagonal elements.

If the PRINT = E option was requested on the $COVAR step, the eigenvalues of the variance–covariance matrix will be provided after the other output from the covariance step (Beal et al. 1989–2011). Generally, the eigenvalues are used to compute a condition number to associate with the model fit. Large values of the condition number, say, greater than 1000, indicate ill conditioning of the model (Bonate 2006). The condition number is calculated by dividing the largest eigenvalue by the smallest eigenvalue. The eigenvalues are always printed in order, from the smallest to the largest. The condition number can be used in many contexts, as an additional piece of information to assist in discriminating between candidate models. During model development, condition numbers should be calculated as complexity is added incrementally to the model. In this way, any step that is taken which is associated with a large increase in the condition number might be viewed cautiously or reconsidered.

6.3.6 Additional Output

If any additional output such as table files or scatterplots was requested by the user in the control stream, this output would be provided in the report file immediately after the covariance step output. Tables of output requested via the $TABLE record without specifying the FILE=option will be printed directly in the report file.

Scatterplots will also be provided in the report file. Note that the scatterplot functionality, available in NONMEM, is quite limited (see also Section 3.9). While options exist for various subsets and stratifications of the data, as well as additional graphing features such as lines of identity, the graphs themselves are low-resolution ASCII graphs. The x axis is presented along the top of the plot, and there is no control over axis settings. As such, NONMEM scatterplots provide a quick and rough look at the data, but the user would be well served to output the table file data to a separate file and read that file into another program with additional graphics capabilities for better control and resolution of graphics.

6.4 ERROR MESSAGES: INTERPRETATION AND RESOLUTION

There are several types of errors that may occur in NONMEM runs, some of which are described in detail in the following: syntax (NM-TRAN) errors, estimation step failures, covariance step failures, PREDPP errors, other types of NONMEM errors, and FORTRAN compiler or run-time errors. Each of these errors manifests itself in a slightly different way, in terms of where to find out that the error occurred in the first place and what information is provided about the error.

6.4.1 NM-TRAN Errors

The first, and perhaps easiest, type of error to resolve is an NM-TRAN (syntax-type) error. When NM-TRAN detects an error, either from the syntax used in the control stream or from processing of the dataset, the message provided by the program describing the error is usually reasonably explicit and decipherable. Examples of such errors include:

```
AN ERROR WAS FOUND IN THE CONTROL STATEMENTS.

   THE CHARACTERS IN ERROR ARE:
   CL
   196  $PK: NO VALUE ASSIGNED TO A BASIC PK PARAMETER.
```

This message indicates that the user forgot to include a definition for CL, a required parameter based on the selected ADVAN and TRANS subroutine, or that the CL parameter was misspelled so as to not be identified by NM-TRAN.

```
AN ERROR WAS FOUND IN THE CONTROL STATEMENTS.

   135  $PK: INITIAL ESTS. REQUIRED FOR THETAS USED IN
   COMPUTATIONS.
```

This error message indicates that the user forgot to include an initial estimate for one of the THETA parameters specified in the code.

```
(WARNING  31) $OMEGA INCLUDES A NON-FIXED INITIAL
ESTIMATE CORRESPONDING TO AN ETA THAT IS NOT USED IN
ABBREVIATED CODE.
```

```
(WARNING  41) NON-FIXED PARAMETER ESTIMATES CORRESPONDING
TO UNUSED PARAMETERS MAY CAUSE THE COVARIANCE STEP
TO FAIL.
```

This message indicates that NM-TRAN has detected a mismatch between the number of initial estimates provided in $OMEGA and the number of ETA parameters included in the code.

```
AN ERROR WAS FOUND IN THE CONTROL STATEMENTS.

THE CHARACTERS IN ERROR ARE:
dataset-9.csv
  33  INPUT DATA FILE DOES NOT EXIST OR CANNOT BE OPENED.
```

This final example error message is indicating that the data file specified in the code in $DATA does not exist or cannot be opened, often the result of a typographical error in specifying either the file name or the path to the file.

When in doubt, a careful review of the online help files relating to the record associated with the error or the user's manual describing the particular feature may help (Beal et al. 1989–2011). Of course, other resources are also available, such as the NONMEM User'sNet, an online listserv for users of NONMEM who post messages describing problems they are experiencing, in the hope that someone in the broader user community might provide some help or advice regarding the situation. A searchable archive of the posts to this listserv is also available.

6.4.2 $ESTIMATION Step Failures

Estimation step failures are perhaps the most troubling of all errors, for if a model fails to converge, it is not always clear what to change in order to achieve success. An error statement is printed in the report file where the monitoring of the search output is provided when these types of errors occur. A run that converges will include the text MINIMIZATION SUCCESSFUL at the end of the monitoring of the search section of the report file. This is an indication that, based on the user settings (such as SIGDIG or NSIG), the necessary convergence criteria have been met with the final parameter estimates that are provided. Runs that fail to minimize successfully will include alternate text, such as MINIMIZATION TERMINATED, followed by some indication as to the reason, such as MAXIMUM NUMBER OF FUNCTION EVALUATIONS EXCEEDED or DUE TO ROUNDING ERRORS. When the maximum number of function evaluations has been exceeded, the user can simply increase the maximum number selected with the MAXEVAL option on the $EST record and restart the run. If a maximum number was not selected by the user, a new maximum can be chosen and set using the MAXEVAL option, increasing the threshold considerably from the value selected (and exceeded) by NONMEM. Recall that use of the model specification file (described in more detail in Chapter 3) can be particularly useful in this situation, to avoid starting the run from the initial estimates again, especially when model run times are long and/or the timeline for the project is short.

In some situations, when the run fails due to rounding errors, the number of significant figures achieved for each of the parameters estimated is provided. With this information, the user can identify the parameter associated with the smallest number of significant figures as well as the parameters associated with a smaller number of significant figures than requested with the SIGDIG or NSIG option on $EST. A closer look at the coding associated with this parameter(s) or a simple adjustment of the initial estimate for that parameter may be the key to getting past such a difficulty. Alternatively, if the lowest number of significant figures obtained is very close to the requested number (say, 2.9 are obtained when 3 were requested), one may choose to overlook such a warning and continue on with model development, accepting the results of this model and moving on to other improvements or changes to the model.

6.4.3 $COVARIANCE Step Failures

In other situations, a successful convergence may be achieved, but conditions of which the user should be aware are revealed following the declaration of a successful minimization. Examples of this situation include two types of errors regarding parameter estimates nearing boundary conditions:

```
ESTIMATE OF THETA IS NEAR THE BOUNDARY AND IS PROBABLY
UNINTERPRETABLE
```

and

```
PARAMETER ESTIMATE IS NEAR ITS BOUNDARY
THIS MUST BE ADDRESSED BEFORE THE COVARIANCE STEP CAN BE
   IMPLEMENTED
```

The first of the messages provided above is an indication that the final parameter estimate for a given parameter is extremely close to or equal to either the lower or upper bound set by the user on $THETA. It is likely that during the search, a value beyond this bound was tried or determined to be preferable to the final estimate provided. In this case, if the bound at issue is not a system constraint, extension of the bound or removal of the bound entirely might be considered and the model retried. The second of the messages regarding boundary conditions provided above refers to a warning provided based on a user-selectable feature of the program. NONMEM contains a mechanism to warn users when final parameter estimates become more than 2 orders of magnitude different from their initial estimates. When this condition is tripped, the second warning message above (i.e., PARAMETER ESTIMATE IS NEAR ITS BOUNDARY...) is output and the covariance step is not executed. This message may also be output in some situations when an element of the correlation matrix becomes very close to 1. If the user does not wish to be warned of such situations, this feature may be disabled via additional options on the $EST record. As described in Chapter 3, separate options are available to disable this boundary test for each type of parameter. The options are as follows:

```
$EST NOTHETABOUNDTEST NOOMEGABOUNDTEST NOSIGMABOUNDTEST
```

Each may also be abbreviated as follows:

```
$EST NOTBT NOOBT NOSBT
```

These options may be set individually or all together, as in the example. A common situation in which this error is tripped is when a particular estimate of interindividual variability is not estimable with the model and dataset and the estimate of ω^2 that is returned is very close to 0. Because this estimate of nearly 0 is likely more than 2 orders of magnitude lower than the chosen initial estimate, this warning will be generated. In this case, either a reparameterization of the model or a reduction in the size of the omega matrix by removing the particular interindividual variability parameter may be considered.

There are many other types of COVARIANCE step failures as well. Most common among these may be those referring to various conditions of the matrices that underlie the calculation of the COVARIANCE step output. Messages indicating that the R MATRIX is singular, and/or nonpositive but semi-definite, or that the S MATRIX is singular are among the messages of this type that are issued. In almost all of these cases, the COVARIANCE step output is not obtained, even though the minimum value of the objective function and the final parameter estimates may be provided. Although the importance of COVARIANCE step success is a somewhat controversial issue among NONMEM users, many pharmacometricians use key elements of output from the COVARIANCE step to fully vet a model and to compare the characteristics of candidate models. As such, understanding what these messages imply may provide some insight as to what to do to overcome them.

The R matrix, sometimes referred to as the Hessian matrix, is a matrix of the second derivatives of the objective function with respect to each of the parameters. A nonpositive semi-definite R matrix is an indication that the minimum value that has been reached is likely not a global or even local minimum and may be what is considered to be a saddle point. When a saddle point is reached, the search does not continue as a step in either (opposite) direction is equally good. A singular (although sometimes positive semi-definite) R matrix implies that the objective function is flat in a *neighborhood* of parameter estimates; this implies that the minimum is not unique. Both of these situations may be the result of overparameterization of the model (Beal et al. 1989–2011). Therefore, a reasonable action might be to simplify the model in some way (perhaps by removing some parameters or estimating less by fixing the value of one or more parameters) or to test a different structure that may prove to be more appropriate for the data.

The S matrix is referred to as the sum of the cross-product gradient vectors, referring to the contribution to the objective function from each individual subject in the final parameter estimation. When the S matrix is found to be singular, strong overparameterization is likely (Beal et al. 1989–2011). A change to the model that would simplify it and result in the estimation of fewer parameters is definitely warranted in this case.

6.4.4 PREDPP Errors

When PREDPP is called, it is assumed that PK parameters such as clearances and volumes cannot be negative. This condition is a bit different than that which is controlled by setting appropriate lower bounds on elements of the THETA vector. In almost all cases, a reasonable lower bound for a PK parameter is 0. But remember that the THETA (fixed-effect term) on which we may set a lower bound is merely the estimate of the typical value of the parameter in most cases. PREDPP is not concerned with this typical value, but the individual-specific (or Bayesian) value of the PK parameter instead. It is this parameter value (e.g., *CL, V2, KA,* etc.) that must remain positive. When a situation occurs that a PK parameter is either equal to 0 or a negative value, a PREDPP error will result. In this case, the coding for that parameter should be carefully reviewed. Such an error is often the result of either the choice of interindividual variability model or of a relationship between the parameter and a covariate. Remember that use of the proportional model for interindividual variability (i.e., `CL = TVCL*(1 + ETA(1))`) will frequently result in negative PK parameters, especially with large negative values for ETA(1). The exponential model (e.g., `CL = TVCL * EXP(ETA(1))`) has similar behavior to the proportional model, implying a log-normal distribution of parameter values, but will never allow for a negative estimate of the parameter (assuming the typical value is positive). Other situations like the use of linear, centered models relating covariates to PK parameters (e.g., `CL = (THETA(1) + THETA(2) * (WTKG-MDWT)) * EXP(ETA(1)))` can result in negative PK parameters, especially for subjects with extreme values of the covariates. In this case, a different selection of initial parameter estimate values for THETA(1) and THETA(2) to avoid proximity to the values that result in a negative parameter may work to alleviate the problem. In some difficult cases, the linear form for the relationship may need to be abandoned in favor of an alternative functional form, or the centering coded in a different way.

6.4.5   Other Types of NONMEM Errors

Errors from certain subroutines may result in termination of the estimation as well. With certain residual variability models, predictions of 0 will result in a termination, so carefully checking the dataset for zero-valued or missing DV values on observation-type event records (which will be interpreted by NONMEM as 0) is essential. Furthermore, with certain parameterizations, such as the use of the absorption lag time parameter (*ALAG1*), certain types of errors are more likely. When ALAG is modeled, data points measured prior to the initial estimate of the lag time will result in a prediction of 0 and may be associated with one of the following messages:

```
PROGRAM TERMINATED BY OBJ, ERROR IN CELS
WITH INDIVIDUAL 1 (IN INDIVIDUAL RECORD ORDERING)
INTRAINDIVIDUAL VARIANCE OF DATA FROM OBS RECORD 1
  ESTIMATED TO BE 0
```

or

```
VAR-COV OF DATA FROM INDIVIDUAL RECORD ESTIMATED TO BE
  SINGULAR
```

If this message is the result of a 0 prediction arising from a sample observed prior to the initial estimate for the absorption lag time, a simple fix is to set the initial estimate for the lag time to a value that is slightly lower than the time of the earliest measured sample.

6.4.6 FORTRAN Compiler or Other Run-Time Errors

It is advisable to learn a bit about the FORTRAN compiler you will be accessing to run NONMEM on your system. There are various compiler settings, usually invoked and set with the installation of NONMEM, which are called *behind the scenes* but may have a great deal of influence on how your models converge (or fail to converge). Important settings include those that deal with numerical underflow and overflow situations and those that determine how to deal with divide by 0 errors. Recommendations are provided by ICON regarding appropriate settings with various operating systems and FORTRAN compilers.

It is also important to be familiar with how NONMEM is installed on the system you will be using. Ways to check on the status of your run prior to completion, ways to check on the status of the machines on which you may run jobs, and learning how to differentiate where errors may be coming from are among the more important features with which to concern yourself. It would be important to know, for instance, whether a particular message regarding termination was issued from NONMEM or PREDPP, indicating a problem with the model, or whether the message was issued from the software system you may be using to facilitate NONMEM processing; the latter may be indicative of a hardware or other system-related problem, unrelated to NONMEM or your model.

6.5 GENERAL SUGGESTIONS FOR DIAGNOSING PROBLEMS

There will always be circumstances when it seems you have exhausted your entire bag of tricks, tried everything you can think of, and still experience difficulty in getting a particular model to fit a set of data. In this section, guidance is offered regarding other things to check or to try.

First off, begin with the dataset. If you haven't thoroughly checked the dataset, this is the time to do so. It is the authors' experience that most of the baffling problems and seemingly unexplainable findings can be traced to a problem with the dataset. Whether it be that the dataset construction is at fault in terms of a programmatic problem with the variables NONMEM needs, errors in how the variables have been created, or how the dataset is structured, or that the data collected in the study(ies) contain features or values that were unexpected, an error in the data is not only possible but likely.

Outlier points or high influence values can sometimes be found during EDA, although some outlier points are difficult to discover with typical EDA plots. Such points may be discovered as extremely high (conditional) weighted residuals. When one or more points exhibit either very high weighted residual values or values that are very different when compared to most other points, this is an indication that the observed values are somehow unusual in comparison to the corresponding predicted values based on the model. A review of all of the data for an individual subject with one or more high weighted residual points may reveal an inconsistency over time within that subject's data. If no within-subject inconsistencies are noted, then this subject should be compared to other subjects similar to this one either in terms of dose and study design features or, if covariates are included in the model under consideration, then to subjects with similar covariate characteristics.

As discussed earlier in this chapter, the values of the gradients may provide some clues as to particular parameters in the model under consideration that are difficult to estimate. If a parameter results in a zero gradient at any point during the search, this is a parameter to investigate carefully. Perhaps a different parameterization could be tried, or this parameter could be eliminated from the model by fixing it to a known value or choosing a different structure entirely.

Because of its tremendous impact on the fit of a population model, the residual variability error structure should be carefully examined for its appropriateness. Scatterplots of individual weighted residuals versus individual predictions provide insight as to whether the selected model for residual variability is appropriate. If the selected model has the right characteristics, these plots should exhibit a lack of trend or pattern across the range of individual predicted values.

A variety of other changes to the model could also be considered. Changing the initial estimates for all parameters to values thought to be either further from the anticipated estimates or closer to such estimates might be considered. If the initial estimate values are either the same as the final parameter estimates or extremely different, problems with minimization can result. Attempting a different estimation method may also be warranted, especially if the data are likely not to support estimation with a more complex method. Finally, changing the requested number of significant figures or tolerance allowed might also be considered.

If the estimates obtained are orders of magnitude different than expected, first examine the scaling factor. Remember that a scaling factor is needed to convert the amounts, starting with the dose, input into the various compartments, into concentration values. Also, recall that the scaling factor must work in conjunction with the units of the various related fields: concentration, dose, and dose-related parameters such as rate, duration, and interdose interval. If the scaling factor is not appropriately set, the parameter estimates may be in different units than expected.

On occasion, and commonly with pediatric data, covariate factors are needed in what is considered the base structural model in order to achieve convergence. If the influence of a certain covariate is large enough, it can be difficult to obtain convergence without including such an effect in the model. Plotting the frequency distributions of each of the ETA terms in the model can also be informative. A very skewed or bimodal distribution may provide some insight into a possible problem. If the tails of a skewed distribution are representative of subjects with a particular covariate or an extreme value of a covariate, that factor may be helpful to incorporate into the model as a predictor of one or more parameters. Otherwise, in the case of the apparently bimodal distribution, if none of the available covariates explain the bimodality, a mixture model may be incorporated into the model to assist in fitting the data.

Mixture models allow for the estimation of two or more (sets of) parameters for different subpopulations of subjects without a specific variable to assign subjects into the relevant groups. A simple example of the incorporation of a mixture model might involve estimating two clearance values for two subpopulations of subjects, when no factor can be identified in the data to assign subjects to one or the other subpopulation. For example, let's say that we have conducted a large study on our drug, which is metabolized by CYP 2D6 enzymes, yet we failed to collect any data to identify the CYP 2D6 metabolizing status of the subjects under study. We might expect to observe different clearances in those subjects who would be classified as poor metabolizers as compared to those subjects classified as extensive metabolizers. With no specific data available regarding metabolizing status to explicitly assign subjects to a particular subpopulation, we can incorporate a mixture model into our pharmacostatistical model, allowing NONMEM to estimate one or more clearances in the different subpopulations based on the observed concentration–time data. Furthermore, using a mixture model framework, NONMEM will assign subjects to a particular group in order to obtain these estimates and provide each subject's assignment along with the final parameter estimates and probability of assignment into each subpopulation. Additional detail regarding NM-TRAN control stream syntax for mixture models is included in Appendix 6.1.

Finally, in those situations when there are known and expected parameter values, but the model is predicting very different estimates, an alternative approach could be considered. Using the current dataset and model structure, a control stream could be crafted with all parameter estimates fixed to the expected values. Instead of estimating the parameters, the $ESTIMATION record would include the MAXEVAL = 0 option. By setting the maximum number of function evaluations to 0, and performing this deterministic simulation of sorts, you are requesting that predictions be generated for all data points based on the model and the fixed parameter values. A comparison of these predictions to the observed values in diagnostic scatterplots, stratified various ways, may provide some insight into how the current data differ from that expected based on the fixed parameter estimates.

When all else seems to fail, reducing the model to a simpler structural form and systematically adding complexity and additional components to the model may provide some clues as to where things start to behave differently than expected. It is always good practice to make one change to the model or the dataset at a time, instead of making multiple changes at once. A systematic approach is likely to result in a better understanding of the data and the system.

APPENDIX 6.1   MIXTURE MODEL EXAMPLE CODE

```
$PROB Mixture Model Example Code - 2 sub-populations of CL

; Purpose: Test a MIXTURE model to estimate two
   sub-populations for CL
;   *possibly* due to unknown CYP2D6 metabolizing status

$DATA datafile.nmdat IGNORE=#
$INPUT ID TIME AMT DV EVID MDV LNDV TSLD WTKG AGE SEXF
```

```
$SUBROUTINES ADVAN1 TRANS2
$PK
        CALLFL=1
; indicates to call the PK subroutine with the first
  event record of
; each individual record
        EST=MIXEST
; define EST variable, which will take on the values
  assigned to
; MIXEST, thus identifying the sub-population to which
  each individual
; is assigned and output EST in TABLE file
        IF (MIXNUM.EQ.2) THEN
           CL=THETA(2)*EXP(ETA(2))
; theta(2) and eta(2) are the CL and IIV in CL for the
  sub-population
; with a relatively slower estimate of clearance
        ELSE
           CL=THETA(1)*EXP(ETA(1))
        ENDIF
; theta(1) and eta(1) are the CL and IIV in CL for the
  reference
; sub-population with the higher (faster) estimate of
  clearance
           V=THETA(3)*EXP(ETA(3))
        ENDIF
        S1=V/1000
$ERROR
        Y=F*EXP(EPS(1))
$MIX
        P(1)=THETA(4)
        P(2)=1.-THETA(4)
        NSPOP=2
; NSPOP indicates that there are 2 sub-populations
; P(1) and P(2) are the estimated proportions of the
  population
; assigned to each group
$THETA   (0,4.0)        ;--th1- Clearance in reference
  sub-population (L/h)
```

```
        (0,1)              ;--th2- Clearance in the
   sub-population with slower clearance (L/h)
        (0,60)             ;--th3- Volume of distribution (L)
        (0,0.9,1)          ;--th4- Proportion of individuals
in the reference sub-population

 $OMEGA  .05               ;--eta1- IIV in CL in the reference
sub-population
         .01               ;--eta2- IIV in CL in the sub-
population with slower clearance
         .03               ;--eta3- IIV in V

 $SIGMA  .02               ;--eps1- RV

 $EST METHOD=1 INTER MAXEVAL=9999 PRINT=5 MSFO=mixture.msf
 $TABLE ID EST TIME TSLD DOSE WTKG AGE SEXF FIRSTONLY
        NOAPPEND ONEHEADER NOPRINT FILE=mixture.tbl
```

REFERENCES

Beal SL, Sheiner LB, Boeckmann AJ, Bauer RJ, editors. *NONMEM 7.2.0 Users Guides*. (1989–2011). Hanover: Icon Development Solutions.

Bonate PL. *Pharmacokinetic–Pharmacodynamic Modeling and Simulation*. New York: Springer Science+Business Media, LLC; 2006. p 65–69.

Neter J, Wasserman W, Kutner MH. *Applied Linear Statistical Models: Regression, Analysis of Variance, and Experimental Designs*. Homewood: Irwin, Inc; 1985. p 98–99.

CHAPTER 7

APPLICATIONS USING PARAMETER ESTIMATES FROM THE INDIVIDUAL

7.1 INTRODUCTION

Bayesian estimation is an analytical technique that allows one to use previously determined information about a population in conjunction with observed data from one or more individuals to estimate the most likely value of a property of interest in the specific individuals from whom the data were obtained. Prior knowledge about the population enhances the understanding of data collected in the individual. Bayesian methods in pharmacometrics provide tools to obtain individual subject parameter estimates (e.g., CL_i or V_i) for a pharmacokinetic (PK) or pharmacodynamic (PD) model when only sparse data are available from the subject. Sparse data in this sense means that there are too few samples from the subject for the estimation of the parameters of the relevant model in the individual alone. Of note, a population analysis dataset may be sparse for some subjects and full profile or *rich* for other subjects.

Bayesian methods in pharmacometric applications require the assumption of a prior population model structure and population parameter values, possibly including measures of uncertainty of the parameter values. With this information in hand, one may estimate the PK or PD model parameters for the individual. From the individual Bayesian model parameter estimates, one may then use the assumed model to *reconstruct* the concentration–time or effect profile for an individual and construct an estimate of the total exposure in the individual. This process is illustrated in Figure 7.1 and described later in this chapter.

A conceptual example of the power of this approach is illustrated here. Suppose one is exploring correlations between drug exposure and the occurrence of an adverse event (AE) to assess the safety profile of a drug product in clinical trials. If sparse concentration–time samples were collected from an individual in the trial and his dosing history is known, then Bayesian methods of individual parameter estimation can be used to reconstruct the concentration–time profile for the individual at any time in the trial. This is true even for cases of nonstationarity in PK such as

Introduction to Population Pharmacokinetic / Pharmacodynamic Analysis with Nonlinear Mixed Effects Models, First Edition. Joel S. Owen and Jill Fiedler-Kelly.
© 2014 John Wiley & Sons, Inc. Published 2014 by John Wiley & Sons, Inc.

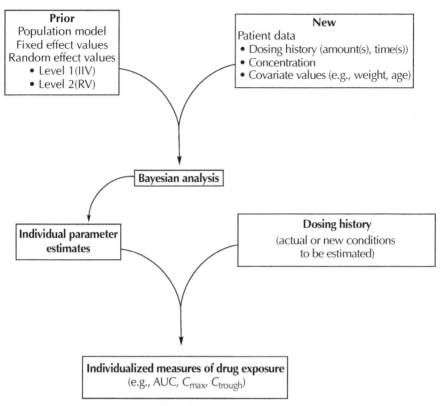

FIGURE 7.1 Overview of Bayesian parameter estimation in a typical PK project.

enzyme induction or cases of nonlinearity such as capacity-limited absorption or metabolism, assuming the model adequately accounts for these processes. Using the individual PK parameter estimates, the dosing history, and the model, drug exposure on the day of an AE can easily be estimated. Estimated exposures at the time of the AE can be used along with estimated exposures in individuals not experiencing the AE to look for correlations between exposure and probability of occurrence of the AE.

Bayesian techniques are also useful in clinical practice settings. Much like traditional therapeutic drug monitoring (TDM) of certain drugs, population-based methods can be used to estimate PK parameters based on a single sample, a population model, and the patient's dosing history. Where some traditional TDM approaches use simplifying assumptions or require sample collection to occur in a certain dosing interval or at a certain time within the dosing interval, population modeling methods with Bayesian parameter estimation may use data collected from an individual at any time during any dosing interval. Of course, collection of samples at some timepoints can be more informative to parameter estimation than others, but the availability of a model can even help in assessing this relative information content. Specialized software for TDM using population PK models and Bayesian techniques is available for clinical application. One such program is called BestDose® (Laboratory of Applied Pharmacokinetics, University of Southern California; (www.lapk.org)).

Individual PK parameter estimates also play an important role during model development for the purpose of identifying relationships between model parameter values and measurable covariates. This approach was previously described in Chapter 5.

This introductory chapter will not deal extensively with the theoretical aspects of Bayesian estimation, but after a brief introduction will focus instead on practical applications and methods used in drug development. The chapter presents methods for obtaining and using individual Bayesian or conditional parameter estimates when a population model is available using either the POSTHOC or the classical conditional estimation methods in NONMEM. The chapter does not focus on newer techniques available in the most recent versions of NONMEM that allow the specification of Bayesian priors when estimating the population parameters of a model, nor does it address $ESTIM BAYES method for parameter estimation.

7.2   BAYES THEOREM AND INDIVIDUAL PARAMETER ESTIMATES

Bayes theorem was developed by Reverend Thomas Bayes and was published posthumously in 1763 (Bayes 1763). A review of Bayes theorem and its subsequent development and application in medicine was published on the 25th anniversary of *Statistics in medicine* (Ashby 2006).

In the context of PK, Bayes theorem can be considered as follows:

$$P(\phi \,|\, C) = \frac{P(C \,|\, \phi)P(\phi)}{P(C)}$$

where ϕ represents the model parameter values and C represents the observed concentrations in the dataset. The probabilities in this equation are defined as:

$P(\phi \,|\, C)$ is the conditional probability of ϕ given C or the posterior probability.

$P(C \,|\, \phi)$ is the conditional probability of C given ϕ or the likelihood.

$P(\phi)$ is the prior or marginal probability of ϕ.

$P(C)$ is the prior or marginal probability of C.

We are seeking the most likely set of parameters, given the observed concentrations in the individual $[P(\phi \,|\, C)]$. These are technical statistical concepts and beyond the focus of this text. However, conceptual relationships important to Bayesian parameter estimation are illustrated in the following weighted least squares objective function, which can be considered to be a Bayesian objective function (Sheiner and Beal 1982; Bourne 2013):

$$\text{OBJ}_{\text{Bayes}} = \sum_{i=1}^{p} \frac{\left(\theta_i - \hat{\theta}_i\right)^2}{\hat{\omega}_i^2} + \sum_{j=1}^{n} \frac{\left(C_j - \widehat{C}_j\right)^2}{\hat{\sigma}_j^2}$$

where θ_i is the estimate of the individual's parameter value; $\hat{\theta}_i$, $\hat{\omega}$, and $\hat{\sigma}$ are the fixed and random effects in the population model; and C_j and $\widehat{C}_j$ represent the observed and model-predicted concentrations.

Since the goal of the numerical estimation method is to minimize the objective function value, a few things can be noted about this Bayesian objective function. The first is that movement of an individual parameter away from the mean value (by increasing $\theta_i - \hat{\theta}_i$) is discouraged unless there is a corresponding improvement in model fit $C_j - \widehat{C}_j$ to offset the increase in the objective function due to parameter value differences. If an individual has more observed data points, there is more opportunity to support moving a parameter away from the typical value in a direction that improves the fit of the model. When there are few or no data points that inform the estimation of a particular parameter, the value of that parameter will often *shrink* toward the typical value, since altering that parameter may have little influence on the values of individual predicted concentration values. The framework of this equation is also useful for illustrating the parsimony of this approach. Increasing the number of parameters without improving the fit of the model either increases the objective function or results in θ_i values that are essentially equal to $\hat{\theta}_i$ so that $\theta_i - \hat{\theta}_i = 0$.

Another observation related to this function is that when the variance of a parameter in the population ($\hat{\omega}_i^2$) is small, the change in the objective function with movement of the individual parameter from the typical value ($\theta_i - \hat{\theta}_i$) is magnified. Thus, if the underlying population variance in a parameter is small, a more substantial amount of improvement in the fit of the concentration data is required for each unit shift of the individual parameter away from the typical value. Conversely, if the variance of the parameter in the population is large, there is relatively less *penalty* in moving the individual parameter value away from the typical value.

A practical point is that one often finds that when there are too many parameters in a model so that the data are not informative regarding one or more parameters, the gradient estimation methods, such as FOCE, may *wander*, since they can change the parameter values without altering the objective function significantly. This can increase run times and lead to numerical problems in the estimation or covariance steps. We encounter this frequently when too many random-effect parameters are included and the data are insufficient to characterize them or when a model is over-parameterized in fixed effects.

When we estimate individual subject parameters of the model (e.g., Cl_i), we are actually estimating the individual η values for the parameters that define the differences between the individual subject parameters from the typical population values of the parameters. For an individual then, we are drawing one instance of η from the distribution of η values defined with mean of zero and variance of ω^2. An example of individual PK model parameter definition is illustrated in the sample control code as follows:

```
$PK
TVCL = THETA(1)
CL = TVCL * EXP(ETA(1))
```

The typical value of the parameter (TVCL) and the individual subject η-parameter value (ETA(1)) together define the value of CL (CL_i) for the individual subject. Also, note that Bayesian parameter estimates are only available for those parameters that include a defined η term. If only a typical value is included for a parameter in a model, then no individual-specific η may be obtained. Frequently, no η is included on one or more parameters when the data are not informative enough to define the individual-specific values of the parameter. For example, when few samples are collected during the absorption phase of an orally administered, immediate-release medication, the ability to estimate individual subject values of k_a is limited. At best, one might get a good estimate of the typical value of k_a for the population. In this case, the model might best be expressed without an η on k_a, and each subject's individual model (i.e., the set of individual parameters) uses the typical value of k_a.

Clearly, obtaining individual parameter estimates using the Bayesian approaches implemented in POSTHOC or conditional estimation methods in NONMEM makes strong assumptions about the population model structure and parameter estimates. Confidence in the individual parameter estimates is predicated on the appropriateness of the model and the experimental circumstances of the individual (e.g., is the dose the individual received outside the dose range used to develop the model?). Even with this strong reliance on prior information, obtaining individual subject Bayesian parameter estimates for pharmacometric models can be a very powerful tool in drug development. The use of Bayesian parameter estimates to reconstruct the concentration–time profile for an individual based on a small number of samples and a prior model has become a common practice in modern PK contributions to the development of a drug product.

Individual-specific parameter estimates can be either empiric or nonempiric Bayesian estimates of the η values. Empiric Bayesian estimates (EBEs) result when the estimation of the population parameters includes the individual subject data for which the Bayesian parameter estimates are obtained. Nonempiric Bayesian estimates use population parameters that were determined without the inclusion of the data for the subject for which the Bayesian estimates are produced. In either case, when the data are very sparse or noninformative for a particular parameter, the η parameter will *shrink* toward the typical value of the population as previously described.

7.3   OBTAINING INDIVIDUAL PARAMETER ESTIMATES

The approach used to obtain individual parameter estimates in NONMEM depends on the estimation method used in the analysis. Individual subject parameters can be obtained using a post hoc procedure after the population model parameter values have been estimated, or they may be computed during the estimation of population parameters using a conditional estimation process.

When first-order estimation is used in NONMEM, individual parameter estimates are requested by adding the POSTHOC option to the $ESTIMATION record, for example:

```
$ESTIMATE METHOD=0 POSTHOC
```

The first-order estimation method only produces population estimates for the elements of THETA, OMEGA, and SIGMA. Individual parameter estimates are not produced by default. Adding the POSTHOC command instructs NONMEM to use Bayesian techniques to obtain individual subject parameter estimates (η-values) after estimation of the population parameters has completed. In this case, the individual η-values do not influence the estimation of the typical parameter values.

Conditional estimation methods in NONMEM produce individual parameter estimates as a by-product of the estimation method. Any of the following estimation methods will generate individual η values during the population parameter estimation step:

```
$ESTIMATION METHOD=COND
$ESTIMATION METHOD=COND LAPLACIAN
$ESTIMATION METHOD=HYBRID ZERO=(...)
```

Use of the hybrid method will generate η values for those parameters not included in the ZERO=(...) statement. Those parameters listed in this option are fit using first-order estimation only and do not generate individual subject η values, unless the POSTHOC option is also requested.

Regardless of the approach used to generate the individual parameter estimates, the individual parameter estimates are made available to the analyst by output from a $TABLE statement. For example, to obtain a table file that contains the final parameter estimates, the following statement might be used:

```
$TABLE ID TIME TRT CL V KA ETA1 ETA2 ETA3 NOAPPEND NOPRINT
ONEHEADER FILE='.\patab01.tab'
```

This command produces a table file with one header row, followed by one row for each record in the analysis dataset. NOAPPEND keeps NONMEM from executing the default action of adding columns for data items DV, PRED, RES, and WRES. NOPRINT keeps NONMEM from the default action of printing the table inside the report file. Including the table in the report file is generally not helpful since it is not easily machine readable, nor is it convenient for the analyst when working with large datasets.

The FILE='...' option directs the table file to be saved as a separate text file with the given path and file name, and the ONEHEADER command inserts one additional row at the top of the file containing the names of the data items. Inclusion of the header row makes the file more useful for the human reader, but it must be either imported or skipped by programs importing data in the file for other uses.

Each row in the output file includes the current value of the parameters or data items listed in the $TABLE statement. The meaning of the parameters depends on how they were defined in the $PK statement. For instance, if:

```
CL = THETA(1)*EXP(ETA(1))
```

then CL in the output file is the individual subject value of CL. With this definition, CL is stationary, having a constant η_1 for the individual and a constant θ_1 for the population, and thus will have an identical value on every record for the subject in the output file.

If, however, CL is defined as a nonstationary parameter, such as:

```
TVCL = CLMAX-(CLMAX-CLBASE*EXP(-(TIME-TILAG)*KI))
  CL = TVCL*EXP(ETA(1))
```

then the individual value of CL will change with TIME across records. Here, CLMAX is the maximum clearance attained, CLBASE is the baseline clearance, TILAG is the lag time for beginning induction, and KI is the first-order rate constant describing the rate of induction. A constant valued η_i is present, but the inclusion of TIME in the definition of TVCL causes the value of CL to vary with TIME.

When parameter values are stationary (i.e., not changing over time), one may need to subset the table output to one record per subject before doing further analysis such as regression of the individual parameters versus covariates. With the exception of one option of the $TABLE record, subsetting and other postprocessing of the output files must be done with programs other than NONMEM. Facility with a programming language or programs designed for that purpose is very useful for controlling the content and quality of the postprocessed files. The $TABLE option that requests that the data file be subset to include only one record per individual is the FIRSTONLY option, which was described previously in Section 3.9.

One may define multiple output files for a given NONMEM run. Output tables with different content may be useful for various postprocessing goals. Some useful arrangements for output files are to include model parameters in one file, concentration-related items in another file, continuous covariates in a file, and categorical covariates in a file.

7.4   APPLICATIONS OF INDIVIDUAL PARAMETER ESTIMATES

There are numerous applications for subject-specific exposure estimates based on individual Bayesian parameter estimates. Individual parameter estimates following a single-dose study might be used to predict steady-state exposure. Individual exposure estimates from sparse data in a Phase 3 trial can be used for comparison with exposure estimates in Phase 1 or Phase 2 trials. Individual estimates of concentration values can be used for model evaluation through computation of IPRED, IRES, or IWRES as discussed in Chapter 5. As part of covariate model building, individual estimates of model parameters can be plotted against covariate values to explore measurable sources of intersubject variation in parameters. Individual exposure estimates might be merged with biomarker, safety, or efficacy data for PK/PD analyses or to explore potential relationships during exploratory analysis. Model-based estimates of exposure represent one of the most valuable assets to the pharmacometrician. Perhaps no other analysis approach carries the ability to make such efficient use of pharmacometric data.

7.4.1   Generating Subject-Specific Exposure Estimates

Computing subject-specific exposure estimates can be accomplished using various approaches depending upon the context of the model and the parameters sought. When a closed-form algebraic solution to the exposure estimate is available, one can compute the value of the exposure estimate through statements in the control file. For example, if CL and $F1$ are constructed to provide individual subject estimates, then individual exposures such as the area under the concentration versus time curve (AUC) or the average concentration at steady-state (C_{ss}) can be calculated as follows:

```
AUC = F1*DOSE/CL
```

Or,

```
CSS = DOSE*F1/(CL*TAU*1000)
```

Here, TAU is the dosing interval, and the value of 1000 is included to remind the reader to pay attention to units. Depending upon the units of the other terms, adjustments may need to be included to express the concentration computed in the customary units. The major limitation of this approach is the requirement for a closed-form solution for the exposure value sought. These are available for estimates of exposure in relatively simple linear models, but will not be available for many of the more complex models.

The exposure estimate computed with a closed-form equation can be output to a file using a $TABLE statement such as:

```
$TABLE ID CL F1 AUC CSS ONEHEADER NOPRINT NOAPPEND
FILE=expos01.tbl
```

The table file will have the same computed exposure value on each record for the individual where values of DOSE, TAU, and the PK parameters (in this case) are constant. This method computes the exposure based on the current value of the variable DOSE in the dataset. Here, DOSE is not the AMT data item that NONMEM used as the dose amount for computations, but is instead an additional data item in the dataset. This value may be different on different records in the data file to reflect changes in dose and, unlike AMT, would be present on all records within an individual record; and the computed exposure value would depend on the DOSE value on that record.

There are many creative ways to address these computations and the arrangement of data items. For instance, if the PK parameters are stationary and there is a closed-form solution for the exposure parameter of interest, one might use the AMT variable instead of DOSE in the aforementioned equations at the beginning of this section. In that case, the exposure value would be nonzero only on the dose event records. One could then subset the table file to unique occurrences of subject and AMT to obtain the unique estimates of exposure.

Like closed-form solutions to the total exposure measures presented earlier, partial AUC values or other record-dependent methods can be used if an equation can be crafted within the control file to compute the value of interest. One can set a variable to *lag* certain values from one record to the next, making calculations such as a linear trapezoidal partial AUC possible.

7.4.1.1 Example: Calculated Subject-Specific Exposure Parameters

Suppose a 100-mg orally administered dose of drug is given once daily for 5 days to 100 patients in a Phase 2 clinical trial. Sparse samples are collected at the following times across the 5 days.

Day 1: predose and at 1, 3, 5, and 8 hours postdose

Days 2, 3, and 4: predose

Day 5: predose and at 1 and 3 hours postdose

Suppose the data are fit using ADVAN2 TRANS2 and the PK of the drug can be described by a one-compartment model with the following parameters.

Cl: 3.5 L/h with 35%CV IIV

V: 42 L with 25%CV IIV

K_a: 1.73 with 80%CV IIV

Residual variability: 21%CV with a CCV model

Data records of the first subject might appear as shown in Table 7.1.

Here, the $AUC_{0-\infty}$ following a single dose and, equally, the AUC for the dosing interval at steady state can be computed in the control file during estimation using the following line of code:

```
IF (AMT.GT.0) AUC = AMT/CL
```

This individual AUC estimate and individual parameters can be output using a $TABLE statement.

```
$TABLE ID TIME KA CL V AUC ONEHEADER NOPRINT NOAPPEND
FILE=expos01.tbl
```

Table records from the first subject might then appear as shown in Table 7.2.

One might also wish to compute other exposure variables such as T_{max}, C_{max}, or C_{min} for comparison with NCA results from Phase 1 trials for instance. Again, for simple models, one might be able to calculate these parameters algebraically in

TABLE 7.1   Example dataset records for one subject

ID	TIME	AMT	DV	EVID	MDV
1	0	100	0.00	1	1
1	1	0	72.77	0	0
1	3	0	102.91	0	0
1	5	0	81.30	0	0
1	8	0	83.69	0	0
1	24	0	30.76	0	0
1	24	100	0.00	1	1
1	48	0	28.58	0	0
1	48	100	0.00	1	1
1	72	0	45.66	0	0
1	72	100	0.00	1	1
1	96	0	36.55	0	0
1	96	100	0.00	1	1
1	97	0	97.98	0	0
1	99	0	119.24	0	0

TABLE 7.2   Example table file output
records, including AUC, for one subject

ID	TIME	K_a	CL	V	AUC
1	0	1.28	2.80	51.58	35.77
1	1	1.28	2.80	51.58	0.00
1	3	1.28	2.80	51.58	0.00
1	5	1.28	2.80	51.58	0.00
1	8	1.28	2.80	51.58	0.00
1	24	1.28	2.80	51.58	35.77
1	24	1.28	2.80	51.58	0.00
1	48	1.28	2.80	51.58	35.77
1	48	1.28	2.80	51.58	0.00
1	72	1.28	2.80	51.58	35.77
1	72	1.28	2.80	51.58	0.00
1	96	1.28	2.80	51.58	35.77
1	96	1.28	2.80	51.58	0.00
1	97	1.28	2.80	51.58	0.00
1	99	1.28	2.80	51.58	0.00

the control stream. As the complexity of the equations increases, stating the equations might be possible but inconvenient. For instance, computing an estimate of C_{max} at steady state first requires computing T_{max} in that interval. For some simple models, this can be accomplished but can become tedious to do so.

In some models, an explicit solution for the desired exposure measures will not be achievable. For example, C_{max} at steady state for a drug that is modeled using a complex absorption model might not have an explicit solution. One approach to estimating exposure measures in these cases, or when one simply finds it more convenient, is to add additional frequent other-type event records to the dataset with DV having a missing value and EVID = 2. The granularity of the time interval for these additional records has to do with the precision desired in the estimate. If it is important to obtain a very precise estimate of C_{max}, it might be necessary to add records at times corresponding to every 5 minutes over the first several hours following dosing. Predicted concentrations will be computed at these timepoints. To have access to these values, the table file must include the individual predicted value without residual error, which can be obtained as follows:

```
$ERROR
IPRED = F
Y = ...
$TABLE ID TIME ... IPRED ... FILE=conc.tbl
```

The table file can then be imported into a postprocessing tool, such as SAS®, R®, Phoenix WinNonlin®, or Excel® and the desired exposure measures computed directly from the individual predicted concentrations.

TABLE 7.3 Example table file output
records with individual parameters,
subset to one record per subject

ID	K_a	CL	V
1	1.278	2.796	51.584
2	1.048	3.664	44.894
3	1.475	5.000	38.266
4	1.259	3.780	44.176
5	2.317	2.744	52.080
6	0.890	3.427	46.462
7	0.812	2.950	50.177
8	0.790	3.826	43.907
9	1.612	3.303	47.346
10	0.382	2.957	50.117

7.4.1.2 Example: Individual PK Parameters in the Dataset The afore-mentioned methods assume the exposure measures are being computed in the same NONMEM run that the parameter estimates are obtained. The dataset contains the AMT, TIME, and DV items needed to estimate the individual parameters, and these parameters are used to compute the exposure measure.

One might alternatively estimate the individual subject parameters in one run and then use these values for subsequent NONMEM runs in which the sampling or dosage regimen circumstances may be changed from those of the dataset in which the parameters were estimated. In this case, in the estimation run, a table file should be produced that outputs the individual subject Bayesian parameter estimates, as illustrated earlier. These individual parameter estimates are then merged with a dataset containing the postulated doses and sample collection times, from which concentration predictions will be estimated and exposure measures computed.

If the individual parameters for each subject are constant, the parameter dataset can be subset to one record per subject. Using the example given earlier, a few records of the parameter file might be structured as shown in Table 7.3.

If one wished to predict the concentration–time profile for each individual subject on day 5 assuming once daily administration of a 75-mg dose for 5 days, a template set of records could be created with the necessary items to describe the situation for a NONMEM dataset. An example template could be given as shown in Table 7.4.

This template gives a single dosing record that brings the subject to the fifth day of dosing using ADDL and II records. Subsequently, frequent sample collection records are included at each time that it is desired to compute a concentration value. A DV data item is required by NONMEM, but in this template file, for the purpose at hand, all values of DV are set to missing, and MDV = 1 on all records. Note that ID is not included, and this template set of records is present without repetition. This template file is then merged to the individual parameter file so that each subject is included in the dataset with each of the dose and sample records in the template file. This is a *one-to-many* merge. Dose and concentration records for the first subject in the merged file would appear as shown in Table 7.5.

TABLE 7.4 Example of template records for simulation of the administration of five doses and prediction of concentration values from 96 to 120 hours

TIME	AMT	ADDL	II	DV	EVID	MDV
0	75	4	24	.	1	1
96	.	.	.	.	0	1
96.5	.	.	.	.	0	1
97	.	.	.	.	0	1
97.5	.	.	.	.	0	1
98	.	.	.	.	0	1
98.5	.	.	.	.	0	1
99	.	.	.	.	0	1
100	.	.	.	.	0	1
104	.	.	.	.	0	1
108	.	.	.	.	0	1
112	.	.	.	.	0	1
116	.	.	.	.	0	1
120	.	.	.	.	0	1

TABLE 7.5 Example of template records following the *one-to-many* merge to include individual parameters and sufficient records for prediction of concentration values from 96 to 120 hours

ID	K_a	CL	V	TIME	AMT	ADDL	II	DV	EVID	MDV
1	1.278	2.796	51.584	0	75	4	24	.	1	1
1	1.278	2.796	51.584	96	.	.	.	.	0	1
1	1.278	2.796	51.584	96.5	.	.	.	.	0	1
1	1.278	2.796	51.584	97	.	.	.	.	0	1
1	1.278	2.796	51.584	97.5	.	.	.	.	0	1
1	1.278	2.796	51.584	98	.	.	.	.	0	1
1	1.278	2.796	51.584	98.5	.	.	.	.	0	1
1	1.278	2.796	51.584	99	.	.	.	.	0	1
1	1.278	2.796	51.584	100	.	.	.	.	0	1
1	1.278	2.796	51.584	104	.	.	.	.	0	1
1	1.278	2.796	51.584	108	.	.	.	.	0	1
1	1.278	2.796	51.584	112	.	.	.	.	0	1
1	1.278	2.796	51.584	116	.	.	.	.	0	1
1	1.278	2.796	51.584	120	.	.	.	.	0	1

The control file that reads this dataset will have an input line that assigns a name to the parameter data items that one used to assign the actual parameter values in the $PK block, such as the following:

```
$INPUT ID IKA ICL IV TIME AMT ADDL II DV EVID MDV
$DATA ...
$SUBROUTINE ADVAN2 TRANS2
$PK
```

```
KA = IKA
CL = ICL
V = IV
```

This assigns individual Bayesian parameter values tabled from the prior run to the required variables for the ADVAN TRANS model. Individual concentrations can then be computed by assigning the model-predicted concentration value at each timepoint for each subject to a variable in the $ERROR block and then computing the values without estimation of the model as follows:

```
$ERROR
Y = ...
IPRED = F
$ESTIM MAXEVAL=0 ...
$TABLE ID TIME IPRED ...
```

This approach can be used in sequential PK/PD modeling when the individual subject parameters are estimated in one run and their values are used in the PD model in a subsequent run. This approach allows one to easily predict the concentration value at the time of every PD event record, if needed.

This approach allows us to evaluate exposure in subjects with unusual responses (e.g., serious AE and lack of response). For instance, this approach would allow one to compute the concentration 5 hours after the second dose in patient 34, if that were the time at which a particular serious AE was observed.

This approach allows access to the parameters of the individuals for resampling applications such as leverage analysis or bootstrapping. Depending upon the purpose, these parameters can be used for predicting concentrations or exposure for the resampled populations, with or without random residual error.

Using a prior fitted model and postulated doses or sample collection times, concentrations of almost any scenario can be predicted based on the assumptions of the model. One must of course be cautious about extrapolating outside of experimental conditions and be clear in stating the assumptions on which these applications of models and parameters are based. For instance, using parameters from a set of healthy volunteers and predicting into pharmacokinetically different patients would lead to a wrong understanding of drug behavior in those patients.

7.4.2 Individual Exposure Estimates for Group Comparisons

When sparse samples are collected from patients in a clinical trial, the methods discussed in this chapter might be used to obtain individual estimates of exposure for comparison between groups and with historical data such as that from Phase 1 studies.

Phase 1 special population studies, such as renal and hepatic impairment studies, commonly present NCA exposure estimates such as AUC and C_{max} summarized by special population group or by levels of covariates. To compare results in the patients of a Phase 3 study in which only sparse samples are collected could be difficult or impossible without approaches like those presented in this chapter. Using these approaches, however, individual Bayesian parameter estimates can be obtained and used to generate exposure measures that are appropriate for comparison with Phase 1 results.

The summarization of exposure estimates by special population subgroups can be particularly informative in guiding clinical decision making regarding the need for dose adjustment.

REFERENCES

Ashby D. Bayesian statistics in medicine: a 25 year review. Statis Med 2006;25:3589–3631.

Bayes T. An essay towards solving a problem in the doctrine of chances. Philos Trans R Soc Lond 1763;53:370–418.

Bourne D. Bayesian analysis of clinical data. In: *Basic Pharmacokinetics.* 2013. p 314.

Sheiner LB, Beal SL. Bayesian individualization of pharmacokinetics: simple implementation and comparison with non-Bayesian methods. J Pharm Sci 1982;71 (12):1344–1348.

CHAPTER 8

INTRODUCTION TO MODEL EVALUATION

8.1 INTRODUCTION

Much has been written about the appropriateness of the terminology used to denote those activities performed after establishing a model that convey a sense of the appropriateness of the model for its intended use. Terms such as model evaluation, model qualification, and model validation, among others, have been used. Yano et al. define the goal of model evaluation as the objective assessment of the predictive ability of a model for domain-specific quantities of interest or to determine whether model deficiencies have a noticeable effect on substantive inferences (Yano et al. 2001). The FDA's Population PK Guidance devotes several pages to the description of several methods of *model validation*, including internal and external validation through predictive performance assessment, objective function mapping and leverage analysis, visual (and numerical) predictive checks, and posterior predictive checks (FDA 1999). In this chapter, we will discuss the typical aims and methodology for these and other techniques for what will be referred to herein globally as model evaluation.

8.2 INTERNAL VALIDATION

Internal validation methods require careful upfront planning and should ideally be specified at the time of analysis plan development to avoid concerns over biased findings. With internal validation techniques, a portion of the analysis dataset is randomly selected and set aside prior to model development (sometimes referred to as the test or the validation dataset). Model development then proceeds with the remainder of the data (usually about 70–80% of the original dataset or original number of subjects, termed the index or development dataset). Once a final model has been established with the model development dataset, the model is used to predict the observations in the validation dataset. With this methodology, the theory is that if the model is an appropriate characterization of the data, the predictions of the randomly selected validation data will be relatively unbiased and precise.

Introduction to Population Pharmacokinetic / Pharmacodynamic Analysis with Nonlinear Mixed Effects Models, First Edition. Joel S. Owen and Jill Fiedler-Kelly.

Clearly, the procedure for selecting the validation data subset requires careful planning. If the validation subset is not representative of the remainder of the data, no matter how appropriate or predictive the model, this procedure will fail to *validate* the model. Several factors should therefore be considered in selecting the validation subset. First and foremost, when selecting a portion of the data for a validation subset, the random procedure should select data at the subject level; that is, all of the data for a particular subject should be either included or set aside. Secondly, the design of the study(ies) that comprise the analysis dataset should be considered, and if substantial differences in design exist within or between studies, the random selection procedure should be stratified so as to maintain similar proportions of the different types of data in each subset. This is particularly important as it relates to the sampling strategy(ies) employed. If a portion of the data was collected according to a sparse sampling strategy and a portion followed a richer sampling design, one could imagine that the internal validation procedure may fail if all of the sparsely sampled data were *randomly* selected for the development dataset and all of the full-profile data were *randomly* selected for the validation dataset. Finally, when drafting the analysis plan, it may also be advisable to plan for stratifying the subset selection based on particular covariate factors expected to be important (if any) in explaining intersubject variability in PK or pharmacodynamics (PD). Alternatively, after the model validation subset is selected, the characteristics of the subset can be compared to those of the model development subset; if major differences are found, the random selection process could be repeated until the datasets are found similar.

The predictive performance assessment that is completed following the selection of data for internal validation is described in Section 8.4.

8.3   EXTERNAL VALIDATION

External validation procedures are similar to internal validation procedures in that a portion of the data are used to develop the model and then the model is applied to a separate dataset for prediction purposes. As such, the term *external validation* can be applied to any number of specific procedures that involve using a separate and distinct set of data in which model predictions are compared to observed data in order to assess model performance. The essential difference between internal and external validation procedures lies in the dataset used for prediction of the model. With external validation, the validation dataset typically arises from data that were collected from a study separate from the one(s) used for model development. The very idea of using the data from a different study to validate a model may generate some rational concerns in that there may be some uncontrollable factor that differs between the two studies, which would render the validation results negative and yet not necessarily be an indication of model inappropriateness. While this is a valid concern, if the predictive performance of the model is good based on an external validation procedure, one would have increased confidence that the model may adequately predict the results of another new study as yet to be performed.

As with internal validation procedures, the choice of the study or dataset to be used for the validation dataset should be made carefully, considering differences in study design, sampling, and patient population characteristics. Of practical interest may be the advantage to utilizing an external validation technique when study time-lines are delayed for a particular study including PK or PD sampling and of interest for predictive purposes. In this way, model development efforts can proceed with other available data, and the delayed study can still be utilized for external validation of the model.

The predictive performance assessment that is completed following the selection of data for external validation is described in Section 8.4.

8.4   PREDICTIVE PERFORMANCE ASSESSMENT

Sheiner and Beal proposed methods for assessing the predictive performance of models using easily calculated statistics (Sheiner and Beal 1981). By comparing the model-based predictions to the observed values (in the validation dataset), one can assess and summarize both the bias and precision of the model across all of the data. A typical measure of bias involves calculating the prediction error (PE_j) using the following formula:

$$PE_j = pred_j - obs_j$$

where $pred_j$ = the jth predicted value and obs_j = the jth observed value.

It is readily apparent that such PEs will have either a positive or negative sign, indicating that the prediction is greater or less than the observation, respectively. Typically, the MPE, or mean prediction error, is reported as a measure of the overall bias in the model-based predictions (i.e., how biased do the predictions tend to be and in what direction?), which involves taking the mean of the PEs calculated for each observation in the dataset. Similar to the interpretation of the PEs themselves, a positive MPE would indicate a tendency to overpredict the observations, on average, while a negative MPE would indicate a tendency to underpredict the values in the dataset, on average. Note also that the PE can be calculated for the population (typical value) predictions from the model as well as for the individual predictions (accounting for between-subject variability). The reporting of such statistics should always indicate which predicted value (population or individual) is used in the calculation.

There are at least two different methods to essentially remove the sign from the PEs, thereby gaining an understanding of the precision of the predictions through the magnitude of the typical deviation (i.e., how far off do the predictions tend to be?). One statistic that is very easily calculated from the PEs is the absolute prediction errors (APEs). Absolute prediction errors address the precision or accuracy of the model-based predictions and can be calculated based on the population or individual predictions, similar to the PEs. To calculate the APE, one would simply take the absolute value of the PE, as follows:

$$APE_j = |PE_j|$$

As with the PEs, taking the mean of all of the APEs in the dataset (the mean APE) provides an indication of how accurate or precise the predictions from the model are on average. Another method for removing the sign from the PEs involves taking the square of each PE, prior to computing the mean. The mean of the squared PEs is often referred to, logically, as the mean squared error (MSE) and is computed as follows:

$$\text{MSE} = \frac{1}{N} \sum_{j=1}^{N} \left(\text{PE}_j^2 \right)$$

A related statistic sometimes computed to address precision is the root mean square error (RMSE), calculated as follows:

$$\text{RMSE} = \sqrt{\text{MSE}}$$

The RMSE may be more easily interpreted than the MSE, since it is expressed in the units of the predictions and observations. Furthermore, such statistics are often reported in percentage units. If one wishes to express the accuracy or precision of predictions as a percentage, it should be clearly stated whether the PEs are expressed as a percentage relative to the observed value or relative to the predicted value, as examples of both are found in practice. The following equation illustrates the calculation of the mean APE as a percentage of the observations:

$$\text{MAPE} = \frac{1}{N} \sum_{j=1}^{N} \left[\left(\frac{\left| \left(\text{pred}_j - \text{obs}_j \right) \right|}{\text{obs}_j} \right) \times 100 \right]$$

The interpretation of such statistics may be facilitated by expression as a percentage (i.e., if the MAPE % based on population predictions is equal to 21% and based on individual predictions is equal to 13%, we would say that, on average, typical value model predictions tend to be within 21% of the observed values and individual predictions [accounting for between-subject variability] tend to be within 13% of the observed values).

When used in practice to compare models, a priori criteria for each statistic (say, < ±10% for MPE, <25% for MAPE) can be specified in the analysis plan to determine the appropriateness or validity of the model. Then, if the calculated statistic based on the internal or external validation exceeds the prespecified criteria, further model refinement may be warranted. On the other hand, if the calculated statistics based on the (internal or external) validation data do not exceed the prespecified criteria, we may consider the model fit for purpose based on the validation procedure.

The calculation of standardized PEs is also described in the FDA Guidance for Industry, Population Pharmacokinetics (FDA 1999). The standardization of such PEs has been proposed to take into account both the variability in the predictions as well as the correlation that exists between PEs arising from the same individual. The reader is referred to Vozeh et al. for a detailed description of this standardization approach (Vozeh et al. 1990). The weighted residuals (WRES) provided by NONMEM obtained using the first-order approximation and those obtained using the first-order conditional estimation approximation (CWRES) are standardized PEs, which are commonly used and take into account the correlation of the observations within an individual.

Several alternatives to the standardized PEs have been proposed, and much work has been done to explore and compare the statistical properties of these metrics. In 2006, Mentré and Escolano proposed a criterion and test for a new metric called prediction discrepancies (pd), which are based on the whole predictive distribution (obtained via simulation) as a means of evaluating nonlinear mixed effect model performance (Mentré and Escolano 2006). The pd for each observation is defined as the percentile of the observation in the whole marginal predictive distribution under the null hypothesis that the model is appropriate. If the model is *valid*, these pd should be uniformly distributed over [0, 1], an assumption that can be tested using a Kolmogorov–Smirnov test. Furthermore, these pd can be plotted versus various independent variables to identify whether trends are present, which might be indicative of deficiencies in the model. Mentré and Escolano show that these pd exhibit better statistical performance than the standardized PEs.

However, since pd did not take into account the correlation of the observations within an individual, subsequent work by Brendel and colleagues proposed the decorrelation of this metric through the calculation of normalized prediction distribution errors, or npde, a statistic shown to have even better properties than the pd (Brendel et al. 2006). The npde, as with most of the other metrics described, can be used for either internal or external validation, depending on whether computed on the dataset used to build the model (internal validation) or on an external dataset. Furthermore, following the decorrelation and if the model is *valid*, the npde are shown to follow a $N(0, 1)$ distribution, which can be tested in several ways. First, to test whether the mean is significantly different from 0, a Wilcoxon signed-rank test can be performed; second, to test whether the variance is significantly different from 1, a Fisher test for variance can be used; and, finally, to test whether the distribution is significantly different from a normal distribution, a Shapiro–Wilk test can be performed.

In their work, Brendel et al. discussed several techniques for external model evaluation methodologies, differentiating their recommendations for methodology selection based on the intended use of the model (Brendel et al. 2006). Among the techniques they explored are those based on PEs or variations of same (deemed appropriate if the aim of the model is simulation), population parameter estimates or hyperparameters (parameters of a prior distribution) which are preferred when the goal is to compare two populations, and objective function-based methods (found useful during model building). In 2008, Comets and colleagues described an add-on package for the open-source statistical package R, designed to compute npde, thus facilitating the use of this metric (Comets et al. 2008). In NONMEM version 7.1.2 and later, npde can be simply requested in the $TABLE file output using the variable NPDE.

Brendel, Comets, Laffont, and Mentré published a simulation-based comparison in 2010 of the statistical properties of npde, pd, standardized prediction errors (SPE), numerical predictive check (NPC), and decorrelated NPC (NPC$_{dec}$) for the external evaluation of a population pharmacokinetic (PK) analysis (Brendel et al. 2010). The authors recommend the use of npde over SPE for external model evaluation (and therefore for internal model evaluation) since npde do not depend on an approximation of the model and have good statistical properties. Moreover, the authors considered interpretation of npde to be less subjective compared to NPC, as NPC does not account for within-subject correlation. The exact binomial test applied to NPC$_{dec}$ was proposed as an alternative to computing a statistic, but the choice of the prediction interval(s) to study remains an issue for the modeler.

8.5   OBJECTIVE FUNCTION MAPPING

Objective function mapping, sometimes also referred to as likelihood profiling or log-likelihood profiling, is a technique that aims to assess whether or not a global minimum was obtained with respect to each model parameter during model convergence. In addition, objective function mapping procedures are commonly used to obtain nonasymptotic confidence intervals (CI) around model parameters.

With objective function mapping, for each estimated parameter of the model (elements of θ, Ω, and Σ alike), a graph is generated illustrating the objective function values associated with the surface around each parameter's final estimate. To obtain these values, a series of models is fitted for each parameter by fixing each parameter estimate to values of varying degrees larger and smaller than the final parameter estimate obtained when the full model was fit. Values over a range such as ±5%, ±10%, ±20%, and ±40% might be evaluated. To obtain each point in the graph for each parameter, a new control stream is generated and run. The only modification to each control stream is to fix the value of (only) the given parameter to successively larger and smaller values over the desired range. To ensure that a valid assessment of the surface with respect to each parameter can be made, it is important that the control stream remains the same as for the comparator model fit and that only the value of the fixed parameter changes. Each of the control streams for each parameter is then run and the results carefully reviewed.

For those models with successful convergence, the minimum objective function value obtained with each model is recorded and plotted on the y axis corresponding to the associated fixed parameter value on the x axis. The final parameter estimate obtained when the full model was fit is also plotted against the minimum value of the objective function obtained from the same fit. When values far from the final estimate for a given parameter are tested, one may encounter difficulties in obtaining a successful minimization. If necessary, the initial estimates of other parameters of the model may need to be altered to attempt to obtain successful convergence. When and if all such efforts to obtain successful convergence fail, the corresponding point may be left off the plot.

As such, for each parameter of the model, a parabola-like curve is generated when the points of this graph are joined or when a smoothing function or fitted polynomial is employed to illustrate the *surface* or likelihood profile with respect to that parameter. As expected, typically, the lowest point of this curve is associated with the fitted parameter estimate, and the minimum value of the objective function increases in both directions as larger and smaller values of the parameter are tested. An example of such a graph is provided in Figure 8.1; in this case, the objective function values are plotted as the difference between the minimum value associated with the final parameter estimates and each new value.

Based on the likelihood ratio test that can be performed to compare hierarchical or nested models (as discussed in Chapter 5), the parameter estimate values (smaller and larger) associated with an increase in the objective function of 3.84 ($\chi^2_{a=0.05, \text{df}=1}$) over the minimum value correspond to a 95% CI around that parameter estimate. The horizontal line on Figure 8.1 is drawn at an objective function value 3.84 units higher than the minimum value; if vertical lines are drawn at the intersection of the horizontal line and the fitted line on this plot, their x axis values would represent the 95% CI around the parameter estimate shown, based on the objective function mapping procedure. In the Figure 8.1 example, the 95% CI about the apparent volume of distribution would be approximately 63.1 and 82.8 L. If a fitting function was employed to illustrate the objective function map, the function can be easily solved for the exact parameter estimate values corresponding to objective function values 3.84 greater than the overall minimum obtained from the full model fit. If a fitting function was not used, either a linear approximation between the two values on either side can be utilized or alternative values can be tested in NONMEM until the desired level of precision of the interval is reached.

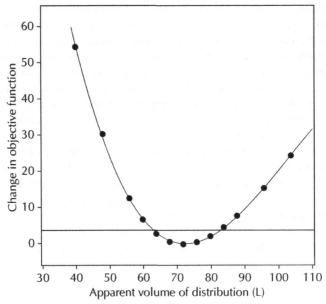

FIGURE 8.1 Example plot illustrating objective function mapping for the apparent volume of distribution.

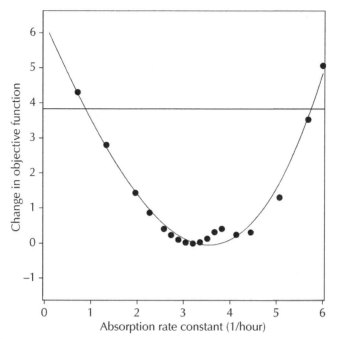

FIGURE 8.2   Example plot illustrating objective function mapping for the absorption rate constant, where an apparent local minimum was obtained.

The possibility exists that the objective function mapping will indicate that a global minimum was not originally obtained with the full model fit. Figure 8.2 illustrates the case of an apparent local minimum associated with the final parameter estimate for the absorption rate constant of 4.15 per hour. Note that through objective function mapping, when lower values were tested, an even lower objective function value was obtained, the lowest with an absorption rate constant value of 3.2 per hour. Now, in this case, considering the magnitude of difference in the objective function values associated with the final estimate of 4.15 per hour and the global minimum value of 3.2 per hour, there is no practical or statistical difference between these two values (i.e., objective function values are different by <0.2). However, if this model were to be considered the basis for simulations, the global minimum for the absorption rate constant may be the better choice.

On occasion, but especially when alternative initial estimates are not tested throughout the model building process, a model building exercise may result in a local minimum with respect to one or more parameters. If this knowledge is gained through the performance of objective function mapping, then the time and effort involved in implementing the procedure was well worth it. In this situation, a more thorough and rigorous evaluation of alternative initial estimates should be performed, followed by a re-evaluation and refinement of the various model components to ensure that previous decisions with respect to model structure are still appropriate at the new lower (and, hopefully, now global) minimum.

8.6 LEVERAGE ANALYSIS

A second technique called cross-validation or leverage analysis is often employed following objective function mapping if all parameters are deemed to be at appropriate minima, the associated CIs around each parameter are reasonable, and the evaluation of model robustness based on objective function mapping was determined to be a success. Cross-validation procedures or leverage analyses provide an assessment of the influence of the data from particular individuals in the analysis dataset on the overall fit. This (internal validation) assessment is accomplished by systematically excluding subsets of subjects from the dataset (in a manner that allows each subject to be excluded exactly once), then refitting the model to each resulting dataset, and comparing the results. A detailed list of steps to perform what would be referred to as a (10×) cross-validation or (10%) leverage analysis is provided as follows:

1. Programmatically assign a random uniform variate to each subject in the dataset (e.g., using the *ranuni* function in SAS or the RAND() function in Excel).

2. Sort the dataset by the random uniform variate.

3. Create 10 new subset datasets, each containing approximately 90% of the total number of subjects, by excluding a different 10% of subjects from each one, such that each subject is excluded from exactly one subset dataset.

   a. For subset dataset number 1: exclude subjects whose random uniform variate is between 0 and 0.1, inclusive.

   b. For subset dataset number 2: exclude subjects whose random uniform variate is greater than 0.1 but less than or equal to 0.2.

   c. For subset datasets number 3–10: exclude subjects whose random uniform variate is greater than 0.2 but less than or equal to 0.3, greater than 0.3 but less than or equal to 0.4, and so on, up to 1.0.

4. If needed, re-sort each of the 10 subsets by ID and TIME or whatever sort variables are required to arrange the subset for NONMEM estimation.

5. Fit the final model to each of the 10 subset datasets (each one containing approximately 90% of the original dataset) and record the final parameter estimates for elements of theta, omega, and sigma.

6. Repeat steps 1–4 one or more times (typically, the procedure is repeated at least twice) based on new randomizations.

7. Generate separate plots for each parameter of the final parameter estimate from each subset (y axis) versus the subset number and iteration (x axis), overlaying the CI for each parameter obtained from the objective function mapping procedure.

An example of the results of a cross-validation procedure for two parameters is provided in Figure 8.3. Ideally, of course, all parameter estimates from the subset fits fall within the established CI for each parameter. However, when one or a small number of the subsets result in disparate estimates (outside the CI bands), then an investigation into the possible differences between the excluded and included subjects

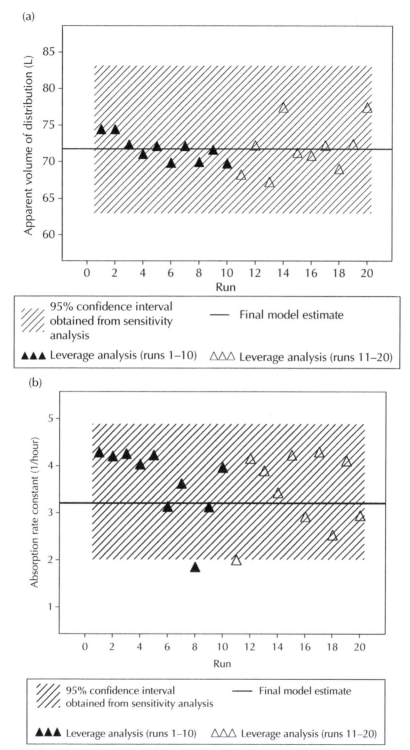

FIGURE 8.3 Example cross-validation scatterplots for the apparent volume of distribution and the absorption rate constant. Panel (a) illustrates a successful cross-validation result for volume where all estimates fall within the CI and Panel (b) illustrates a cross-validation exercise, which resulted in two subsets whose parameter estimates fall outside the CI.

in the particular subset(s) may be warranted. If several subsets result in parameter estimates outside the established CI, then a more thorough investigation is warranted. Many times, minor discrepancies with a given parameter in one or two subsets are easily explainable; for instance, an E_{max} or EC_{50} estimate outside the established CI for a given subset may be the result of an unusual distribution of dose or exposure in the random subset (i.e., perhaps most or all of the subjects with the highest dose were excluded in the subset). As such, cross-validation or leverage analysis techniques provide additional insight into the influence or leverage particular subjects have on the population parameter estimates.

8.7 BOOTSTRAP PROCEDURES

Another (internal) model evaluation technique involves fitting the model to multiple datasets, each consisting of subjects resampled from the original dataset, and then summarizing across the model fits. A typical bootstrap procedure involves the following steps:

1. Generate a bootstrap dataset of the same size as the original dataset by resampling with replacement from the original dataset (with the subject as a unit). In other words, assuming an original dataset of size is equal to n subjects, randomly select one subject from the original dataset to include in the first bootstrap sample dataset. Repeat the selection of an individual a total of n times (each time considering the entire original dataset as a source) until a total of n subjects are included in the bootstrap dataset. For an example dataset of 10 subjects, by sampling with replacement, the first bootstrap sample may consist of the data from subjects 9, 6, 2, 4, 9, 7, 3, 1, 4, and 8. Note that (based on the random nature of the resampling process) subjects 5 and 10 were not selected for inclusion in this sample at all and subjects 9 and 4 were each selected more than once.

2. Repeat this process hundreds or thousands of times to generate a large number of resampled bootstrap datasets (typically at least 500).

3. Fit the model of interest to *each* bootstrap replicate dataset. Assuming covariance step output is not of interest for the purpose of the bootstrap procedure, each of these runs can be done without $COV (this will save a great deal of run time).

4. Summarize information regarding the convergence characteristics of the model results in the bootstrap datasets (e.g., the model converged in 953/1000 bootstrap samples represents a 95.3% convergence rate). If specific convergence criteria were set a priori for acceptance of the bootstrap procedure, compare this statistic to those criteria and stop if the criteria are not met; otherwise, continue on with Step 5.

5. Using the models that successfully minimized, calculate summary statistics for each final parameter estimate across the bootstrap datasets (e.g., mean, median, minimum, maximum, 90% prediction interval based on 5th and 95th percentiles of the distributions, etc.).

6. Compare the summary statistics for each parameter estimate (in particular, perhaps, the 90% prediction or bootstrap CI) to the original model fit results.

TABLE 8.1   Example table comparing bootstrap
results to the final parameter estimates

Parameter	Final parameter estimate	90% CI based on bootstrap procedure
CL (L/hour)	26.7	19.3–38.9
V (L)	5.32	3.67–7.05
K_a (1/hour)	0.761	0.698–0.847
IIV CL	0.109	0.0702–0.156
IIV V	0.135	0.0831–0.217
RV	0.0431	0.0328–0.0569

Presentation of bootstrap results can take on many forms but should always include the convergence rate of the model in the bootstrap samples. A tabular view of the results can be prepared by presenting the final parameter estimates in a table column next to the CI obtained from the bootstrap procedure as shown in Table 8.1.

Another option for presentation of bootstrap results involves presenting histograms of the distributions of the bootstrap results for each parameter. This type of display could include vertical lines superimposed at the lower and upper limits of the CI in addition to a differently colored line at the final parameter estimate. *Success of a bootstrap technique is typically two pronged: meeting a prespecified convergence rate in addition to the CI for each parameter encompassing the original final parameter estimate.*

8.8   VISUAL AND NUMERICAL PREDICTIVE CHECK PROCEDURES

The visual predictive check (VPC) and NPC procedures originally proposed by Karlsson and Savic are simulation-based methods developed based on the theory that simulations based on the model will produce simulated data that are similar (in features and distributional characteristics) to the original data upon which the model was developed if the model is an appropriate characterization of the data (Karlsson and Savic 2007). In part, the VPC technique relies on a graphical presentation of results (albeit typically combined with some statistical summaries), while the NPC technique reduces the simulation results to statistical comparisons of expectations of the simulated data to calculations based on the observed data.

8.8.1   The VPC Procedure

More specifically, to perform a VPC on a given model, the first step is to simulate a large number of datasets based on the model. Typically, variability is introduced into the simulated replicate datasets through random sampling from the OMEGA and SIGMA matrices. Keeping the model structure intact (i.e., making no changes to the $PK or $PRED block), the $THETA, $OMEGA, and $SIGMA blocks are either replaced by an $MSFI statement calling the model specification file from the final model or the estimates in these blocks are fixed to the final parameter estimates from the fit of the model to be evaluated. Note that if $MSFI is used, the additional option TRUE=FINAL should be used on the $SIM record to ensure that the final estimates from the run generating the MSF are used as the starting point for the simulations (as opposed to the initial estimates from that run, which would be the default behavior without this option). The $EST and $COV statements are replaced by the following record:

```
$SIMULATION ONLYSIM (seed) SUBPROBLEMS=xxx
```

where *seed* is a random seed value to be used as a starting point for the random number generation and *xxx* is the number of replicate datasets to be simulated. In general, as large a number as possible should be specified for the number of replicates. VPC procedures are often done with at least 1000 replicates. Later, we will discuss typical comparisons of the observed and simulated predictions; for now, it is important to understand that we often compare the 50th percentile (the median) of the observed data and the simulated predictions, along with the 5th and 95th percentiles, corresponding to a 90% prediction interval. If the original sample size of the data is quite small, a smaller prediction interval may be a better choice for comparison purposes (say, an 80% or even a 50% prediction interval) because the behavior in the tails of a small sample will generally not be as well behaved as with a larger sample. The final point related to this subject is that if the performance of the model near the tails of the distribution is of particular interest, as opposed to the behavior near the median, then a larger number of replicates, say 2000, might be chosen instead of the typical 1000.

The simulation procedure then selects *realizations* or *random draws* from the OMEGA and SIGMA matrices for each subject and observation in the dataset, respectively. The predictions from each simulation are concatenated, one following another, until the requested number of replicate datasets (*xxx*) is reached. The resulting table file contains the requested number of replicate datasets in one giant table file, with the DV column values replaced by the simulated values. Due to the sheer size of this file, especially when a large number of SUBPROBLEM replicates is requested, care should be taken to include only those variables in $TABLE, which will be useful in fully exploring and evaluating the results of the VPC procedure. See additional information regarding the presentation of VPC results in Section 8.8.2.

One specific addition to the VPC simulation run may be considered to facilitate postprocessing of the table file. A new variable may be defined in the $PK or $PRED block, set equal to the NONMEM IREP variable as follows:

```
REP = IREP
```

This new variable (REP) may then be appended to the table file output to indicate the particular replication number of the dataset (e.g., 1 through the number of SUBPROBLEMS requested, *xxx*) for each record in the table output.

8.8.2   Presentation of VPC Results

Visual predictive check results are typically presented in the form of a figure or series of figures illustrating the original raw data (say, concentration or dose-normalized concentration vs time) with a prediction interval derived from the simulations overlaid. Since the table file from a VPC simulation with 1000 subproblems contains 1000 simulated values for each observed concentration, the table file must be processed and manipulated in order to generate the desired prediction interval. Furthermore, with many datasets used for population PK modeling, concentrations are collected at random times following dosing and not at specific (nominal) and/or consistent sampling times across subjects. *Binning* or grouping of simulated concentrations or observations within small intervals of time following dosing is often performed to prevent a very erratic-looking profile that may result from potentially vastly differing sample sizes at each true time following dosing. To facilitate the generation of a prediction interval (band) that can be easily plotted across time and used to facilitate the identification of possible model misspecification, time bins, or ranges of sampling times relative to the last dose of drug, may be specified (Karlsson and Holford 2008). There are several different objectives that may be considered in the selection of such bins: (i) to provide a fairly equal distribution of points in each bin, (ii) to provide evenly spaced intervals of time in each bin, and (iii) (manual selection) to include points that tend to cluster together *naturally* across the distribution of time, perhaps loosely based on the defined sampling strategy but allowing for variability around each window. Additionally, automated methods for bin selection are available such as those proposed by Lavielle et al. and implemented in MONOLIX and PsN (Lavielle and Bleakley 2011).

Then, the prediction interval bounds for the specified bin can be calculated based on all of the points falling within the bin (i.e., collected or simulated at times following dosing within the time bin, say, between 0.75 and 1.25 hours postdose or around a nominal sampling timepoint of 1 hour). For graphical presentation purposes, the prediction interval is typically plotted at the midpoint of the time bin (on the x axis), and a shaded box may be used to illustrate the CI about the prediction interval bound within the time bin. An example VPC presentation for a PK dataset is provided in Figure 8.4; in this VPC display, the raw data points are plotted, along with the median and 90% prediction interval based on the simulations from the model (dashed lines); the CI bands about the prediction interval are included as shaded regions; and the corresponding percentiles based on the raw data are also included (solid lines).

In addition to the VPC presentation style that shows all of the observed data overlaid on the simulation-based prediction interval, other display styles are often used. Since plots like Figure 8.4 can become very busy and it can be difficult to assess model misfit via the VPC prediction interval with all of the data points from a large dataset included, another option is to present a simpler display with only the corresponding prediction interval based on the observed data and the simulation-based prediction interval. Thus, with this style, 6 lines are typically displayed: the 5th, 50th, and 95th percentiles of the distribution of observed data in each bin (using one line style) and the same percentiles of the distribution of simulated predictions in each bin (using a different line style). This plot often provides a cleaner view of the

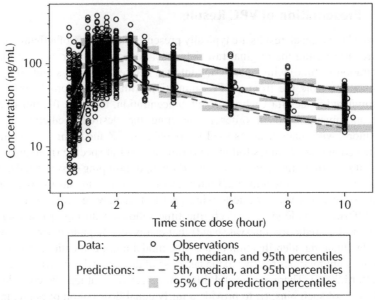

FIGURE 8.4 Example VPC plot illustrating the simulation-based prediction interval overlaid on the raw data, the corresponding percentiles based on the observed data, and the CI about the median and 90% prediction interval bounds as shaded regions. Medians and percentiles are plotted at the mean time since dose of the data observed within each time since dose interval.

areas (bins) where there may be considerable discrepancy between the observed and simulated data. A third display style involves calculating a CI around the simulation-based prediction interval bounds and the simulation-based 50th percentile. When these three intervals are plotted, the simulation-based lines around which they are derived can be dropped from the plot and the plot constructed to include the three bands (presented as three shaded areas for each bin on the graph) and the corresponding 5th, 50th, and 95th percentiles based on the observed data. With this display style, it is easy to identify the areas of potential concern with regard to possible model misspecification because, in those areas, the lines based on the observed data will fall outside the corresponding CI bands around the simulation-based percentile. Figure 8.5 provides an example of this type of cleaner VPC display. For this example, the VPC results are supportive of the model in that the median of the simulated predictions tracks very well with the median of the observed data, across the entire dosing interval, and the 90% prediction interval is also fairly consistent with the corresponding percentiles based on the data. In only a handful of time bins does the 5th percentile of the data fall outside the CI around the lower prediction interval.

As is evident from Figure 8.4, a quantification of the number of observed data points falling outside the simulation-based prediction interval (above and below) is clearly of interest. Ideally, $100 - n\%$ of points should fall outside an $n\%$ prediction interval. Clearly, many more than $100 - n\%$ of points falling outside the prediction interval provide an indication that there is a problem with the model; however,

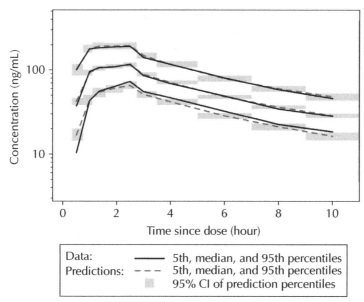

FIGURE 8.5 Example VPC plot illustrating the CI about the median and 90% prediction interval bounds as shaded regions with the corresponding percentiles based on the observed data overlaid. Medians and percentiles are plotted at the mean time since dose of the data observed within each time since dose interval.

substantially less than $100 - n\%$ of points falling outside the prediction interval similarly provides evidence of a potential issue. For example, if the results of a VPC indicate that only 0.1% of observed data points fall outside of a 90% prediction interval based on the model, this might be an indication of the overestimation of some or all random-effect estimates (variability components) in the model. If, on the other hand, 25% of the observed data fall outside of a 90% prediction interval based on the model, we would need to explore the patterns of behavior in the points falling outside of the interval to understand whether there is a systematic bias in some portion of the model fit or whether there might be a problem with the random-effect terms here as well.

When PK datasets contain data collected following a variety of different dose levels or other important covariates that may affect the prediction in a significant way (such as dosing interval or route of administration), stratification of the VPC plots by dose (or other relevant covariates) is often performed in order to get a fair view of each dose level and to not be misled into overinterpreting what may not be model misfit at all, but a simple imbalance in the data. On the other hand, with such sources of variability contributing significantly to the predictions within each bin, the VPC results (prediction intervals) may be less sensitive to true model misspecification as they are relatively less reflective of the unexplained variability introduced in the VPC simulation. For a simple factor such as dose amount, the VPC plots discussed earlier may be dose normalized by dividing both the observed concentrations and the simulated concentrations (prior to calculating the prediction interval) by dose. However, when the model is not linear with respect to dose, this particular technique is not appropriate to use. Furthermore, when there are many more factors (covariate or design related) that would warrant consideration of stratification, another slightly more complex alternative may be appropriate.

While the VPC has considerable intuitive appeal, there are several situations for which it is not appropriate and some conditions that limit its usefulness in certain circumstances. Karlsson et al. describe adaptive dosing trials and dose adjustment scenarios, especially when the PK or PD model is nonlinear, as examples of scenarios where the typical VPC may not be appropriate (Karlsson and Savic 2007). Models with significant covariate effects, requiring stratification of plots and a small number of data points in each plot, and situations where the study design varies among subjects, or within a study, are other situations that may limit the usefulness of VPC plots. Furthermore, the reader is referred to Post et al., who studied some specific extensions to the VPC (i.e., the quantified visual predictive check (QVPC) and the bootstrap visual predictive check (BVPC)) to facilitate its use in objective model performance evaluation, specifically focusing on the consideration of information relating to missing or unobserved data in the interpretation of VPC results (Post et al. 2008). To address some of these limitations of the VPC, Bergstrand and colleagues proposed the prediction-corrected VPC in 2011 and Wang et al. proposed the standardized VPC in 2012 (Bergstrand et al. 2011; Wang and Zhang 2012).

Wang's standardized visual predictive check (SVPC) is an attempt to standardize the calculation of the prediction intervals based on subject-specific design features in order to improve the ability of this diagnostic to identify structural model misspecification or inadequate estimation of random effects. The predicted value versus time plots produced with this methodology are thus presented with a (standardized) y axis ranging from 0 to 1; the authors describe this aspect as a feature that facilitates the review and interpretation of the findings as the ideal plot would have a lack of trend with a balanced distribution of points between 0 and 1 over time. Wang proposes that the standardization employed with the SVPC makes it applicable to all situations (Wang and Zhang 2012).

The prediction-corrected VPC aims at addressing the lack of sensitivity of the typical VPC, which may result from not accounting for the expected within-bin variability that arises from significant covariate effects or systematic design differences within the dataset. Alternative calculations for both the observed and simulated predictions are used to calculate the prediction intervals for comparison. These calculations attempt to normalize the values within a bin by the ratio of the prediction $(PRED_{ij})$ to the average prediction within the bin $(PRED_{avg,bin})$. Through case studies, the authors illustrate the improved ability of the prediction-corrected VPC to correctly diagnose model misspecification (Bergstrand et al. 2011).

Also of note, a recent paper by Lavielle et al. examined the consequences of various strategies that may be used to select bins for use in VPC procedures. The authors propose an automated strategy for the selection of bins (implemented in MONOLIX and PsN) to avoid possible problems with VPCs that may be performed by selecting bins of equal width or equal size. The reader may be interested in exploring this issue further in order to understand and appreciate the impact that bin selection may have on model misspecification conclusions drawn from VPC results (Lavielle and Bleakley 2011).

It should also be noted that the VPCs, along with several different options for binning and presentation of graphical results, are implemented in the PsN software, thus facilitating use of this procedure (Lindbom et al. 2005).

8.8.3   The Numerical Predictive Check (NPC) Procedure

The NPC is an alternative model diagnostic tool that is closely related to the VPC procedure. In fact, although some of the computations associated with the NPC are specific to the method, the basis for the method (simulations based on an appropriate model will mimic the observed data) and the file upon which the calculations are performed is the same as the simulated output that is processed for the VPC graphs previously described (PsN 2013).

With an NPC, a variety of different prediction intervals of varying widths can be constructed. Intervals can be constructed based on the distribution of simulated data points (across replicate datasets) around an individual data point or based on the distribution of simulated data points in the corresponding bin. For each possible prediction interval, it may be noted whether or not the observation falls inside or outside the prediction interval bounds, thus generating a count of false negatives (points that are outside the PI for the point but inside the PI based on the bin), false positives (points that are inside the PI for the point but outside the PI for the bin), true negatives (points that are both inside the PI for the point and the PI for the bin), and true positives (points that are both outside the PI based on the point and the PI based on the bin). Comparisons may then be made to the expected number of points falling above or below the interval based on the selected interval width; for example, 10% of points would be expected to fall outside (5% above and 5% below) a 90% prediction interval, and 40% of points would be expected to fall outside a 60% prediction interval.

8.9   POSTERIOR PREDICTIVE CHECK PROCEDURES

Yano, Beal, and Sheiner described another simulation-based technique, fundamentally similar to the VPC and NPC techniques, called the posterior predictive check (Yano et al. 2001). With this technique, a particular summary feature (statistic) is computed from the raw data and compared to its posterior predictive distribution generated from model-based simulations. In these simulations, the distribution of the statistic for comparison and the corresponding p-value are derived from the simulated replicate datasets. Since the choice of which statistic to calculate and use for a PPC procedure is critical to the interpretation of the results of this technique and the ultimate conclusion regarding the qualification of the model, oftentimes more than one statistic, each summarizing a different feature of the data that is important to predict, are used in a PPC. Examples of statistics that might be relevant for a particular dataset would be drug concentration at a particular time following dosing, EC_{50} (concentration at which 50% of effect is achieved), or E_{max} (maximum effect). Based on the comprehensive simulation study performed by Yano et al. to thoroughly explore this technique, the authors concluded that based on their "admittedly limited study,…if a PPC 'invalidates' a model, one can be reasonably certain that the model has serious

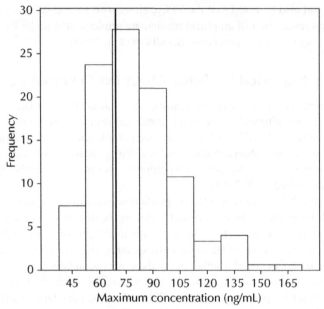

FIGURE 8.6 Example posterior predictive check plot illustrating the distribution of simulated estimates of the (dose-normalized) maximum concentration with the mean observed maximum concentration (vertical line) overlaid.

deficiencies..." but also that "...the failure of the PPC to invalidate a model offers little assurance that the model is correct" (Yano et al. 2001). Due in part to its computational complexity and in part to the paucity of applications of this technique to a variety of real data problems, this technique remains a lesser-used option in the arsenal of model evaluation and qualification techniques (Jadhav and Gobburu 2005). Figure 8.6 provides an example of a posterior predictive check plot for the (dose-normalized) maximum concentration.

REFERENCES

Bergstrand M, Hooker AC, Wallin JE, Karlsson MO. Prediction-corrected visual predictive checks for diagnosing nonlinear mixed-effects models. AAPS J 2011;13 (2):143–151.

Brendel K, Comets E, Laffont C, Laveille C, Mentré F. Metrics for evaluation with an application to the population pharmacokinetics of gliclazide. Pharm Res 2006;23 (9):2036–2049.

Brendel K, Comets E, Laffont C, Mentré F. Evaluation of different tests based on observations for external model evaluation of population analyses. J Pharmacokinet Pharmacodyn 2010;37:49–65.

Comets E, Brendel K, Mentré F. Computing normalised prediction distribution errors to evaluate non-linear mixed-effect models: the npde add-on package for R. Comput Methods Programs Biomed 2008;90:154–166.

Food and Drug Administration (FDA), Guidance for Industry, Population Pharmacokinetics. Rockville: Food and Drug Administration; 1999.

Jadhav PR and Gobburu JVS, A new equivalence based metric for predictive check to qualify mixed-effects models. AAPS J 2005;7(3):E523–E531. Article 53.

Karlsson MO, Holford NH. A tutorial on visual predictive checks; 2008. PAGE 17. Abstr 1434. Available from www.page-meeting.org/?abstract=1434. Accessed December 16, 2013.

Karlsson MO, Savic RM. Diagnosing model diagnostics. Clin Pharmacol Ther 2007;82:17–20.

Lavielle M, Bleakley K. Automatic data binning for improved visual diagnosis of pharmacometric models. J Pharmacokinet Pharmacodyn 2011;38 (6):861–871.

Lindbom L, Pihlgren P, Jonsson EN. PsN-Toolkit—a collection of computer intensive statistical methods for non-linear mixed effect modeling using NONMEM. Comput Methods Programs Biomed 2005; 79 (3):241–257.

Mentré F, Escolano S. Prediction discrepancies for the evaluation of nonlinear mixed-effects models. J Pharmacokinet Pharmacodyn 2006;33:345–367.

NPC/VPC user guide and technical description 2013 PsN 3.6.2. Available at http:\\psn.sourceforge.net/pdfdocs/vpc_npc_userguide.pdf. Accessed December 16, 2013.

Post TM, Freijer JI, Ploeger BA, Danhof M. Extensions to the visual predictive check to facilitate model performance evaluation. J Pharmacokinet Pharmacodyn 2008;35:185–202.

Sheiner LB, Beal SL. Some suggestions for measuring predictive performance. J Pharmacokinet Biopharm 1981;9 (4):503–12.

Vozeh S, Maitre PO, Stanski DR. Evaluation of population (NONMEM) pharmacokinetic parameter estimates. J Pharmacokinet Biopharm 1990;18:161–173.

Wang DD, Zhang S. Standardized visual predictive check versus visual predictive check for model evaluation J Clin Pharmacol 2012;52(1):39–54. Erratum in J Clin Pharmacol 2012 Apr;52(4):NP1–NP3.

Yano Y, Beal SL, Sheiner LB. Evaluating pharmacokinetic/pharmacodynamic models using the posterior predictive check. J Pharmacokinet Pharmacodyn 2001;28 (2):171–192.

CHAPTER *9*

USER-WRITTEN MODELS

9.1 INTRODUCTION

Nonlinear mixed effect models are useful for the construction of an immense variety of pharmacometric models. The PRED and PREDPP routines of NONMEM provide flexibility to describe complex models and are not limited to the set of prebuilt models provided in the specific ADVAN routines (ADVAN1, 2, 3, 4, 10, 11, and 12) or to a limited set of numbers of compartments or functional forms for rate and transfer processes. Our use of the expression *user-written model* does not simply mean writing a control file. The use of any model in NONMEM requires a user-written control file that includes elements such as code to call the dataset, the names of the parameters to be estimated, specification of the fixed- and random-effect parameter structures, and initialization of parameter values. The expression *user-written models* in this chapter refers to control files in which the complete mathematical structure of the model must be specified by the analyst. We will focus on the expression of these user-written models using PREDPP, including models not specified with the specific ADVANs, which must be defined specifically by the analyst using the general ADVANs (5, 6, 7, 8, 9, and 13). For pharmacokinetic (PK) analysis, perhaps the most common need for user-written models is to describe the complex nature of drug absorption rather than an unusual arrangement or number of compartments in a model. Recirculation, transit compartments, and nonlinear elimination or transfer processes are other settings in which the need for more complex PK models is frequently encountered. For the analysis of pharmacodynamic data, user-written models are generally required except in the simplest cases.

Chatelut et al. (1999) provide an interesting example of a PK scenario that we will use to demonstrate various ways to code user-written models. The authors describe a variety of models that were tested in the PK model development process for alpha interferon, one of which described the PK properties with a one-compartment model disposition with simultaneous first-order and zero-order absorption without a lag time. One way to describe this model is to describe an absorption, or depot, compartment for each rate process and estimate the fraction absorbed through each process. Figure 9.1 depicts the schematic diagram of a model that can be used to describe these simultaneous processes, where the

Introduction to Population Pharmacokinetic / Pharmacodynamic Analysis with Nonlinear Mixed Effects Models, First Edition. Joel S. Owen and Jill Fiedler-Kelly.
© 2014 John Wiley & Sons, Inc. Published 2014 by John Wiley & Sons, Inc.

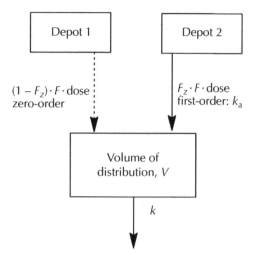

$(1 - F_z) \cdot F \cdot$ dose
zero-order

Depot 1

Depot 2

$F_z \cdot F \cdot$ dose
first-order: k_a

Volume of
distribution, V

k

FIGURE 9.1 Simultaneous absorption model. (Adapted from Chatelut et al. (1999). Copyright © 2001, John Wiley & Sons. All rights reserved.)

variable F_z is the fraction of the dose absorbed by the first-order rate, $1 - F_z$ is the fraction of the dose absorbed by the zero-order rate, V is the volume of distribution in the body, and k is the first-order elimination rate constant. With this basic compartmental model structure, a variety of absorption processes can be described, including:

- One or more zero-order and/or first-order absorption processes
- Serial or parallel absorption from two or more sites
- Absorption lag times on either or multiple compartments
- Known or unknown fractions being absorbed through each route.

Some arrangements of the model features listed can be dealt with using the specific ADVANs (e.g., ADVAN1 or ADVAN2), while other arrangements require user-defined model structures in the general linear or nonlinear ADVANs. Some of these aspects will be briefly described here, with more detailed description and code examples to follow later in this chapter.

If two sequential first-order absorption processes are to be modeled, a single absorption compartment in a specific ADVAN might be used to describe both processes, using the model-change-time parameter (MTIME) in NONMEM. However, the specific ADVANs include at most one absorption site with a single first-order input rate constant. When two or more parallel first-order absorption sites with different rates of input are to be modeled, a separate absorption compartment is needed to account for the mass transfer from each site. Each depot compartment will have a first-order absorption rate constant (e.g., KAFAST and KASLOW). This scenario can be described using a general ADVAN and a model with two depot compartments.

The fraction of the dose entering each of two (or more) depot compartments must be constrained using an approach like that shown in Figure 9.1 using the parameter F_z. Without such constraints, it would be possible for the system to have

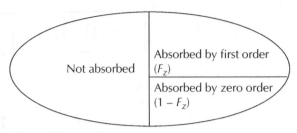

FIGURE 9.2 Illustration of the partitioning of the administered dose.

errors such as adding more drug to the depot compartments than the actual dose amount. This error can occur because using this approach requires that two dosing records be included in the dataset, one for each absorption compartment. The full dose amount must be included in the AMT variable for each depot compartment. As illustrated in Figure 9.2, the F_z and $1 - F_z$ parameters partition the absorbed dose between the two depot compartments.

Individually, F_z and $1 - F_z$ do not represent the absolute bioavailability fraction, F, that we usually consider. F is the total fraction of the administered dose that will be absorbed by any route. F_z represents that fraction of F that will be absorbed through the first-order absorption process. Intravenous data and an alternate coding method would be required to accomplish the simultaneous estimation of the true absolute bioavailability fraction and the fractions of the absorbed dose that are absorbed by each oral absorption process, whether those are both by first order, or by first- and zero-order processes.

In this model, the volume of distribution, V, is the proportionality between observed concentrations in the plasma and the concurrent amount of drug in the body (excluding the absorption sites). The first-order elimination rate constant is denoted k. This modeling approach will be explained in greater detail later in this chapter. At this point, the example is included to demonstrate an occasion in which a user-written model is needed to express a particular PK model.

The standard ADVAN2 routine can be used to model data following the administration of both oral and intravenous doses, another example of a combination of first- and zero-order processes similar to the Chatelut et al. (1999) example explained earlier. Use of ADVAN2 is possible in this case because the specific dose amount administered by the oral and intravenous routes would be known. In the alpha interferon example given earlier, a single dose is administered subcutaneously, yet the dose is absorbed by two different absorption rate processes. Since the fraction absorbed by each rate process is not known and must be estimated, this problem is somewhat more complex. Similar scenarios arise when a dose is administered by nasal or oral inhalation, and part of the dose is absorbed locally, while part is swallowed and absorbed at a different rate in the gastrointestinal (GI) tract. Estimating the fraction absorbed at the two sites is important for an accurate description of the absorption process.

9.2 $MODEL

When using PREDPP, the implementation of user-written models is achieved using one of the PREDPP subroutines ADVAN5, 6, 7, 8, 9, or 13. Use of each of these ADVANs requires a $MODEL block to define the number and properties of the compartments of the model. Compartments are named and properties given using a COMP statement for each compartment in the model. For example, a two-compartment model with parallel zero-order and first-order absorption compartments could be specified as shown in Figure 9.3.

Specification of the $MODEL statement for this scenario might be coded as follows:

```
$MODEL
      COMP(DEPOT1, DEFDOS)
      COMP(DEPOT2)
      COMP(CENTRAL, DEFOBS)
      COMP(PERIPHERAL)
```

Here, DEPOT1, DEPOT2, CENTRAL, and PERIPHERAL are arbitrary names, while DEFDOS and DEFOBS are NONMEM-defined terms with specific meaning. Any alphanumeric name that is not a reserved name can be used to name the compartments, though the use of meaningful names will avoid confusion for the analyst. DEFDOS and DEFOBS define the default compartments for the dose and observation events, respectively. Defining these default properties is needed when the compartment (CMT) data item is not included in the dataset and NM-TRAN must assign the compartment for these events. DEFDOS and DEFOBS can be overridden by the use of CMT in the dataset. By specifying the appropriate compartment number on each dataset record, doses may be entered into and observations made from any compartment. The EVID item is used as it is with any specific ADVAN routine, to describe the type of record. Other compartment options exist, such as defining a compartment that can be turned off or on by default, but these are not used as frequently.

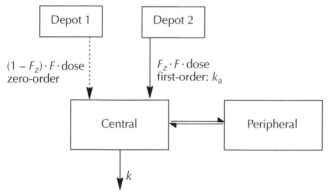

FIGURE 9.3 Two-compartment model with parallel zero-order and first-order drug absorption.

Through PREDPP, NONMEM accounts for the *mass* in each compartment over time. Here, *mass* is used in a mathematical sense and may represent any dependent variable (DV), such as drug concentration, amount, or pharmacodynamic effect. For PK models, the units of predicted values (i.e., mass or concentration) are defined by the relationship of the dose units and the scale parameter of the observation compartment. The analyst must always take care to confirm that the scale parameter appropriately balances the units of predictions and the units of the observations in the dataset, for each compartment in which observations are made. Use of the scale parameter was discussed in detail in Section 3.5.2.2.

9.3 $SUBROUTINES

After the definition of the compartment structure of the model, the relationships between those compartments must be defined, as well as the general numerical analysis methodology that will be used to evaluate the model. The general methodology employed to specify and evaluate the model is governed by the ADVAN routine selected. The relationships and transfer between compartments are generally defined by the parameters and equations in the $PK, $DES, $AES, and $ERROR blocks, if present. The $PK and $ERROR blocks also have been described in Chapter 3 to some extent, but we will elaborate here on the use of these and other blocks for the construction of user-written models.

Selection of a particular ADVAN is accomplished using the $SUBROUTINES statement. When differential equations are used (ADVAN 6, 8, 9, and 13), the number of significant digits to be carried to be accurate in the computation of the compartment amounts must also be specified. This value can be defined using the variable TOL on the $SUBROUTINES statement, for example, $SUBROUTINES ADVAN6 TOL=4. One may consider changing the value of TOL when numerical difficulties are encountered during estimation, when run times are excessively long, or when greater precision in the results is required. The optimal TOL value for a particular problem is a balance between the informativeness of the data, the complexity or nonlinearity of the model, and the precision of the final parameter estimates required.

Alternatively, a $TOL statement may be used to define this value. If needed, with ADVAN9 and 13, separate values can be assigned to the different compartments of the model. TOL is not the number of significant digits in the final parameter values but is related to the number of significant digits used internally for computation of the mass in the compartments.

9.3.1   General Linear Models (ADVAN5 and ADVAN7)

ADVAN5 and ADVAN7 allow the expression of multicompartment models composed of exclusively first-order transfer between compartments. These ADVANs require the control file to state the number of compartments and to define the transfer links between compartments. Models using ADVAN5 and ADVAN7 generally execute more quickly than those that require the expression of the model as differential equations. While model compartments are defined using the $MODEL

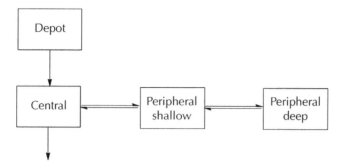

FIGURE 9.4   Catenary compartment model with first-order absorption.

statement, links between compartments are defined in the $PK block using first-order rate constants with the letter K followed by numerical index values defining compartment numbers of the source and destination of mass transfer. For example, the parameter $K12$ defines first-order transfer from compartment 1 to compartment 2. The first index value is the source compartment, and the second index value is the destination compartment. When greater than nine compartments are present, causing the compartment numbers to increase to two-digit numbers, the index values are separated by the capital letter T. For example, transfer from compartment 1 to compartment 10 would be coded as $K1T10$. Elimination of drug from the body is coded with an index value of 0 for the output compartment. Thus, $K20$ represents the first-order transfer of drug from compartment 2 out of the body (e.g., into the urine).

Consider a three-compartment model with first-order absorption with a catenary arrangement of compartments as shown in Figure 9.4.

ADVAN5 and ADVAN7 require that the microrate parameters of transfer be defined as described earlier. However, these may be transformed into any other set of parameters desired. The code below could be used to describe the model in Figure 9.4 in parameters of clearance and volume terms using ADVAN5:

```
$PROBLEM Catenary 3-compartment model with first-order
  absorption
$INPUT ID TIME AMT DV CMT EVID MDV
$DATA filename
$SUBROUTINES ADVAN5
$MODEL                          ; define the parameters of the
  COMP (DEPOT, DEFDOS)          ; model
  COMP (CENTRAL, DEFOBS)
  COMP (PSHALLOW)
  COMP (PDEEP)
$PK
  KA = THETA(1)*EXP(ETA(1))   ; Modeled using Cl & V terms
  V2 = THETA(2)
  CL = THETA(3)*EXP(ETA(2))
  Q1 = THETA(4)
```

```
Q2 = THETA(5)
V3 = THETA(6)
V4 = THETA(7)

K12 = KA              ; Micro-rate parameter
K20 = CL/V2           ; definitions are required
K23 = Q1/V2           ; for ADVAN 5 & 7
K32 = Q1/V3
K34 = Q2/V3
K43 = Q2/V4
```

Through the simple constructs of ADVAN5 and ADVAN7, using only the $MODEL statement and the definition of first-order rate constants in the $PK block, a wide variety of mammillary, catenary, or other models may be easily defined. However, the analyst must always consider whether the model defined is reasonable for its purpose, whether it is identifiable, and whether the data collected are sufficient for the estimation of the model parameters.

9.3.2   General Nonlinear Models (ADVAN6, ADVAN8, ADVAN9, and ADVAN13)

The general nonlinear ADVANs use differential equations to describe the properties of the model and allow nonlinear relationships for mass transfer. A differential equation describing the rate of change of mass in the compartment must be included for each compartment of the model. In addition to the use of differential equations, ADVAN9 also allows the expression of the compartment mass using algebraic equations. Some of the NONMEM literature refers to these as equilibrium compartments. The use of differential equations to express the model gives almost limitless freedom to define the system and is at the heart of the great flexibility of NONMEM.

The major difference between these ADVANs is the particular differential equation solvers used by each for the estimation of model parameters. Some of the methods are optimized for stiff versus nonstiff differential equations (ADVAN8 versus ADVAN6) or use various other numerical methods to solve the differential equations (ADVAN9 and ADVAN13). A discussion of these differences is beyond the scope of this text. However, one approach to selecting the preferred ADVAN method for a particular model and dataset was suggested to the authors in personal communication with Dr. Beal. The method entails writing a control file for each method one wants to compare. The next step is to set MAXEVAL=1 on the $ESTIMATION record line and run the models. Based on comparison of the output from each method, the method that gives a successful first iteration most quickly is likely the method to be preferred for the particular model and dataset combination.

9.3.3 $DES

In pharmacometric applications, systems of differential equations are used to express the instantaneous rate of change of *mass* (i.e., mass, concentration, or effect) in each compartment of a model. The $DES block contains the system of equations, with one equation for each compartment. Each equation is stated using an indexed expression, DADT(i), where i is the compartment number. For example, the first-order disappearance of drug from the depot compartment might be expressed as DADT(1)$=-KA*A(1)$. Here, $A(1)$ is the mass in compartment 1 at the current instant in time.

Equations can be expressed where the rate of change of drug in the compartment is dependent upon the amount of drug in more than one compartment. For instance, the rate of change in concentration in the central compartment of a two-compartment model with first-order absorption and elimination might be expressed as DADT(2)$=KA*A(1) - (K23+K20)*A(2)+K32*A(3)$. A differential equation must also be written to describe the transfer of drug in and out of the peripheral compartment. Thus, a two-compartment disposition model with first-order absorption will actually be expressed as a model with three compartments that are typically numbered as (1) depot, (2) central, and (3) peripheral. The complete system for the model could be stated in the $DES block as:

```
$DES
    DADT(1)  =  -KA * A(1)
    DADT(2)  =   KA * A(1)  -  (K23 + K20)  * A(2)  + K32 * A(3)
    DADT(3)  =   K23 * A(2)  -  K32 * A(3)
```

Inclusion of the absorption, or depot, compartment leads to a renumbering in the NONMEM code of index values from the typical numbering that might be used in the literature to describe a model. For instance, we typically define the transfer of drug from the central to the peripheral compartment of a two-compartment model as $K12$, regardless of the route of administration. Thus, in our aforementioned example, the value $K23$ corresponds to the traditional parameter $K12$. Care must be used in the presentation of final parameter values so their meaning is clear to the reader. Parameterization of models in terms of clearance and volume does not remove this problem since these terms are also indexed based on the index values of the NONMEM compartments, which may vary depending upon the route of drug administration. This issue is not necessarily specific to NONMEM, but is common to any full expression of the PK system to include compartments for absorption.

In this example of a two-compartment model, KA, $K23$, $K20$, and $K32$ are fixed-effect parameters that must be defined in the $PK or $DES blocks and assigned initial values in the $THETA block. NM-TRAN does not have expectations for the parameters of models written with any of the general ADVANs, and the analyst must be careful to correctly define each parameter needed in the model. It is not always necessary, or possible, to estimate every parameter in a model. Some parameters may be fixed to a certain value and not estimated (Wade et al. 1993). The implications of this parameter value assignment to the questions being addressed should be specifically assessed by the analyst where appropriate.

The two-compartment model with first-order absorption is specifically implemented in ADVAN4. When appropriate, the use of ADVAN4 is preferable over the statement of the same model using $DES in a general ADVAN since it may be coded more easily and will execute much more quickly. However, the ability to express the model using the $DES block allows one to easily modify the model and express other models with modifications to this basic structure. For instance, a more complex model might be required to describe the absorption process of a particular drug. Use of ADVAN4 allows for either first-order or zero-order drug input. In both cases, the amount of each dose must be specified using the AMT variable. First-order input is invoked by defining the parameter k_a. Zero-order input can be achieved using the RATE and AMT data items in the dataset and by defining the duration parameter in $PK, as discussed previously in Chapter 4. Beyond simple first- and zero-order input, some absorption models will require the use of multiple absorption compartments with a variety of expressions of the transfers between these compartments.

When modeling in a $DES block, the current value of time is available in the variable T. This value is *more continuous* in nature than the discrete steps of time (i.e., TIME) in the records of the dataset. The step size for T is a function of the numerical algorithm in use. Sometimes in the $DES block, the use of T, rather than TIME, can improve the stability of a nonlinear model, particularly one with time-dependent parameters.

9.4 A SERIES OF EXAMPLES

Several examples will be used to illustrate a variety of approaches for the coding of user-written models. The first examples do not require a general ADVAN to state the problem, although there is unique coding required for each case. The later example demonstrates the use of the general nonlinear ADVANs. The general examples of user-written models presented in this chapter include complex absorption patterns and a nonlinear metabolite model.

9.4.1 Defined Fractions Absorbed by Zero- and First-Order Processes

Consider a hypothetical example where a 300-mg dose of a drug is orally administered in a controlled-release formulation. For the sake of simplicity, we will assume that the first 100 mg undergoes immediate release with no lag time for absorption, the remaining 200 mg is released via a controlled-release formulation, and bioavailability of the compound is complete (i.e., 100%). The formulation is designed such that the second portion of the dose is released beginning at two hours after administration with a controlled-release mechanism that imparts a slower, zero-order absorption process for the remainder of the dose. The first portion of the dose is considered as a bolus administered into the first-order depot compartment (CMT=1), while the second portion of the dose can be thought of as an infusion directly into the central compartment. A conceptual diagram of this scenario is shown in Figure 9.5. The zero-order depot is conceptual and need not be explicitly included in the model. The zero-order dose can simply be coded as a zero-order infusion directly into the central compartment (CMT=2).

Note that the fractional split of the dose between compartments and the time of release for the second compartment are assumed to be known. With these simplifications, the expression of this model can be achieved using ADVAN2. To code

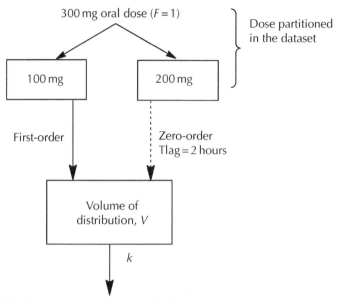

FIGURE 9.5 One-compartment model with first-order and zero-order absorption, dose fractions known and complete bioavailability.

TABLE 9.1 Example dosing records for simultaneous bolus and zero-order input: fixed amounts through each route

ID	TIME	DV	AMT	EVID	RATE	MDV	CMT
1	0	.	100	1	0	1	1
1	0	.	200	1	−2	1	2

the model, the total dose of the drug is divided between two compartments, one with a *fast* first-order absorption rate and one with a *slow* zero-order absorption rate. In this simple example, the fraction of the dose absorbed according to each rate is assumed based on the design of the dosage form. When the fraction for each component is known, splitting the dose into two compartments is a simple step implemented during dataset construction. Two dosing records are needed for each individual dose administered, and the doses would be assigned to CMT = 1 (AMT = 100) for the *fast* portion and CMT = 2 (AMT = 200) for the *slow* portion. The first single dose for the first subject might be coded in the first two dosing records as shown in Table 9.1.

A portion of the control file must consist of defining the model parameters. The delay in the beginning of the *slow* drug absorption process could easily be included using an indexed lag-time parameter, ALAG(*i*), which is available within PREDPP for every compartment. If we assume we know the time the second absorption process begins, we can fix the value of ALAG in the control file (e.g., ALAG2 = 2, since absorption is expected to begin two hours after the dose). Alternatively, if the lag is anticipated to differ between doses based on treatment differences, we can include the lag time (e.g., LAGT) as a data item, then set ALAG2=LAGT in the control file. LAGT in the dataset would contain the value specific to the treatment.

For this example, the initial portion of the control file might be constructed as follows:

```
$PROBLEM First- and Zero-Order Abs.; Known Fractions; F=1
$INPUT ID TIME DV AMT EVID RATE MDV CMT
$DATA    filename
$SUBROUTINES ADVAN2 TRANS2
$PK
     KA = THETA(1)*EXP(ETA(1))
     ALAG2 = 2                  ; Lag for start of zero-order
     D2 = THETA(2)              ; Duration of zero-order input
     CL = THETA(3)*EXP(ETA(2))
     V  = THETA(4)              ; Central compartment volume
     K  = CL/V                  ; Elimination rate constant
```

Use of the RATE data item and $D2$ parameter allows the duration of the zero-order input process to be estimated. The process begins at time ALAG2=2 and continues until the entire drug amount from this process has been absorbed. The duration of that process is estimated through the D2 parameter, based on the best fit of the data. The rate of absorption can be calculated as Rate=AMT/D2. The units of the zero-order rate of input are mass per unit time.

In more common situations, when we do not assume we know the time the second absorption process begins, we can use ALAG2=THETA(i). Here, the estimate of THETA(i) gives the value of the lag time, and no drug absorption from the second compartment begins until time is greater than ALAG2. In this simple example, drug absorption continues from the *fast* first-order compartment until the entire amount of drug that will be absorbed from that compartment has been absorbed. Absorption from the *slow* zero-order compartment begins at TIME=ALAG2 and continues until the entire drug amount that will be absorbed from this route has been absorbed. The two processes may continue simultaneously after TIME reaches ALAG2.

9.4.2 Sequential Absorption with First-Order Rates, without Defined Fractions

Another example includes a change in rate of absorption, but without specifically modeling the fraction absorbed at each rate. This change might occur because the solubility or permeability of the drug changes substantially as the drug proceeds down the GI tract. Consider a case where the absorption rate decreases with time because there is relatively faster absorption in the upper GI tract than the lower. This situation can be expressed using ADVAN2. The time of the change in rate can be defined using *model-event-times* (MTIME(i)) in PREDPP. Multiple model-event-times can be used, and these times are indexed sequentially. If there is only one event time, then MTIME(1) is the estimated time that (in this example) the absorption rate decreases. The event time is estimated by setting it equal to a fixed-effect parameter to be estimated, for example, MTIME(1)=THETA(1). The change in *KA* is implemented using a block of code to estimate each *KA* (e.g., KAFAST and KASLOW), using the logical indicator variable MPAST(1) to test whether the current time has passed the event time. Here, *KA* is a NONMEM-reserved name in ADVAN2. KAFAST and KASLOW are user-defined variable names. MPAST(i), a NONMEM-reserved word, is an indexed NONMEM-defined logical variable having the following values: MPAST(1)=0 if TIME≤MTIME(1), and MPAST(1)=1 if TIME>MTIME(1). The current value of *KA* is set based on the value of MPAST(1). For example:

```
KAFAST = THETA(1)
KASLOW = THETA(2)
MTIME(1) = THETA(3)
KA = KAFAST*(1-MPAST(1)) + KASLOW*(MPAST(1))
```

At times less than or equal to MTIME(1), MPAST(1) has the value *0*, so *KA*=KAFAST. At times greater than MTIME(1), MPAST(1) has the value *1*, so *KA*=KASLOW. Using this approach, this model too can be coded using ADVAN2. Also, only a single dosing record for each dose administered is needed, unlike the case above where a separate dosing record was needed for each depot compartment. Here, since we are using ADVAN2, there is only one depot compartment, and the change in absorption rate is mediated through a change in the absorption rate parameter.

9.4.3 Parallel Zero-Order and First-Order Absorption, without Defined Fractions

A more interesting challenge arises when the amount of the dose absorbed at each rate and the time at which absorption begins are not known. This is similar to the Chatelut et al. (1999) model described in Section 9.1. We can address this problem using a model with each dose administered in full into two compartments, and in which the fraction of the dose entering through each compartment is estimated. To implement such a model, two dosing records must be included in the dataset for each actual dose administered. One dose record is assigned to each of the two dosing compartments. However, the AMT variable on both dosing records should equal the entire dose amount. This scenario can be modeled using ADVAN2 where the depot compartment, CMT=1, is associated with first-order input, and the zero-order input process directly enters the central compartment, CMT=2, like an intravenous infusion. Dosing records might be structured as demonstrated in Table 9.2 for the first subject.

TABLE 9.2   Example dosing records for simultaneous bolus and zero-order input: estimated amounts through each route

ID	TIME	DV	AMT	EVID	RATE	MDV	CMT
1	0	.	300	1	0	1	1
1	0	.	300	1	-2	1	2

The fraction of the absorbed dose that enters through the depot compartment is estimated by defining the NONMEM bioavailability parameter for that compartment as a parameter to be estimated, $F1$ (e.g., $F1$=THETA(1)). The fraction of the absorbed dose entering through the second dosing compartment (i.e., the central compartment) is calculated by subtraction, $F2 = 1 - F1$, and thus partitions the administered dose between the two dosing compartments. If the bioavailability fraction were not used to partition the dose, the two dosing records could imply the absorption of twice the administered dose. These fractions, $F1$ and $F2$, are not the true bioavailability fractions, but are instead the fraction of the absorbed dose that is absorbed by each route. This distinction is illustrated in Figure 9.2. The following code demonstrates how this model can be implemented using ADVAN2 and is one way to code the scenario introduced in Figure 9.1:

```
$PROBLEM Parallel first-order and zero-order absorption
        ; with the fraction absorbed by each route to be
        ; estimated
$INPUT ID TIME AMT DOSE DV EVID RATE MDV CMT
$DATA study01.csv

$SUBROUTINE ADVAN2

$PK
    F1     = THETA(1)          ; DEPOT fraction (first order)
    F2     = 1-F1              ; CENTRAL fraction (zero order)
    ALAG2  = THETA(2)          ; Lag on slower z.o. process; h
    D2     = THETA(3)          ; DURATION Z.O.;   h
    KA     = THETA(4)          ; First-order absorption; 1/h
    TVV2   = THETA(5)
    V2     = TVV2*EXP(ETA(1))  ; Central CMT volume; L
    TVK    = THETA(6)
    K      = TVK*EXP(ETA(2))   ; F.O. elimination rate; 1/h
    S2     = V2/1000           ; DOSE = mg; DV = ng/mL

$ERROR
IPRED = F
Y = F*(1+EPS(1))

$THETA
(0, 0.3, 1)   ; First-order fraction of the dose
(0, 2)        ; Lag for z.o. absorption:    h
(0, 8)        ; Duration of z.o. absorption
(0, 0.35)     ; First-order absorption rate: 1/h
(0, 50)       ; Volume of distribution: L
(0, 0.085)    ; First-order elimination rate constant: 1/h

$OMEGA
0.08
0.08
```

```
$SIGMA
0.04
$ESTIM …          ; Add other code as needed
$TABLE …
```

9.4.4   Parallel First-Order Absorption Processes, without Defined Fractions

A similar situation, but one that changes the coding approach, arises when the two input processes are both first order. In this case, two compartments are needed that can transfer drug by first-order rates of transfer into the central compartment. There is no specific ADVAN that includes this possibility, so one must use one of the general ADVANs and code the structure of the model in the control file. If all transfers in the entire model are first order, then we can use one of the general linear model subroutines (ADVAN5 or ADVAN7).

The dataset for this scenario with two parallel first-order absorption processes must have a dose record into each depot compartment for each administered dose. Since both absorption processes are parallel first-order processes, the RATE data item is not needed, but like the example in Section 9.4.3, the AMT variable should equal the total administered dose amount. Example dosing records for the first subject are shown in Table 9.3.

Assuming two first-order absorption rate processes, this model can be implemented with the following code using a general linear model expression (ADVAN5 or ADVAN7):

```
$PROBLEM Parallel first-order absorption
$INPUT ID TIME DV AMT EVID MDV CMT
$DATA filename
$SUBROUTINE ADVAN5
$MODEL
   COMP (DEPOT1, DEFDOS)
   COMP (DEPOT2)
   COMP (CENTRAL, DEFOBS)

$PK
   F1    = THETA(1)
   F2    = 1 - F1
   ALAG2 = THETA(2)          ; Lag on slower process
   K13   = THETA(3)          ; DEPOT1 -> CENTRAL
   K23   = THETA(4)          ; DEPOT2 -> CENTRAL
   TVV3  = THETA(5)
   V3    = TVV3*EXP(ETA(1))  ; Central CMT volume
   TVK   = THETA(6)
   K30   = TVK*EXP(ETA(2))   ; First-order elim. rate
   S3    = V3/1000           ; DOSE = mg; DV = ng/mL
```

TABLE 9.3 Example dosing records for parallel absorption processes, with estimated amounts absorbed through each route

ID	TIME	DV	AMT	EVID	MDV	CMT
1	0	.	300	1	1	1
1	0	.	300	1	1	2

```
$ERROR
Y = F * (1 + EPS(1))
$THETA ...                      ; Add other code as needed
$OMEGA ...                      ;
$SIGMA ...                      ;
$ESTIM ...                      ;
$TABLE ...                      ;
```

This example is also similar to the scenario in Figure 9.1, except both absorption processes are first order. With two parallel first-order absorption steps, the model cannot be described using a specific ADVAN, and one of the general linear (link models) or nonlinear (differential equation models) ADVANs must be used.

9.4.5 Zero-Order Input into the Depot Compartment

A final model structure we will mention with these sorts of mixed rate absorption processes is one that has a zero-order input into the depot compartment. This is simply an infusion of the drug into the depot, which is then absorbed by a first-order process. This model has some nice properties, giving a *sigmoidal* shape to the absorption profile. The approach has certain advantages over a simple first-order absorption model with lag time. Frequently, the inclusion of lag time parameters can lead to numerical difficulties during estimation. The infusion of drug into the depot can sometimes avoid these numerical issues. With this model structure, the entire dose goes through both input processes, the zero order, followed by the first order. There is only one dose record needed per actual dose administered, that being the infusion dose into the depot. The dose record can have RATE = −2 and the duration of input estimated in the control file with a fixed-effect parameter. Since there is only one dosing record used and the entire dose goes through both input steps, there is no need to divide the dose into separate fractions through each route as with some of the models described earlier.

There are many other drug absorption models that can be constructed, including the transit compartment models, mechanistic absorption models, enterohepatic recycling models, Weibull function models, and many others. Each of these can be expressed in NONMEM using user-written models that extend the properties available in the specific ADVANs. The flexibility of model expression in NONMEM has hopefully been illustrated in this series of absorption models, along with some of the specific coding features of the datasets and control stream code that are needed to implement these models.

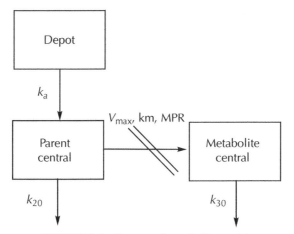

FIGURE 9.6   Parent and metabolite model.

9.4.6   Parent and Metabolite Model: Differential Equations

For a more complex modeling scenario, consider that a drug compound in development is eliminated both renally and by a saturable metabolic process to a single metabolite. Suppose a 100-mg single dose of the parent compound is administered orally, and concentration data are collected for both the parent compound and the metabolite. Simultaneous description of the concentrations of the parent and metabolite for this nonlinear model requires the expression of the model using differential equations. The model is illustrated in Figure 9.6, where MPR is the metabolite-to-parent ratio of molecular weights, k_a is the first-order absorption rate, and $k20$ and $k30$ are the first-order elimination rates for the parent and metabolite, respectively. $A(1)$ is the amount of parent compound in the central compartment at time, t. Saturable elimination is defined via the Michaelis–Menten model parameters V_{max}, the maximum rate of elimination, and k_m, the second compartment amount $(A(2))$ at which the metabolism rate is half maximal. Differential equations to define the model in terms of rates of change in compartment amounts are listed below:

$$\frac{dA(1)}{dt} = -k_a \cdot A(1)$$

$$\frac{dA(2)}{dt} = k_a \cdot A(1) - k20 * A(2) - \frac{V_{max} \cdot A(2)}{k_m + A(2)}$$

$$\frac{dA(3)}{dt} = -k30 * A(3) + \frac{V_{max} \cdot A(2)}{k_m + A(2)} \cdot \text{MPR}$$

Since this model involves the conversion of mass from parent to metabolite, a correction of mass must be implemented between compartment 2 (parent in the central compartment)

TABLE 9.4   Example dosing and observation records for simultaneous modeling of parent and metabolite concentrations

ID	TIME	DV	AMT	EVID	MDV	CMT	
1	0	.	100	1	1	1	◄─── Dose record
1	0.5	46	.	0	0	2	◄─── Parent record
1	0.5	156	.	0	0	3	◄─── Metabolite record

and compartment 3 (metabolite in the central compartment). This can be implemented in the dataset directly, by scaling the metabolite concentrations to the mass equivalent of the parent compound. Alternatively, appropriate terms in the transfer equations can be multiplied by the ratio of molar masses in the differential equations.

The dataset structure for this model requires that the parent and metabolite concentrations be listed in the same DV column, and the type of observation is indicated by the compartment number (CMT=2 for parent and CMT=3 for metabolite). A few example records are shown in Table 9.4.

Here, the DV item indicates observed concentration values, while CMT=2 indicates that the concentration is in the central compartment for the parent compound and CMT=3 indicates that the concentration is in the central compartment for the metabolite.

This model could be implemented using the following code in a control file:

```
$PROBLEM Model of Parent and Metabolite Concentrations
$INPUT ID TIME DV AMT EVID MDV CMT
$DATA filename
$SUBROUTINE ADVAN6 TOL=4
$MODEL
   COMP (DEPOT, DEFDOS)
   COMP (CENTPRNT, DEFOBS)
   COMP (CENTMETB)
$PK
   K20  = THETA(1)*EXP(ETA(1))
   V2   = THETA(2)*EXP(ETA(2))
   KA   = THETA(3)
   VMAX = THETA(4)
   KM   = THETA(5)
   K30  = THETA(6)
   V3   = THETA(7)
   S2   = V2/1000
   S3   = V3/1000

$DES
   DADT(1) = -KA*A(1)
   DADT(2) = KA*A(1) - K20*A(2) - (VMAX*A(2))/(KM + A(2))
   DADT(3) = -K30*A(3) + ((VMAX*A(2))/(KM + A(2)))*MPR
```

```
$ERROR
   IF (CMT.EQ.2) TYPE=0            ;Parent concentration
   IF (CMT.EQ.3) TYPE=1            ;Metabolite concentration

Y = F*EPS(1)*(1-TYPE) + F*EPS(2)*TYPE

$THETA ...                        ; Add other code as needed
$OMEGA ...                        ;
$SIGMA ...                        ;
$ESTIM ...                        ;
$TABLE ...                        ;
```

A parent and metabolite model like this is not uniquely identifiable for the metabolite since both the fraction of the parent converted to the metabolite and the volume of distribution of the metabolite are not simultaneously known. In other words, neither the mass in the metabolite compartment nor its volume is known specifically if only the parent compound is administered, even though metabolite concentrations are observed. The model can be uniquely identified, only if the extent of conversion is characterized from a prior ADME study or if the clearance or volume of distribution of the metabolite is measured by administration of the metabolite directly. Regardless of the unique identification of the metabolite parameters, the model can be useful to characterization of observed concentrations and other purposes.

Other common applications of the general ADVANs certainly include the mechanistic enzyme induction models, transit compartment absorption models, target-mediated models, and the specification of most PK/pharmacodynamic models. These models are not included in any of the specific ADVANs and can require a wide array of structures. The coding of pharmacodynamic models is addressed in detail in Chapter 10.

REFERENCES

Chatelut E, Rostaing L, Grégoire N, Payen J-L, Pujol A, Izopet J, Houin G, Canal P. A pharmacokinetic model for alpha interferon administered subcutaneously. Br J Clin Pharmacol 1999;47:365–371.

Wade JR, Kelman AW, Howie CA, Whiting B. Effect of misspecification of the absorption process on subsequent parameter estimation in population analysis. J Pharmacokinet Biopharm 1993; 21 (2):209–222.

CHAPTER 10

PK/PD MODELS

10.1 INTRODUCTION

Most of the discussion up to this point in our text has been in regard to pharmacokinetics (PK) alone. However, PK considerations in the development and clinical use of drugs generally have a supportive role. Primary questions of interest to the physician and pharmacist, once a particular drug has been selected for use, are *how much* and *how often* should the drug be administered to a particular patient. Though these are specifically kinetic concepts of extent and rate, the clinician is essentially asking questions of safety and efficacy, which when considered quantitatively we call pharmacodynamics (PD). PK questions are generally not primary, though they are an essential piece of the landscape over which the clinical decisions must be made.

Definitions of acceptable safety and adequate efficacy are specific to each drug and indication. Defining these and determining the questions of primary interest during drug development require significant input from a multidisciplinary team including clinicians and thought leaders in the field. The team must understand the clinical context of the disease to be treated and of currently available drug therapy to effectively assess the potential for a new drug. Considerations of pharmacology, chemistry, pharmaceutics, regulatory, pharmacoeconomics, and other disciplines contribute valuable input to the team in constructing the questions of primary importance for the development of the product. Defining the primary questions to be addressed in the development program is often enabled by preparing a target product profile early in the development process. Crafting the target product profile encourages disciplined thought regarding the questions of interest and the data needed to address those questions.

The pharmacometrician must translate these questions of interest into quantitative expressions and ensure that sufficient data are collected to allow the successful use of pharmacostatistical models to address these important questions. Perhaps of equal or greater importance to the value of their contribution, the pharmacometrician must be able to communicate the findings of modeling results to the team in clear terms that inform the decision-making process. Graphical representation of models and their implications can be of great benefit to that communication. A clinician does not need to understand the mathematical details of a complex system of differential equations in order to appreciate the behavior of a model and the extent to which this model answers

Introduction to Population Pharmacokinetic / Pharmacodynamic Analysis with Nonlinear Mixed Effects Models, First Edition. Joel S. Owen and Jill Fiedler-Kelly.
© 2014 John Wiley & Sons, Inc. Published 2014 by John Wiley & Sons, Inc.

interesting questions about drug effects. The pharmacometrician should compose the presentation of modeling results in a way that directly supports decision making by the project team.

Pharmacometricians must have excellent modeling skills as well. Disease processes and drug action are complex in nature and require significant skill to model quantitatively. Frequently, PD models must consider issues of baseline response, relationship to PK, disease progression, development of tolerance, and many other factors. In addition, PD data may be continuous or discrete (e.g., binary or categorical). These considerations make PD models inherently more complex than most PK models. As an introduction to PK/PD modeling with NONMEM, this chapter will focus primarily on typical PD models of continuous data.

10.2 IMPLEMENTATION OF PD MODELS IN NONMEM

The particular approach to implementation of PD models depends on the characteristics of the data and the questions to be answered. Direct linear or nonlinear regression can be performed between dependent and independent variables using $PRED. Alternatively, the PD model may be expressed using PREDPP in a couple of ways. If the PK model can be described by one of the specific ADVANs (i.e., ADVAN1–4 and 10–12), and the PD model is simple enough to be expressed algebraically, a specific ADVAN may be used with the PD model expressed in the $ERROR block. For more complex PK or PD models, the general ADVANs (i.e., ADVAN5–9 or ADVAN13) may be used. We will consider examples of each of these approaches in this chapter.

In addition to considerations of which algorithms to use, there are a variety of modeling processes that may be followed in fitting PK and PD models. Since PK/PD models can be quite complex, the data and modeling process requirements must be considered carefully. PK/PD models can be developed by either simultaneously fitting the PK and PD parameters or by sequentially fitting the PK followed by the PD parameters. The selection of the process to use is at least in part, a balancing of the precision of the final parameter estimates against the substantial time requirements for execution of some processes.

Simultaneous fitting of a PK/PD model is the most computationally intensive approach and typically the most time consuming. When a large number of parameters are being estimated simultaneously, models may suffer from stability problems in estimation, which will additionally prolong the run times. When the data are sufficient to estimate all the parameters simultaneously, this approach is considered the *gold standard* since there is interplay between the parameters of PK and PD in both directions (Wade and Karlsson 1999; Zhang et al. 2003).

Sequential fitting is a two-step process. First, PK model parameters are estimated using a PK model and only the PK data. From these results, PK parameters or estimates of exposure are subsequently used as input in the PD model. This approach is easier to implement, and run times will generally be much shorter when compared to a simultaneous approach. Once the PK model has been estimated and parameters or exposure measures have been determined, there are at least three options for estimation of the PD model as shown in Table 10.1. First, the individual

TABLE 10.1 Three options for estimation of the PD models

Option	Parameters that have fixed values	Dataset for estimating PD model contains
1	PK = Individual estimates	PD observations
2	PK = Population estimates	PD observations
3	PK = Population estimates	PK and PD observations

conditional estimates of parameters of the PK model can be fixed, while the PD model parameters are estimated using only the PD data. Second, the typical values of the population PK parameters can be fixed, while the PD model parameters are estimated using only the PD data. And finally, the typical values of the population PK parameters can be fixed, while the PD model parameters are estimated and have both the PK and PD data present in the dataset.

These PK/PD modeling approaches were described and compared by Zhang et al. (2003). These authors observed that sequential approaches minimize more quickly and more often, at least when using the classical estimation methods in NONMEM. In addition, when comparing the fitting options, sequential approaches that fixed the PK parameters to the population values, but included both the PK and PD data in the dataset were preferable, in that they yielded PD model parameter estimates that were similar in value and precision to those of simultaneous fitting, and did so in about 40% of the time required for simultaneous fitting.

10.3 $PRED

Using the $PRED block is efficient with relatively simple models such as some direct-effect models. Unlike PREDPP, PRED does not account for the context of the model; it does not have an internal representation of time or compartment amounts as PREDPP does. Thus, each record in the dataset must contain all of the information required for evaluation of the model, and no *missing* values are permitted, as these would be interpreted as zero values. Dataset construction for this type of model can be relatively simple since there are no dosing- or *other*-type records, and there is no continuity between records that must be built into the dataset, except that the records of an individual subject must be kept together. Other independent variables (e.g., treatment group, dose, concentration, exposure measure, sex, age, and weight) may be included in the dataset but must not be missing on any record if they are used in the model. These independent variables may be stationary or time varying. Sometimes, it is useful to include the subject's baseline PD value as a separate (constant valued) data item. In this way, the baseline may be used as a covariate in the model, when appropriate, or it may be used for graphical or data summarization purposes.

When using $PRED to implement a PD model, the control file must define the observed value of the dependent variable (Y) in terms of the individual predicted value (F), and a residual error term (EPS(i)). Pharmacokinetics may enter these models if the dataset contains the needed concentration values on each record, or if the concentration is predicted through algebraic equations using only the information available from each record. The latter is sometimes more complex in multiple-dosing situations since PRED does not account for the dosing history of a patient. The algebraic equations must themselves include the multiple dosing nature of the data. This is achievable for some circumstances, but will generally require the assumption of constant dose amounts given in equal and precise dosing intervals, since no dosing records are included in the dataset for a model specified through $PRED.

10.3.1 Direct-Effect PK/PD Examples: PK Concentrations in the Dataset

An example of the utility of the PRED approach is the exploration of a relationship between maximum drug concentration (C_{max}) and maximum change from baseline in corrected QT interval of the electrocardiogram (ΔQTc). This example is not put forward as an endorsement of this approach to the analysis of such cardiac data but is simply used as a demonstration of how one might code this type of model using $PRED.

Each record in the dataset contains both a PK value (C_{max}) and a PD value (ΔQTc). A few rows of data might be constructed as shown in Table 10.2.

With a single observation per subject, two levels of random effects would be confounded, and the model would not be identifiable. In this simple example, with one observation per subject, one might structure a linear model with a single level random effect (L1) as follows.

```
$PROB    QTc, PRED
$INPUT   ID=DROP DQTC=DV CMAX
$DATA data.csv IGNORE=C      ; Since the header row
                             ; starts with a C, that row
                             ; is dropped
$PRED
   INT = THETA(1)            ; Intercept
   SLP = THETA(2)            ; Slope
   EFF = SLP*CMAX + INT      ; Drug effect model - linear
   Y   = EFF + ETA(1)        ; Residual error model -
                             ; additive

$EST PRINT=5 MAX=9999 SIG=3

$THETA
   0.1                       ; Intercept
   0.5                       ; Slope

$OMEGA
   0.04                      ; Magnitude of Additive error
```

The ID data item is dropped by NMTRAN, since with only one random-effect level all data are treated as if they come from a single subject, or more precisely, there is no subject level in the model. The PD value is the DV under analysis, and thus the DQTC data item is identified in the $INPUT line as the DV data item. The independent

TABLE 10.2   Example of data for use with a model in $PRED

CID	DQTC	C_{max}
1001	3.6	54.9
1002	4.9	48.6
1003	2.1	35.2
1004	6.3	65.1
1005	5.2	55.6
1006	3.5	40.2
...	...	...

variable, CMAX, is an element of the dataset and defined in the $INPUT statement. The model relates these independent and DVs through a linear regression model. INT and SLP are the intercept and slope parameters of the linear model, respectively. EFF is the predicted effect, or ΔQTc.

ΔQTc is identified as the DV data item, and thus is associated by NONMEM with the Y value in the residual error model. This association is made automatically by NONMEM. The residual error model, or the relationship between Y and the predicted value, EFF, is defined explicitly.

Note that because IGNORE=C is included on the $DATA statement and the first character of the first row of the dataset is a C, this header row is dropped by NMTRAN when the data file is read. In this way, the header row can be included for the human reader of the dataset, but the character data are dropped as required when NONMEM reads the dataset.

The following is another example of a direct-effect model coded using $PRED, which in this case uses a PK value from the dataset (CONC) to fit a Hill function with multiple random effects to a set of PD data. Estimating multiple levels of random effects assumes we have multiple observations per subject, at least for many members of the dataset.

```
$PRED
EMAX = THETA(1) * EXP(ETA(1))        ; Emax - maximum effect
EC50 = THETA(2) * EXP(ETA(2))        ; EC50 - conc. of half
                                     ; Emax
GAMMA = THETA(3)                     ; Gamma - shape
                                     ; parameter
BL = THETA(4) * EXP(ETA(3))          ; Baseline PD value
N = EMAX * (CONC**GAMMA)             ; Numerator-Hill
                                     ; Equation
D = (EC50**GAMMA) + (CONC**GAMMA)    ; Denominator-Hill
                                     ; Equation
EFF = BL - (N/D)                     ; Effect of drug is to
                                     ; decrease the baseline
Y = EFF + EPS(1)                     ; residual error model
```

Here, CONC is the simultaneous drug concentration eliciting the immediate reduction in PD response. The ETA terms are level 1 random effects describing intersubject differences in PD parameters. EPS(1) is a level 2 random effect of the residual error model. Level 1 effects are constant for the individual and vary between subjects. Level 2 effects are at the observation level and differ between observations within a subject. No PK model is assumed or estimated in this example. PK is included simply as the concentration measurements obtained simultaneously with the PD measures. Using this approach, a PK value is required with each PD value. If the PK value were not present, either the corresponding PD value would have to be dropped, or a PK value would have to be imputed, perhaps through some interpolation or assumption of the model.

In this example, the PD baseline value is estimated in the model. Even in cases where the baseline is measured, one might want to not only include the measured baseline value as the first record in the dataset for each subject but also estimate the baseline as a parameter of the model. If we use the observed baseline as a fixed value, then we assume we know the value without error. Modeling the baseline as a parameter allows us to estimate the magnitude of variability in the baseline and explore the influence covariates may have in explaining that between-subject variability. As mentioned previously, we may also want to keep the baseline value as a constant valued data item on every record (in a separate column from the DV column) in order to use the baseline as a covariate on other parameters in the model.

10.3.2 Direct-Effect PK/PD Example: PK from Computed Concentrations

Direct-effect PK/PD models can also be constructed where the PK concentrations are computed from individual subject parameters. For example, concentrations at any time-after-dose, tad, in the nth dosing interval of length, τ, for a drug having first-order absorption and first-order elimination can be predicted with the following equation:

$$C(\text{dose}, tad, \tau) = \frac{F \cdot \text{dose} \cdot k_a}{V(k_a - k)} \left[\frac{(1 - e^{-nk\tau})}{(1 - e^{-k\tau})} e^{-k \cdot tad} - \frac{(1 - e^{-nk_a\tau})}{(1 - e^{-k_a\tau})} e^{-k_a \cdot tad} \right]$$

This equation could be coded into a $PRED block to calculate the concentration in the plasma at any time in the dosing interval, whether that interval follows the first dose, n doses, or enough doses to be considered to be at steady state. The equation is constructed on the assumption that all doses were given at the scheduled time and with the constant dosing interval, τ. To use this with $PRED, every record of the dataset must contain values of each of the PK variables, tad, n, and τ, as well as the individual subject PK parameters, k_a, V, and k. If a value is missing on a record, it will be treated as a zero value, which may lead to unanticipated or undesired results. The PD model can be included by including additional code as in the examples described earlier.

It should be noted that each of these models relates the PD response directly to the simultaneous concentration in the plasma. These are not models based on effect site concentrations. Their advantage is relative simplicity in dataset construction and the relative speed at which parameter estimation will occur.

10.4 $PK

While modeling with $PRED has the advantages of relative simplicity and ease of dataset construction, modeling with PREDPP (invoked by $PK) provides power and flexibility that is perhaps not available in any other program. Using PREDPP, one gains access to the tools provided for managing time, compartment amounts, repeated doses, multiple routes of dosing, optimized specific PK models, a variety of differential equation solvers, and so on. These have been discussed previously in the text, and they are just as beneficial for combined modeling of PK and PD.

However, along with this richness, using PREDPP also brings in greater complexity of the dataset structure and control code as were discussed in Chapters 3 and 4. As various PK/PD model approaches are explored during a modeling exercise, sometimes it is necessary to reformat the dataset to accommodate changes in the model to be estimated. Simultaneous modeling of PK and PD requires particular formatting of the dataset. As with PK data alone, the dataset for analysis with PREDPP must specify the time-ordered sequence of all events by individual in the dataset. Each record must correspond to only one type of event, whether a dose, a PK or PD observation, or an *other-type* event such as changing the value of a time-dependent covariate. Dosing records for drug administration are generally required, and in some circumstances, a *dose* record may be used to initialize the amount in the PD compartment. One of the ways the initial condition, or amount in a PD compartment, can be set is as a bolus dose record into that compartment. All DV values (i.e., observations) are placed in the DV data item column of the dataset, both for PK and PD observations. The compartment (CMT) item is used to assign the record to either a PK or a PD compartment. The options that PREDPP provides make it a very flexible tool, but one for which a thorough understanding of the models and the program are required.

10.4.1 Specific ADVANs (ADVAN1–ADVAN4 and ADVAN10–ADVAN12)

When using the specific ADVANs in NONMEM, the system is optimized for PK analysis. NONMEM has certain *expectations* for the compartments and parameters that will be included. There is flexibility with these, but that is primarily in the parameterizations of the models, routes of input, and whether or not there is an absorption or output compartment. These ADVANs were not primarily written for modeling PD effects or for joint PK/PD models. Within a certain range of models though, PK/PD models can be implemented with the specific ADVANs.

One approach that can be used for effect compartment link models, when the PK can be expressed as a one-compartment model, is to use ADVAN3 or ADVAN4 and assign the peripheral compartment interpretation to be that of the effect site concentration. The transfer rate constant from the central into the peripheral compartment must be fixed to a very small fraction of the elimination rate constant so an insignificant mass transfer takes place. The scale parameter for the peripheral compartment is set so that at steady state, the effect site concentration equals the central compartment concentration. The transfer rate constant from the peripheral compartment back to the central compartment then has the usual interpretation of k_{eo} in these models.

Code for the Hill model structure of the PD model is placed in the $ERROR block and includes the concentration in the peripheral compartment as the driver of PD effect.

The dataset for this approach will include a CMT item. If CMT = 1 (i.e., the central compartment for ADVAN3), then the observation is a PK concentration. If CMT = 2, then the observation is a PD concentration. This assignment in itself does not adjust the amount in the second compartment—that amount is the effect site drug concentration, not the effect itself. Instead, the CMT item is used here as a *switch* in the $ERROR block to select between two residual variability models, one for PK and one for PD. If PK and PD data are collected at the same time, the corresponding records should have the same time value. An illustration of this approach is given in the example provided with NONMEM: *PK_PD_ simultaneous_1_example (pkpdsim1.exa)* (Beal et al. 1989–2011). This type of model was first developed by Sheiner et al. to describe the PK/PD properties of D-tubocurarine (Sheiner et al. 1979).

Here the PD model is fully specified algebraically in the $ERROR block. PREDPP has no programmed expectations of the PD component of the model with these specific ADVANs. Also, as will generally be necessary for combined PK and PD models, there are separate residual variability models for PK and PD. As each record is processed during parameter estimation, the appropriate residual variability model is selected by the use of the CMT data item. The value of CMT serves as a logical switch to assign the correct residual error model. The values of CMT must correspond to the definitions given to the compartments defined by the ADVAN.

10.4.2   General ADVANs (ADVAN5–ADVAN9 and ADVAN13)

The general ADVANs give much more flexibility to the implementation of PK/ PD models. Models built using the general ADVANs typically include one or more PD compartments, which are defined in the $MODEL statement. The definition of the PD model may be included in the $ERROR block when it is simple enough or more commonly as a compartment amount defined by the general linear or general nonlinear ADVANs. When a general ADVAN is used, the values of CMT must correspond to the definitions given to the compartments defined by the $MODEL statement.

A nonstandard PK model that does not fit into the specific ADVANs may create the need to use a general ADVAN even though the PD model is simple enough to be included in the $ERROR block. The following example demonstrates the use of ADVAN6 with a differential equation approach to model the PK and effect site concentrations of a drug. The PD model is resolved in the $ERROR block.

10.4.3   PREDPP: Effect Compartment Link Model Example (PD in $ERROR)

The following code example describes a two-compartment PK model, with an effect site concentration in the third compartment. The PK model has first-order elimination from both the central and peripheral compartments, in accordance with a model of Hoffman elimination (Schmith et al. 1997).

```
$SUBROUTINES ADVAN6 TOL=5
$MODEL
  COMP = (CENTRAL, DEFDOSE, DEFOBS)   ;PK-Central
  COMP = PERIPH                       ;PK-Peripheral
  COMP = EFFECT                       ;Effect site conc.
$PK
  TVCL   = THETA(1)*(CRCL/MDCC)**THETA(2)
  CL     = TVCL*EXP(ETA(1))
  TVV    = THETA(3)*(WTKG/MDWT)**THETA(4)
  V      = TVV*EXP(ETA(2))
  Q      = THETA(5)
  VP     = THETA(6)

  K20    = 0.0237                     ;mean in vitro value
  K10    = (CL/V) - (K20*VP)/V
  K12    = Q/V
  K21    = (Q/VP) - K20

  S1     = V1/1000
  TVK30  = THETA(7) + THETA(8)*SEXF
  K30    = TVK30*EXP(ETA(3))

  EMAX   = 100
  GAMMA  = THETA(9)
  TVC50  = THETA(10)
  C50    = TVC50*EXP(ETA(4))

$DES
  DADT(1)=K21*A(2)-(K12+K10)*A(1)     ;Central CMT PK
  DADT(2)=K12*A(1)-(K21+K20)*A(2)     ;Peripheral CMT PK
  AA=A(1)*1000
  DADT(3)=K30*(AA/V-A(3))         ;Effect site concentration

$ERROR
  Q = 1                               ;PK record flag
  IF (CMT.EQ.3) Q = 0                 ;PD record flag
  Y1=F*EXP(EPS(1))                    ;RV model for PK
  NUM = EMAX*(F**GAMMA)
  DEN = EC50**GAMMA + F**GAMMA
  Y2 = NUM/DEN + EPS(2)               ;RV model for PD
  Y = Q*Y1 + (1-Q)*Y2                 ;Assignment of RV model
```

The model gives an example of covariate adjusted PK parameters. Clearance is expressed as a power function relationship based on the median-centered creatinine clearance (MDCC). Volume of the central compartment is a power function centered on the median patient weight in kilograms (MDWT). The values of MDCC and MDWT could be included on every record of the dataset or hard coded into the control stream.

This example demonstrates one way to approach the analysis of data for which the PK properties are not described by one of the specific ADVANs, but the

PD properties are simple enough to be included in the $ERROR block. The code above demonstrates the PK being described using differential equations in ADVAN6. Alternatively, since every transfer rate is first order, the model could have been coded using ADVAN5 or ADVAN7. This exemplifies the variety and flexibility of coding methods available in NONMEM, which allows for the expression of many models. However, the user must understand the implications of the code he writes.

10.4.4 PREDPP: Indirect Response Model Example: PD in $DES

Other PD models require that the PD component of the model be expressed using PD *mass* in one or more compartments of the model. They are too complex to fit within a specific ADVAN or to be expressed algebraically using code for the PD model in the $ERROR block. Experience and an understanding regarding the function of the various components of NONMEM will aid in deciding which approach is most appropriate for a given situation.

The class of indirect-response models, illustrated in Figure 10.1, is an example of a group of models that require the use of PD compartments. Indirect response models include one or more compartments for which the *mass* in the compartments is the magnitude of the PD response or its precursors. There is at least one input to the response compartment, frequently modeled as a zero-order process, and at least one elimination route, frequently modeled as a first-order process. The indirect response component depicts the drug concentration or exposure measures as either stimulating or inhibiting the input or elimination rate of the response.

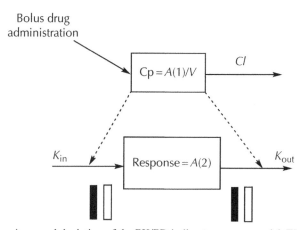

FIGURE 10.1 A general depiction of the PK/PD indirect response model. The black rectangles indicate the inhibition of either input or output rates of the response and the white rectangles indicate the stimulation of the rate of change in response. (Adapted from: Springer, © 1997 Plenum Publishing Corporation, J Pharm Biopharm 1997:25(1):107–123. Figure 1. Mathematical Formalism for the Properties of Four Basic Models of Indirect Pharmacodynamic Responses. Krzyzanski W and Jusko WJ. With kind permission from Springer Science+Business Media B.V.)

The following code demonstrates sequential PK/PD modeling for an indirect response model. The model includes one compartment PK with the drug concentration in the central compartment inhibiting the production of the effect.

```
$PROB Indirect Response Model - One Compartment PK
$DATA ID DV CMT … … BSLN ICL IV    ; Showing only the IDR
                                   ; required data items
$SUBROUTINES ADVAN8 TOL=3
$MODEL
  NCOMP = 2
  COMP = CENTRAL
  COMP = RESPONSE
$PK
  CL = ICL
  V  = IV
  KEL = CL/V
  K0 = THETA(1)*EXP(ETA(1))        ; K0 is the estimate of
                                   ; the zero-order input
                                   ; at baseline.

  KOUT = THETA(2)*EXP(ETA(2))
  IMAX = THETA(3)*EXP(ETA(3))
  IC50 = THETA(4)*EXP(ETA(4))

  S1 = V
  A_0(2) = BSLN                    ; Sets the initial
                                   ; condition of the PD
                                   ; Response

$DES
  CP = A(1)/V
  DADT(1) = -KEL*A(1)
  KIN = K0*(1-IMAX*CP/IC50+CP))    ; The modeled input rate
  DADT(2) = KIN -KOUT*A(2)

$ERROR
  Q = 1                            ; PK record flag
  IF (CMT.EQ.2) Q = 0              ; PD record flag
  Y1=F*EXP(EPS(1))                 ; RV model for PK
  Y2 = F + EPS(2)                  ; RV model for PD
  Y = Q*Y1 + (1-Q)*Y2              ; Assignment of RV model
```

(...plus other code...)

Other code might also be added, including $ESTIM, $COV, or $TABLE steps. Also, the input line only shows the data items relevant to this discussion. Others may be needed as well.

The code above demonstrates a sequential modeling process where the individual subject PK parameters from previous PK modeling are included in the dataset (i.e., ICL and IV). Invoking ADVAN8 indicates the model will be expressed using differential equations and defines the specific differential equation solver that will be used. The $MODEL statement defines two compartments of the model, CENTRAL for PK and RESPONSE for PD.

The PK parameters are assigned to the individual subject estimates stored in the dataset (e.g., CL=ICL). The PD parameters are estimated with exponential intersubject variability for each parameter. K0 represents the zero-order steady-state baseline input rate of PD response and KOUT the first-order elimination of the response. IMAX is the fractional, maximum extent of inhibition of response and IC50 is the drug concentration that elicits 50% of the maximal reduction in response. The scale compartment parameter is set equal to the volume for the PK compartment. Since the *amount* of RESPONSE is modeled directly and in the units of the observations, no scale parameter is needed for the RESPONSE compartment.

BSLN, like ICL and IV, is a user-defined data item, and NONMEM has no understanding of its value until it is defined in the $PK block. The value of BSLN is the individual subject baseline observed PD value. These values are sometimes included on every row of the dataset. The value of BSLN included on the first record of every individual is used to initialize the amount in the PD compartment (via the A_0(2)=BSLN statement), and in addition because it is included on every row of the dataset, BSLN may be used for grouping or summarizing the output data in tables or figures, or it may be used as a covariate of other model parameters, where appropriate.

In the $DES block, the concentration in the PK compartment is defined as the amount in the first compartment (i.e., CENTRAL) divided by the volume of distribution. The instantaneous rate of change of drug in this compartment is given by the first differential equation, DADT(1), which defines the first-order elimination of drug from this compartment. Drug input in this example is by intravenous bolus, the description of which would be included only in the dataset, where dosing records are assigned to CMT=1. The instantaneous input rate, KIN, is defined as an inhibitory Imax model, dependent upon the drug concentration in the first compartment, and the values of Imax and IC50, and the baseline input rate, KIN.

Alternatively, this code might be adapted to include an effect site compartment that would drive the PD response. Or, there might be precursor compartments in the PD model, where drug may first effect changes in precursor amount through inhibitory or stimulatory actions. The flexibility of NONMEM coding allows one to describe a seemingly endless arrangement of models. The user must be careful to evaluate the sufficiency of the data to inform the estimation of the parameters being estimated and the underlying identifiability of the model.

10.5 ODD-TYPE DATA: ANALYSIS OF NONCONTINUOUS DATA

In addition to continuous endpoints, PD analyses can be performed where the endpoint is discrete or categorical using the LAPLACIAN estimation method of NONMEM. Noncontinuous data in the NONMEM literature have been termed *odd-type* data. Examples of the types and analysis methods are given in Table 10.3.

The methods for analyzing odd-type data in NONMEM are beyond the scope of this introductory text. There are excellent chapters with code examples in the book

TABLE 10.3 Examples of noncontinuous data types

Data type	Analysis method	Example
Dichotomous-binomial	Logistic regression	Cure/fail
Multinomial ordered categorical	Proportional odds	Pain scores
Count data	Poisson regression	Adverse event counts

Pharmacometrics (Ette 2007). Just a few brief comments are provided here on some differences between fitting continuous and odd-type data. The LAPLACIAN method is used most commonly for these data. When using the LAPLACIAN estimation method for noncontinuous data, the following estimation options are commonly used in order to specify the model as a likelihood or −2*log-likelihood, respectively: LIKELIHOOD and −2LL. The NONMEM reserved variable F_FLAG has defined values indicating whether F is the typical value (as for continuous data), a likelihood, or a −2LL value. This variable is also useful with the simultaneous estimation of continuous (e.g., PK) and noncontinuous (e.g., PD) data.

If both continuous PK and noncontinuous PD data are to be analyzed together, the dataset should be organized as any other PK/PD dataset and should include an additional indicator variable for the observation type. If PREDPP is not called, the PK or exposure data should be paired with the PD endpoints on every record. There is no DV data item with PRED, so the PK and PD data may be included as separate data items (i.e., in separate columns).

A section of the code that shows the expression of a logistic regression PD model in $PRED is shown here.

```
$PRED
     LOGIT = THETA(1) + THETA(2)*(AUC-118) + ETA(1)
     A = EXP(LOGIT)
     P = A/(1 + A)
     IF (DV.EQ.1) Y = P
     IF (DV.EQ.0) Y = 1 - P

$EST METHOD = COND LAPLACIAN LIKELIHOOD
$COV MATRIX = R
```

This model relates the centered exposure estimate (AUC − 118) to the probability of response using a linear logit.

10.6 PD MODEL COMPLEXITY

Pharmacodynamic processes are subject to a number of effects that may cause the system to change over time. A baseline PD value, such as blood pressure, heart rate, pain score, glucose level, body weight, and so on, may change in response to the presence of a drug, that is, the drug effect, but it may also change for such reasons as progression of disease, biological feedback systems, or the development of tolerance to the effect of the drug. In addition, just the participation in a trial, even when only receiving a placebo treatment, may cause a change in the response variable, that is, the *placebo effect*. In order to account for the time course of drug effect, these factors of nonstationarity in the PD model must be addressed. These are frequently complex models that require the general linear or nonlinear ADVANS of NONMEM.

Frequently, a PD model must account for the effect of placebo treatment in addition to the effect of drug. When drug response is measured over time, particularly when placebo and active treatments are administered in parallel groups, one must make assumptions about the role of the placebo effect in the treated group. It is commonly assumed that the drug treatment is additive to the placebo effect, though other models could be conceived. Over longer periods of study, even disease progression might need to be accounted for in the model. Such models have been developed for the cognitive decline in Alzheimer's patients over the duration of long clinical trials (William-Faltaos et al. 2013).

A broader use of PK/PD models is to balance models of PD response for both safety and efficacy in a clinical utility model to quantitate the benefit versus risk profile and optimize dose selection. The evaluation of a candidate product can be enhanced through such quantitative approaches. The methods introduced in the chapter are some of the building blocks for such models (Poland et al. 2009).

10.7 COMMUNICATION OF RESULTS

An essential skill of the pharmacometrician is the ability to communicate the results and implications of models to the project team, stakeholders, physicians, pharmacists, and even the public. PK/PD models can be quite technical and complex, but their great utility is in the ability to use them to answer questions of clinical interest.

At the beginning of a project, the pharmacometrician must be involved with project team members, management, business development, thought leaders, clinicians, and regulators to establish the important questions the modeling exercise is intended to answer. Starting with clearly formulated questions will improve the effectiveness in the exercise of answering key questions. Clearly formulated questions will also help focus the presentation of conclusions of the modeling. A number of issues that should be considered for the clear communication of PK/PD model results include the following:

- Are the appropriate questions addressed?
- Is the basic behavior of the model explained?
- Are assumptions stated explicitly and the ramifications of violations of the assumptions understood?
- Are there clear graphical representations of models and results?
- Has a meaningful *story line* been used to explain the data, the model, and the implications to the questions of interest?
- Are appropriate summary statistics presented to evaluate the outcome of the model with clinically oriented tabulations of observed effects?

The issue of communication is brought up briefly in this chapter on PK/PD models since this is an area of modeling which frequently addresses the critical clinical issues of safety and efficacy. The pharmacometrician must be able to communicate clearly the implications of the constructed models and perhaps subsequent simulations for the benefit of the decision makers, clinicians, and patients.

PK/PD models provide powerful tools for analysis of data and for simulations for testing and communication of model results. PK/PD simulations are the topic Chapter 11.

REFERENCES

Beal SL, Sheiner LB, Boeckmann AJ, Bauer RJ, editors. *NONMEM 7.2.0 Users Guides*. (1989–2011). Icon Development Solutions, Hanover. Available at ftp://nonmem.iconplc.com/Public/nonmem720/ guides. Accessed December 13, 2013.

Ette EI, Williams PJ. *Pharmacometrics: The Science of Quantitative Pharmacology*. 2007. Wiley-Interscience. Hoboken, NJ.

Krzyzanski W, Jusko WJ. Mathematical formalism for the properties of four basic models of indirect pharmacodynamics responses. J Pharmacokinet Biopharm 1997; 25(1):107–123.

Poland B, Hodge FL, Khan A, Clemen RT, Wagner JA, Dykstra K, Krishna R. The clinical utility index as a practical multiattribute approach to drug development decisions. Clin Pharm Ther 2009; 86 (1):105–108.

Schmith VD, Fiedler-Kelly J, Phillips L, Grasela TH. Dose proportionality of cisatracurium. J Clin Pharmacol 1997; 37(7):625–629.

Sheiner LB, Stanski DR, Vozeh S, Miller RD, Ham J. Simultaneous modeling of pharmacokinetics and pharmacodynamics: application to D-tubocurarine. Clin Pharm Ther 1979; 25(3):358–371.

Wade J, Karlsson MO. Combining PK and PD data during population PK/PD analysis [Abstract] 1999, PAGE 8. Abstr 139. Available at www.page-meeting.org/?abstract=139. Accessed August 31, 2013.

William-Faltaos D, Chen Y, Wang Y, Gobburu J, Zhu H. Quantification of disease progression and dropout for Alzheimer's disease. Int J Clin Pharmacol Therap 2013; 51(2):120–131.

Zhang L, Beal SL, Sheiner LB. Simultaneous vs. sequential analysis for population PK/PD data I: best-case performance. J Pharmacokinet Pharmacodyn 2003; 30(6):387–404.

CHAPTER 11

SIMULATION BASICS

11.1 INTRODUCTION

The use of simulation is a natural extension of model development in that simulation allows us to use our models to ask relevant questions about various study design features or conditions (i.e., simulation scenarios) that we have yet to study and to determine the likely impact of these scenarios on study outcome and subsequent clinical or regulatory decision making. If model development provides us with a quantification of the parameters that govern a (perhaps) mechanistic explanation for a system and the impact of drug on that system, then simulation allows us to ask *what if*?-type questions to more fully explore that system. This use of simulation implies the existence of a *predictive* model and is the main focus of the remainder of this chapter. There are, however, several other important uses of simulation, including the demonstration and visualization of various model features and assessment of model performance. The area of simulation-based diagnostics which utilizes simulation techniques to evaluate model performance has exploded recently, starting with the use of simulations in assessing goodness of fit for models of noncontinuous endpoints and extending dramatically with the concept of visual predictive check (VPC)-type procedures and the numerous variations thereof for model evaluation (see Chapter 8 for more on this topic) (Karlsson and Savic 2007). Given the typical historical increases in computing capacity (a critical factor in the successful implementation of simulation strategies) and the ever-increasing degree of complexity in pharmacometric and systems pharmacology models, it is logical to expect continued expansion of the use of simulations as an integral element of model-based drug development.

11.2 THE SIMULATION PLAN

The implementation of a simulation effort should be treated much like the implementation of a model development or data analysis effort as previously described, with careful planning and forethought. As such, an important first step is the preparation of a formal simulation plan, with review and approval by appropriate team members. The process of thinking through each facet of the simulation effort, from the technical aspects of how the simulation will be performed to the manner in which the results

Introduction to Population Pharmacokinetic / Pharmacodynamic Analysis with Nonlinear Mixed Effects Models, First Edition. Joel S. Owen and Jill Fiedler-Kelly.
© 2014 John Wiley & Sons, Inc. Published 2014 by John Wiley & Sons, Inc.

will be illustrated for interpretation, is a necessary initial step, and one which often eliminates wasted effort (and rework) later.

Furthermore, simulation planning is an ideal opportunity for team members with diverse backgrounds to collaborate in providing valuable and necessary input to make the simulations relevant and useful. Clinicians knowledgeable in the treatment of the disease under consideration should be consulted to ensure that the characteristics of the patient population to be simulated match those of the typical patients for whom the drug is intended. Team leaders and clinical research associates should be consulted to ensure that the assumed study design and execution features, including the data to be collected and sampling schedule, will accurately reflect what can be implemented and expected if a trial like the one to be simulated was actually conducted. Statisticians should be consulted to ensure that the planned study design features such as sample size, endpoint calculations, and the primary statistical analyses can be similarly implemented in the simulation scenarios, so that the estimated probabilities of success with various strategies can be utilized with confidence to facilitate real decision making during a drug development program.

11.2.1 Simulation Components

There are several main components to be considered and specified in the use of simulations in a modeling and simulation framework. These components concern not only the model to be used and the extent of variability to be introduced (often referred to as the input–output model), but *how* the model will be used in terms of assumptions about the population to be simulated (the covariate distribution model), the features of the trial design and expected execution characteristics (the trial execution model), the number of replicates to be generated, and how the simulated data will be analyzed for decision-making purposes (Kimko and Dufull 2007). These components will be discussed sequentially in the subsections that follow.

11.2.2 The Input–Output Model

When simulation is performed following the development of a pharmacometric model, the specification of the input–output model may be one of the easiest steps. The estimated model, including its associated fixed- and random-effect parameter estimates can be directly used for the input–output model of the simulation. When all components are known to the simulation scientist, and the model code is available, this is a trivial step (see example in Section 11.2.2.1). However, when a model described in the literature is to be used in a simulation scenario, portions of the necessary information for complete specification of the model are often missing or uncertain. In this case, assumptions will need to be made in order to execute the simulation strategy. When assumptions are required about model features that are critical to the results and interpretation of findings, these assumptions must be clearly and carefully stated with the presentation of the results. Furthermore, consideration should be given to varying such settings or testing differing assumptions in order to protect against invalid or irrelevant results. For example, if a pharmacokinetic/pharmacodynamic (PK/PD) model to be used from the literature was developed in a different patient population than the population of interest for the simulations, it may be that certain baseline features, critical to the model-predicted outcomes, are not known for the population of interest. Various scenarios could be considered where the baseline was set equal to the baseline distribution in the other patient population, the mean or median of the baseline distribution is set equal to the mean or median of the other population, but the variability around that mean is increased in the new population to be simulated, or the features of the baseline distribution are derived from other publications of similar populations or from publicly available databases of similar patients. Testing of various scenarios with regard to key assumptions is, therefore, recommended in many situations. The results of the various scenarios can then be presented separately or weighted and pooled with appropriate input from key team members.

If a pharmacometric model is intended for use in simulations, the fixed-effect parameters are generally fixed to the final estimates obtained when the model was estimated using the original model development dataset and the variances of the interindividual variability (IIV) in the parameters and the residual variability are fixed to the variance estimates from the model estimation. The assumptions regarding the variability estimates (elements of omega and sigma, or etas and epsilons) are that the random-effect model terms are normally distributed with mean 0 and variance as specified by the user. Thus, when the simulation step is implemented, new realizations are generated for the eta and epsilon terms for each virtual subject (etas for each parameter with IIV; level 1 error) and for each sample from that subject (epsilons for each endpoint or dependent variable (DV) to be simulated according to the specified $ERROR model; level 2 error) based on these assumptions and the parameter estimates specified. Thus, the resulting simulated parameter distributions should roughly mimic the original estimated parameter distributions.

The variability structure is a critically important feature of models to be used as input–output models in simulations. The specification of the random effects in a nonlinear mixed effects model for simulation can play a fundamental role in the output obtained and, therefore, the simulation findings. When pharmacometric models intended for use in simulations are developed using a diagonal structure for the omega matrix, the inherent underlying assumption is that no covariances (correlations) exist between the individual-specific discrepancies (random effects) for various pairs of parameters in the model. While many so-called *final* pharmacometric models rely on this assumption, simple pair-wise scatterplots of the individual eta estimates will reveal that this is often not so. This is not to say that such models are necessarily invalid, however, as the inclusion and precise estimation of such covariance terms in an already complex model without causing overparameterization may be a difficult and elusive task, particularly for the classical estimation methods. One advantage of some of the newer estimation methods is that the full omega matrix is more easily obtained.

If the inclusion of a full omega block structure in a model to be used for simulation can be estimated with successful model convergence, and even if the estimation of some of the off-diagonal terms of the omega matrix are associated with very poor precision, the use of this more complete model in a simulation scenario may be preferable as it should provide a more realistic outcome than the model with the diagonal omega matrix structure. Even if the covariance between some of the pairs of IIV terms is estimated to be moderate or small, incorporation of this assumption instead of an assumption of zero covariance will preclude or limit the simulation of certain pairs of estimates that would be highly implausible. When the covariance between two parameters (say CL and V) is moderate to high, the corresponding IIV in a related parameter (such as $t_{1/2}$, whose calculation is based on the other two parameters) will be appropriately lower if the covariance is accounted for in the simulation versus if it is ignored and the two original parameters are assumed to be independent. For these reasons, the use of a full omega block structure in models to be used for simulations, whenever possible, is recommended.

11.2.2.1 *Coding a Simulation*   In the following example, a simple PK model is to be used for simulation.

```
$PROBLEM sim-example
$DATA /home/user/data/dataset.csv IGNORE=#
$INPUT ID DATE=DROP TIME AMT ADDL II DV LGDV CMT EVID MDV
   TSLD NUM
$SUBROUTINES ADVAN2 TRANS2
$PK

TVKA=THETA(1)
KA=TVKA
TVCL=THETA(2)
CL=TVCL*EXP(ETA(1))
TVV=THETA(3)
V=TVV*EXP(ETA(2))
S2=V/1000

$ERROR

EP1=EPS(1)
IPRED=F
IRES=DV-IPRED
W=F
IWRES=IRES/W
Y=IPRED+EPS(1)*W

$THETA (9.77476E-01)    ;--th1- KA: absorption rate (1/hr)
       (3.06802E+00)    ;--th2- CL: clearance (L/hr)
       (6.01654E+01)    ;--th3- V: volume (L)

$OMEGA (8.17127E-02)    ;--eta1- IIV in CL [exp]
       (6.22633E-02)    ;--eta2- IIV in V [exp]

$SIGMA (4.77067E-02)    ;--eps1- Constant CV [ccv]

$SIMULATION (9784275) ONLYSIM

$TABLE ID TIME CL V KA ETA1 ETA2 EP1
       FILE=sim-example.tbl NOPRINT
```

Note that the $PK and $ERROR blocks in this simulation control stream are largely the same as those in a typical control stream intended for estimation. Furthermore, if the purpose of the simulation is to better understand the features or behavior of a particular model with the features (e.g., number of subjects, doses, and sample collection events) of the analysis datasets, then the analysis dataset may also be used without modification. Using this method, simulated observations, based on the model and parameter estimates, will be generated for each real observation in the original analysis dataset. The lines of code in the control stream shown in bold font are elements that are unique to simulation.

The $ERROR block contains the line "EP1 = EPS (1) ." In order to output the simulated epsilon values, if they are of interest, the EPS(1) variable must be renamed; by doing so, the new variable *EP1* may be output to a table file (whereas EPS(1) may not). Also note that the $THETA record contains no lower or upper bounds for any of the parameters. While the addition of bounds would not change the behavior of this code, they are unnecessary, as only the initial estimates of each parameter are used for the simulation. The use of the FIXED option with each estimate is similarly unnecessary. In this example, the values used for $THETA, $OMEGA, and $SIGMA are the final parameter estimates obtained from a previous estimation of this dataset, although they need not necessarily have been obtained this way.

The power of simulations and the implementation of simulations in a modeling and simulation framework, lies in the ability to ask questions of a model and consider *what-if* scenarios; some of these scenarios may involve considering alternative parameter estimates for some or all parameters. The alternative values would be implemented via the $THETA, $OMEGA, and $SIGMA records as shown in the example. Some changes in scenario may require defining a new dataset structure to change the number of subjects, dose amounts or frequency, timing of sample collections, or other elements of the dataset that reflect alternate events than those described in the original dataset.

In order to invoke the simulation process, the $SIMULATION record is included, in this case, in place of the $ESTIMATION and $COVARIANCE records which would be included in a more typical control stream for estimation. Two options are specified in this example with $SIMULATION, a required seed value provided in parentheses, and ONLYSIM. The seed value initiates the pseudo-random number generator. Details of the seed value and its usefulness will be discussed in more detail in Section 11.3.1. The ONLYSIM option indicates to NM-TRAN that only simulation is to be performed with this control stream, that is, no estimation is to be performed. In addition, by specifying ONLYSIM, the values of the random variables *CL, V, ETA1, ETA2,* and *EP1* that are output to the table file will be the simulated values (those most likely of interest in this situation) and not the typical values, which would be output without the ONLYSIM option (Beal et al. 1989–2011).

While the NONMEM report file resulting from a simulation is not generally of particular interest, the table file output is the primary source of results. The following lines illustrate the information reported from a simulation in the

NONMEM report file, where the monitoring of the search output would be found in an estimation run:

```
SIMULATION STEP PERFORMED
  SOURCE  1:
     SEED1:       747272046    SEED2:                    0
  NONMEM(R) Run Time: 0:00.48
```

As previously discussed, the table file contains the simulated values of the random parameters that are requested for display, such that *CL, V, ETA1,* and *ETA2,* in this example, will contain unique simulated values for each subject in the dataset. Similarly, *EP1* will contain the unique simulated values for each record in the dataset. Typically of most interest, the simulated values for each observation may be found in the DV column in the table file. When DV, PRED, RES, and WRES are appended to the table file output, by default, the DV column will contain the simulated values in place of the original observed values. The PRED column will contain the population predicted values for each subject and sampling timepoint, based on the model and typical value parameters provided. The RES and WRES columns, although provided by default, are generally ignored from a simulation run, as the RES contains the difference between the simulated observation (in DV) and the population prediction (in PRED) and the WRES column consists of only 0 values. Appendix 11.1 provides a portion of the original data file and the corresponding portion of the table file output from the simulation discussed earlier.

With most simulation applications, it is of interest to simulate with replication, that is, to simulate several hundred datasets and explore behavior across the more sizable sample. To accomplish this type of replication, another option is available on the $SIMULATION record: SUBPROBLEMS. The SUBPROBLEMS option, as shown below, indicates that the entire simulation process should be repeated a specified number of times (in this case, 500 times). The table file output then contains the concatenated output of all of the subproblems, listed one after another (Beal et al. 1989–2011).

$SIMULATION (9784275) ONLYSIM SUBPROBLEMS=500

As discussed in Section 8.8.1, when describing the VPC procedure for model evaluation, one may wish to keep track of the particular replication of the simulation. To do so, simply add the code:

```
REP = IREP
```

to the $PK block and request the variable REP in the table file to provide the replication number, which may be useful in postprocessing the output.

11.2.3 The Covariate Distribution Model

Another critical component in any simulation scenario is the covariate distribution model. The covariate distribution model defines the characteristics of the virtual patient population to be simulated. The characteristics that need to be simulated consist of only those which have an impact on the input–output model(s) in some way. Thus, any patient characteristic that is included in either the PK or PK/PD model as a covariate effect will need to be assigned for each virtual patient in the simulation population. If the PK/PD model includes or relies on a baseline effect that is related to a subject characteristic, this will need to be assigned as well. Very careful consideration should be given to simulation of the patient characteristics in order to make the simulation results as meaningful as possible. There are various methods that could be implemented to define the covariate distribution model. These include sampling patient characteristics for each virtual patient from available distributional information, resampling patient characteristics from a set of characteristics or patient covariate vectors in an available dataset, and the use of information available from public databases containing information regarding patient characteristics. Each method has certain advantages and disadvantages, which will be discussed in turn, in the sections that follow.

11.2.3.1 *Sampling of Covariate Values from a Distribution(s)* With a limited set of patient characteristics to be simulated, one could consider simply using the distributional characteristics (mean, standard deviation, range) of the covariates in the model development dataset or some other known and appropriate population or set of data to randomly assign values to the virtual population to be simulated. Many software packages, such as SAS® and R, have functions that permit random sampling from a specified distribution. Similar to the discussion in Section 11.2.2 regarding accounting for the covariance between parameters, consideration of the covariance between patient characteristics is essential. Ignoring such relationships, such as the relationship between weight and height, it would be possible to simulate a highly improbable 40 kg patient who measures 190 cm in height. It is a simple task with most statistical software packages or even Excel® to calculate the covariance between two variables or sets of numbers for use in simulation. With the variances and covariances between variables at hand, the simulation of patient characteristics would be done using the complete variance–covariance matrix, thus providing a simulated population with a more realistic and representative set of patient characteristics. Of course, when many covariates are required, the size of the task grows and consideration of the full variance–covariance matrix for all covariates may be required.

Careful consideration should also be given to covariates that are typically derived or assigned from other covariates, such as creatinine clearance calculated using the Cockcroft and Gault approximation or a classification variable used as an indicator of disease severity such as Child-Pugh score, which is based on total bilirubin, serum albumin, and several other factors (Cockcroft and Gault 1976). For such covariates, the factors from which these covariates are derived should be simulated first, using the appropriate variance–covariance relationships with other covariates, and then the calculation applied to the relevant factors. In this way, the appropriate relationships between the calculated or derived covariates and the factors upon which these relationships are based will be preserved.

While the same principles apply when sampling distributional information about covariates from a publicly available or proprietary database as when sampling from a known distribution, additional consideration should be given to understanding the source and relevance of the data in the database to the simulation study at hand. For example, if the database consists entirely of healthy subjects, would healthy subjects be expected to be similar to the patients to be generated in the simulation study, at least with regard to the subject characteristics of interest? If the database contains patients with the disease or condition of interest, is the severity of the disease the same? Is the history of the disease the same? Are there subjects being treated with concomitant medications that would need to be excluded from the population which would be sampled for the simulation, etc.? Furthermore, if there are factors known to be prognostic for affecting the likelihood of response, these should be carefully considered in the simulation plan. Options for dealing with such factors might include stratified sampling of the factors of interest across specified levels of the prognostic factor, the inclusion of the prognostic factor(s) along with the covariate factors of interest for the model while accounting for the covariance between these factors and the covariates of interest, or simply restricting the population to be sampled within a specified range of the prognostic factor, so as to exclude the most extreme values.

11.2.3.2 *Resampling of Covariate Vectors*   An alternative to sampling of covariates based on distributional characteristics is a technique called resampling which involves randomly selecting covariate values with replacement from the measured values observed in a given dataset. Resampling techniques are sometimes referred to generally as bootstrap sampling (Efron 1979). The process for generating a bootstrap confidence interval about parameter estimates is described in detail in Section 8.7. To illustrate the process of resampling covariate vectors, assume the original dataset consists of 10 patients with the following weight measurements: 71, 79, 89, 87, 73, 91, 77, 75, 84, and 85 kg. Now, to resample a new population of 15 subjects from this population, we might obtain the following values: 84, 77, 89, 71, 85, 75, 73, 84, 75, 71, 85, 84, 87, 91, and 77 kg. Notice that some weight values were selected more than once and the subject with a weight of 79 kg was not selected for the new sample at all. In this way, a new sample is obtained, derived from the original sample and with similar, but not identical, characteristics to the original sample.

When multiple covariates are required for the simulation, resampling is typically performed at the covariate *vector* level. Thus, a string of covariate values observed in a patient are kept together and the entire vector or combination of covariates is selected (or not) with each random pick, as described earlier for a single covariate. For example, if the variables required for the simulation include weight, gender, and creatinine clearance for each virtual subject, combinations of these three variables that are present for subjects in the observed dataset would be resampled as a combination of the three factors. In this way, the covariances between factors are explicitly preserved (thus also preventing unusual or unlikely combinations of covariates). Generally, however, when resampling techniques are used in this way, the resulting variance terms may be smaller in the resampled set as compared to the original population because novel combinations of covariate values will not be obtained in the new sample.

11.2.3.3 *Use of Inclusion and Exclusion Criteria*   With clinical trial simulations, regardless of the method used for the simulation of patient covariates, a final step to consider in the simulation of the virtual population is to apply the inclusion and exclusion criteria that would be used for the trial to be simulated. As an alternative to simulating only patients within strict specifications for various criteria, the simulation of patient characteristics based on a population of similar patients and subsequent application of appropriate criteria to appropriately limit the population under study may result in the generation of a more realistic population.

11.2.4   The Trial Execution Model

The third major component to the simulation effort is the specification of the trial execution model. This may include everything about the actual trial design, such as the dosing regimen(s), the randomization of patients to treatment and placebo, the sampling strategies for PK and PD endpoints or biomarkers, the length of the treatment phase, the use of a placebo run-in phase, etc. but also typically includes other important aspects of trial execution, such as investigator and patient non-compliance, patient dropout due to one or more reasons, and the use of alternative estimates of variability. The application of different study design features, such as sampling strategies and dosing regimens, is commonly cast as the evaluation of different simulation scenarios, while the other features specified with the trial execution model should be considered as a part of each scenario evaluated in order to make the results more representative of reality. After all, it would be highly unlikely that any trial conducted would result in 100% compliance on the part of both the investigators and the patients.

With regard to the evaluation of different dosing regimens (an increasingly common use of simulations), dosing regimens can be handled in three ways (in increasing order of complexity): (i) simple static design features (e.g., 20% of the population is randomly assigned to receive placebo, 40% of the population is randomly assigned to receive the low dose, and 40% is randomly allocated to the high dose), (ii) protocol-specified fixed titration strategies, or (iii) adjusted based on patient response or clinician evaluator judgment (i.e., adaptive trial design). Although the implementation details get more complicated with each of these scenarios and more modeling work is required upon which to base the modifications, dosing adjustments based on simulated patient response can be incorporated into simulation scenarios as well.

For each of the typical trial execution considerations, more or less simple alternatives can be applied. With regard to dropout for instance, if a model to predict study dropout has been developed, then this model and the factors included in the dropout model can be used in a postprocessing step, after the input–output model is applied to the simulation dataset of the virtual population. It may be particularly important to apply this model after the input–output simulation is complete, especially when the value of the endpoint (response) is an important predictor of the likelihood of dropout, as is often the case (e.g., in a pain study where the likelihood of dropout due to receipt of rescue medication is related to the primary pain score endpoint). With model-based predictions of which virtual patients will drop out, the data from those subjects least likely to drop out can be censored as appropriate prior to analysis of the simulated data. On the other hand, if a model to predict dropout is not available and cannot be developed at the time of the simulation effort, information regarding the extent of observed dropout in previous studies can be utilized. For example, if prior studies have indicated that approximately 10% of subjects drop out at some time after the 4-week visit, a simple random assignment of dropout status (yes or no) can be made to the simulated samples collected after 4 weeks based on a probability of 10%.

With regard to compliance, there are many aspects that could be considered, based on the particular trial design. At the very least, there is compliance with regard to dosing as well as with regard to sampling of PK and PD data. Similar to the discussion of dropout in the less informed case described earlier, compliance models are not common and the application of some extent of random noncompliance based on the data observed in previous similar studies may be the best that can be accomplished. If there is particular concern over compliance in the patient population to be studied, differing extents or patterns of noncompliance could be considered in different scenarios so that this factor could be explicitly evaluated. Obviously, the more informed these aspects of the simulation are, the more realistic and relevant the results will be, but even when specific information is lacking, a random assignment with a clear statement of the assumption is better than an assumption of no dropout or perfect compliance.

If the purpose of the simulation effort is to simulate the next phase of development by predicting the probability of success with differing trial designs or dosing regimens, careful consideration should be given to the assumptions surrounding variability. When existing models and estimates of variability are derived from more stringently controlled studies or studies performed in more homogeneous populations, it is reasonable to expect that the between- and perhaps even the within-subject variability estimates would underestimate the variability in the new study. As such, and especially in circumstances where the variability in the response may have a large influence on the projected success of the trial, an inflation of the variability estimates may be considered. In these situations, information can sometimes be derived from other drugs in the class or the study of this drug in another indication to further bolster or support the choice of a particular variability inflation factor.

11.2.5 Replication of the Study

A fundamental concept in simulation applications of all sorts is replication. Replication implies numerous repetitions of the experimental conditions based on the inherent random variability elements introduced (i.e., IIV and RV terms or just IIV, depending on the application). In clinical trial simulation scenarios, trials (as a unit) are replicated hundreds or thousands of times, and the results across all replicates reported to control for the effect of sampling variability. If the purpose of the simulation is merely to get an idea of the range of expectations based on the model, hundreds or thousands of (replicate) virtual patients may be simulated, and the variability across all presented as a prediction interval.

The reason for such replication is straightforward. We would generally not feel comfortable basing a critical decision on a single replicate or realization of a subject in a simulation scenario or even of a single simulated trial, recognizing that it is only a single realization from a distribution. Thinking now as simulation scientists, it may not be nearly as troubling to experience a failed trial or two in the context of a majority of positive results (unless, of course, you are the one funding the trials!). In simulation studies, the concept of replication becomes one of security in numbers— the more replicates we run, the more confident we are that the results are reflective of the true underlying model, parameter estimate central tendencies, and variability upon which the simulation is based. Even though a lone replicate may not be at all coincident with the model expectations, thousands of replicates will give us a better picture of what we can reliably expect.

The choice of the particular number of replicates to implement is not always obvious. While intuitively, more is generally better, whether thousands of replicates are needed over hundreds may be an important consideration in terms of many factors beyond the scientific merits of the results, including the time required, the availability of processing resources, and the disk space required to store the voluminous results. If too few replicates are generated, the results may not be reflective of the true expectation, simply due to variability in the samples obtained. Except in the case of very high variability, 500–1000 replicates are generally quite sufficient for most simulations. The FDA Guidance for Industry, Population Pharmacokinetics mentions the use of at least 200 replicates in a discussion regarding the generation of bootstrap samples (FDA 1999). When resampling observed covariate vectors to simulate the covariate distribution model, however, expansion of the population by up to two- or threefold over the original sample size may be reasonable (i.e., resampling characteristics for up to 150 subjects from an original sample of 50), but expansion to a population that is 10 or more times larger (i.e., characteristics of 500 new virtual subjects resampled from an original sample of only 50) might be questionable.

11.2.6   Analysis of the Simulated Data

If available, a draft protocol or protocol synopsis for the study to be simulated should be studied carefully at the time of simulation planning. In addition to ensuring that the trial design aspects are accurately represented in the trial execution model and that the virtual patient population is accurately represented via the covariate distribution model and the inclusion/exclusion criteria, the statistical analysis of the data should be specified. In order to provide the most accurate projection of the trial results based on the simulation, the simulated data from each trial replicate are analyzed in exactly the same way as the observed trial data will be analyzed. In this way, each replicate trial will be associated with its own p value and determination of success. Looking across the hundreds or thousands of replicate studies, an overall probability of success and confidence interval about that probability can be obtained.

11.2.7   Decision Making Using Simulations

Ultimately, the use of simulation results to support development-related decision making can be greatly facilitated by the consideration of different scenarios under varying reasonable assumptions and by the input of the broader team in interpreting and *validating* the simulation results. The generation of key graphical displays and summaries of the findings can be extremely important in illustrating the differences between various scenarios and the variability and uncertainty in the results. Such displays can become a central focus of team planning meetings, allowing for a more quantitative basis for decision making than the intuition- and past experience-driven alternative which has been historically, and is unfortunately still, commonly used.

Other tools, such as the clinical utility index, have been proposed as an alternative means of facilitating decision making using modeling and simulation results (Poland et al. 2009). This, and other proposed indices attempt to simultaneously take into account the factors most relevant to a decision (say, the primary efficacy endpoint and a key dose-limiting adverse event) and reduce these factors to a single number (Yassen et al. 2008). With the appropriate buy-in from team members regarding the calculation of such indices and the weighting of the various factors that go into the calculation, the use of such measures may allow for a more objective means of evaluating various scenarios under consideration.

Consideration of the questions for which answers are required may provide a framework for an assessment of the usefulness of simulations in decision making. For example, if it is of interest to quantify the expected percentage of subjects that would have a particular cell count below a specified cutoff, this could easily be determined by postprocessing the simulation results. Calculations of similar measures for different scenarios, at different times postdosing, or with different cutoffs may provide an excellent tool for facilitating the selection of a particular development strategy.

11.3 MISCELLANEOUS OTHER SIMULATION-RELATED CONSIDERATIONS

11.3.1 The Seed Value

The incorporation of random variability into any aspect of a simulation effort requires the use of a random number generator or random number lookup feature; this feature, in turn, requires the assignment of a seed value. The string of digits used for the simulation seed value(s) allows for the entire simulation to be reproduced. Using the same seed value, a simulation control stream run twice (with no other changes to the model code or input dataset) would result in identical output. However, the use of a different seed will start the simulation at a new and different place in the random number sequence, producing new and different values for each simulated variable. Appendix 11.2 illustrates the use of an alternative seed value for the simulation described in Section 11.2.2.1. Note that the resulting table file contains different values for all of the random variables, including DV, compared to the original simulation output in Appendix 11.1, while the values of PRED (as expected) do not differ between the two tables.

Certain simulation applications require holding this seed value constant, while for others, it would be more appropriate to use a changing seed. When the purpose of the simulation exercise is to compare different scenarios which are defined by aspects of the trial execution model, say different dosing regimens, for example, one would typically want to essentially hold all other aspects of the trial constant so that the comparison can be made on the basis of the difference in dosing regimen alone. Thus, in this situation, one would use the same seed for each new simulation scenario of another dosing regimen to be considered. In this way, if four different dosing regimens were to be compared, using the same seed value for each simulation, the same virtual patients would be simulated in each scenario. Specifically, the eta on CL assigned to patient #1 would be the same in each scenario, allowing for a fair comparison of the differences due to dose. If different seed values were used with each scenario, then each scenario would essentially consist of a different virtual population and it would be difficult to conclude that the differences could be ascribed only to dose and not also to the particular realization of the random variability.

If, on the other hand, the purpose of the simulation is to understand variability in a large population of subjects, and this is accomplished by performing many small simulations and concatenating the results, one would want to be sure to use different seeds for each simulation. Use of the subproblems option continues the random sequence as the simulation continues from one subproblem to another, and thus each subpopulation is simulated as if with different seeds.

11.3.2   Consideration of Parameter Uncertainty

Most of the simulation scenarios described earlier are based on the utilization of specified point estimates for the theta (fixed effect) terms in the model and specified variance estimates for the random-effect terms. However, there exists uncertainty in the estimation of all parameters of the model, including the fixed-effect terms that are generally simply fixed to a specific value. If desired, and perhaps of particular interest when there is poor precision of parameter estimation, it is possible to introduce this parameter uncertainty into a simulation scenario either in addition to or instead of the between-subject variability.

The inclusion of parameter uncertainty is accomplished by sampling from the variance–covariance matrix of the parameter estimates as opposed to the variance–covariance matrix for the omega and sigma matrices. Either a portion or the entire variance–covariance matrix of the parameter estimates is used in place of the typical omega matrix; this may result in some required recoding of the $PK and $ERROR blocks. In this way, realizations for each parameter are obtained from this distribution of uncertainty about each parameter, resulting in more or less variability about each parameter based on the precision of the original estimate.

When the PK parameters to be simulated with parameter uncertainty are originally modeled using exponential error models for IIV, an initial step of re-estimation after a reparameterization, is required. This reparameterization log-transforms each of the parameters such that the natural log of each is now estimated. Since it is assumed that the underlying distribution of the OMEGA matrix is multivariate normal, the $PK block is recoded to introduce each of the elements of OMEGA as an additive component to the transformed parameter, resulting in the expected log-normal distribution of the individual parameter estimates.

Appendix 11.3 provides a detailed illustration of the various steps involved in running a simulation with parameter uncertainty.

11.3.3 Constraining Random Effects or Responses

Oftentimes when realizations of the omega and sigma matrices are simulated, a handful of values will be generated, based on the specified distributions, that are very unusual and thought to be extremely unlikely. Such values may well be more extreme than any of the values of the estimated distribution upon which the simulation was based. Because this is possible, it may be of interest to either include code in the control stream to not allow for the generation of such values or to exclude such values in a postprocessing step if generated.

In a similar way, it is possible to simulate drug concentration values lower than the limit of quantification of the assay, it is possible to simulate negative concentration values based on the residual variability model selected, or to simulate PD endpoint or biomarker values that are implausible or even impossible. As described earlier for random-effect estimates, code can be inserted in the control stream to disallow the generation of such values or they can be excluded from the analysis of the simulated data in a postprocessing step prior to analysis. An example excerpt of the relevant control stream code to constrain the estimates of sigma to avoid negative simulated observations is included below:

```
$PRED
...(code excluded)...
    Y =  EFFECT + SD
    IF (ICALL.EQ.4) THEN
        DOWHILE (Y.LT.0)
            CALL SIMEPS(EPS)
            Y=EFFECT + SD
        ENDDO
    ENDIF
```

With an appropriate *bound* for a parameter (EBE) or ETA value, similar coding could be developed to constrain a PK parameter between specified limits using the appropriate constraint in the DOWHILE statement and 'CALL SIMETA(ETA)' in place of 'CALL SIMEPS(EPS)' as in the example above.

APPENDIX 11.1   EXAMPLE SIMULATION OUTPUT

Data for first two subjects from original data file for simulation example in Section 11.2.2.1:

ID	DATE	TIME	AMT	ADDL	II	DV	LGDV	CMT	EVID	MDV	TSLD	NUM
1	1	8:30	100	27	24	.	.	1	1	1	0	1
1	14	7:40	.	.	.	1000.8	6.908555	2	0	0	23.17	2
1	22	8:00	.	.	.	874.41	6.773549	2	0	0	23.5	3
1	28	17:10	.	.	.	2338.4	7.757222	2	0	0	8.67	4
2	1	7:00	100	27	24	.	.	1	1	1	0	5
2	14	12:40	.	.	.	1229.2	7.114119	2	0	0	5.67	6
2	20	22:30	.	.	.	1128.2	7.028379	2	0	0	15.5	7
2	28	13:20	.	.	.	1747.6	7.465999	2	0	0	6.33	8

Corresponding table file output for first two subjects for simulation example in Section 11.2.2.1:

TABLE NO. 1

ID	TIME	CL	V	KA	ETA1	ETA2	EP1	DV	PRED	RES	WRES
1.0000E+00	0.0000E+00	2.5408E+00	7.3805E+01	9.7748E-01	-1.8854E-01	2.0433E-01	4.3634E-02	0.0000E+00	0.0000E+00	0.0000E+00	0.0000E+00
1.0000E+00	3.1117E+02	2.5408E+00	7.3805E+01	9.7748E-01	-1.8854E-01	2.0433E-01	3.5388E-01	1.5229E+03	7.6218E+02	7.6070E+02	0.0000E+00
1.0000E+00	5.0350E+02	2.5408E+00	7.3805E+01	9.7748E-01	-1.8854E-01	2.0433E-01	-2.6000E-01	8.2298E+02	7.4946E+02	7.3526E+01	0.0000E+00
1.0000E+00	6.5667E+02	2.5408E+00	7.3805E+01	9.7748E-01	-1.8854E-01	2.0433E-01	3.2583E-01	2.4564E+03	1.5961E+03	8.6029E+02	0.0000E+00
2.0000E+00	0.0000E+00	3.6236E+00	7.9115E+01	9.7748E-01	1.6642E-01	2.7381E-01	1.1079E-01	0.0000E+00	0.0000E+00	0.0000E+00	0.0000E+00
2.0000E+00	3.1767E+02	3.6236E+00	7.9115E+01	9.7748E-01	1.6642E-01	2.7381E-01	-6.4987E-02	1.4292E+03	1.8536E+03	-4.2432E+02	0.0000E+00
2.0000E+00	4.7150E+02	3.6236E+00	7.9115E+01	9.7748E-01	1.6642E-01	2.7381E-01	-1.0547E-01	8.7463E+02	1.1270E+03	-2.5235E+02	0.0000E+00
2.0000E+00	6.5433E+02	3.6236E+00	7.9115E+01	9.7748E-01	1.6642E-01	2.7381E-01	-1.0705E-01	1.3264E+03	1.7952E+03	-4.6889E+02	0.0000E+00

APPENDIX 11.2 EXAMPLE SIMULATION OUTPUT WITH A DIFFERENT SEED VALUE

Table file output for first two subjects for simulation example in Section 11.2.2.1 when a seed value of 1906493 is used in place of the original seed value of 9784275:

TABLE NO. 1

ID	TIME	CL	V	KA	ETA1	ETA2	EP1	DV	PRED	RES	WRES
1.0000E+00	0.0000E+00	2.8225E+00	6.4554E+01	9.7748E-01	-8.3412E-02	7.0409E-02	3.5797E-01	0.0000E+00	0.0000E+00	0.0000E+00	0.0000E+00
1.0000E+00	3.1117E+02	2.8225E+00	6.4554E+01	9.7748E-01	-8.3412E-02	7.0409E-02	-3.6021E-02	8.7347E+02	7.6218E+02	1.1130E+02	0.0000E+00
1.0000E+00	5.0350E+02	2.8225E+00	6.4554E+01	9.7748E-01	-8.3412E-02	7.0409E-02	5.5851E-01	1.3920E+03	7.4946E+02	6.4250E+02	0.0000E+00
1.0000E+00	6.5667E+02	2.8225E+00	6.4554E+01	9.7748E-01	-8.3412E-02	7.0409E-02	3.7435E-01	2.3471E+03	1.5961E+03	7.5093E+02	0.0000E+00
2.0000E+00	0.0000E+00	2.0007E+00	7.4016E+01	9.7748E-01	-4.2754E-01	2.0718E-01	2.9242E-02	0.0000E+00	0.0000E+00	0.0000E+00	0.0000E+00
2.0000E+00	3.1767E+02	2.0007E+00	7.4016E+01	9.7748E-01	-4.2754E-01	2.0718E-01	-1.2442E-01	2.1818E+03	1.8536E+03	3.2821E+02	0.0000E+00
2.0000E+00	4.7150E+02	2.0007E+00	7.4016E+01	9.7748E-01	-4.2754E-01	2.0718E-01	-5.2921E-01	9.0144E+02	1.1270E+03	-2.2554E+02	0.0000E+00
2.0000E+00	6.5433E+02	2.0007E+00	7.4016E+01	9.7748E-01	-4.2754E-01	2.0718E-01	-2.5953E-01	1.8145E+03	1.7952E+03	1.9261E+01	0.0000E+00

APPENDIX 11.3   SIMULATION WITH PARAMETER UNCERTAINTY

Step 1: Reparameterization of the original control stream to estimate the log-transformed PK parameters:

```
$PROBLEM est-lnpk

$DATA /home/user/data/dataset.csv IGNORE=#
$INPUT ID DATE TIME AMT ADDL II DV LGDV CMT EVID MDV TSLD NUM
$SUBROUTINES ADVAN2 TRANS2
$PK

TVKA=EXP(THETA(1))
TVCL=EXP(THETA(2))
TVV=EXP(THETA(3))

IIVCL=EXP(ETA(1))
IIVV=EXP(ETA(2))

KA=TVKA
CL=TVCL*IIVCL
V=TVV*IIVV

S2=V/1000

$ERROR
IPRED=F
IRES=DV-IPRED
W=F
IWRES=IRES/W
Y=IPRED+EPS(1)*W

$THETA (-INF, -2.3)    ;--th1- KA: Ln absorption rate (1/hr)
       (-INF, 1.1)     ;--th2- CL: Ln clearance (L/hr)
       (-INF, 4.09)    ;--th3- V: Ln volume (L)

$OMEGA (0.1)       ;--eta1- IIV in CL [exp]
       (0.12)      ;--eta2- IIV in V [exp]

$SIGMA (0.0625)    ;--eps1- Constant CV [ccv]

$ESTIMATION METHOD=1 INTER MAXEVAL=9999 PRINT=5
$COVARIANCE

$TABLE ID TIME CMT TSLD NUM TVCL TVV CL V KA ETA1 ETA2
       FILE=est-lnpk.tbl NOPRINT
```

Portion of output file from Step 1: log-transformed estimation:

1

****

        FIRST ORDER CONDITIONAL ESTIMATION ERACTION
              COVARIANCE MATRIX OF ESTIMATE

****

	TH 1	TH 2	TH 3	OM11	OM12	OM22	SG11
TH 1							
+	2.24E-03						
TH 2							
+	1.07E-04	6.52E-04					
TH 3							
+	4.88E-04	3.90E-04	1.18E-03				
OM 11							
+	-4.35E-05	1.41E-06	5.41E-05	1.05E-04			
OM 12							
+	....	....	....	....	....		
OM 22							
+	1.13E-04	3.42E-05	1.63E-04	3.15E-05	1.51E-04		
SG 11							
+	1.57E-05	6.47E-06	1.23E-06	-3.75E-06	....	-4.44E-07	4.32E-06

Step 2: Example control stream for a simulation including parameter uncertainty:

```
$PROBLEM sim-parm-uncert-lnpk

$DATA /home/user/data/dataset.csv IGNORE=#
$INPUT ID DATE TIME AMT ADDL II DV LGDV CMT EVID MDV TSLD
  NUM
$SUBROUTINES ADVAN2 TRANS2
$PK

; Use etas as a mechanism for introducing new variables
  for parameter uncertainty
; based on estimates from covar matrix of previous
  estimation run
UNCKA=ETA(1)
UNCCL=ETA(2)
UNCV=ETA(3)
```

```
; add random effects to the ln-transformed parameter
  estimates and back-transform
KA=EXP(THETA(1) + UNCKA)
CL=EXP(THETA(2) + UNCCL)
V=EXP(THETA(3) + UNCV)

S2=V/1000

REP=IREP

$ERROR

IPRED=F
IRES=DV-IPRED
W=F
IWRES=IRES/W
Y=IPRED+EPS(1)*W

$THETA (-0.0226)   ;--th1- KA: Ln absorption rate (1/hr)
       (1.12)      ;--th2- CL: Ln clearance (L/hr)
       (4.10)      ;--th3- V: Ln volume (L)

; use estimates of uncertainty in theta 1-3 from previous
  estimation run
$OMEGA BLOCK(3)
0.00224
-0.000107 0.000652
0.000488 0.000390 0.00118

; do not include residual variability (or IIV) in this
  simulation, only parameter uncertainty
$SIGMA (0 FIX)     ;--eps1- Constant CV [ccv]

$SIMULATION (7562053) ONLYSIM NSUB=100

$TABLE REP ID TIME CMT TSLD NUM CL V KA ETA1 ETA2 ETA3
       NOHEADER FILE=sim-parm-uncert-lnpk.tbl NOPRINT

; output extra table file containing only one record per
  subject to confirm uncertainty
$TABLE REP ID CL V KA ETA1 ETA2 ETA3
       FIRSTONLY ONEHEADER FILE=sim-parm-uncert-lnpk-
         oneper.tbl NOPRINT
```

Table file output for first several subjects from Step 2: simulation including parameter uncertainty:

Excel:	A	B	C	D	E	F	G	H
TABLE NO. 2								
REP	ID	CL	V	KA	ETA1	ETA2	ETA3
1.0000E+00	1.0000E+00	3.0554E+00	5.7727E+01	8.9697E-01	-8.6131E-02	-3.0852E-03	-4.4268E-02
1.0000E+00	2.0000E+00	3.1631E+00	6.2392E+01	1.0007E+00	2.3349E-02	3.1540E-02	3.3438E-02
1.0000E+00	3.0000E+00	3.1261E+00	6.2569E+01	9.6304E-01	-1.5063E-02	1.9790E-02	3.6267E-02
1.0000E+00	4.0000E+00	3.1162E+00	6.1531E+01	9.1610E-01	-6.5032E-02	1.6605E-02	1.9535E-02
1.0000E+00	5.0000E+00	2.9304E+00	5.8710E+01	1.0104E+00	3.2900E-02	-4.4864E-02	-2.7393E-02
1.0000E+00	6.0000E+00	3.1752E+00	6.1751E+01	9.1920E-01	-6.1651E-02	3.5365E-02	2.3107E-02
1.0000E+00	7.0000E+00	3.0780E+00	5.9337E+01	9.0374E-01	-7.8612E-02	4.2881E-03	-1.6769E-02

To confirm the parameter uncertainty, read table file into Excel and calculate the following:

```
VAR(F1:F1470)  =  0.002180
VAR(G1:G1470)  =  0.000615
VAR(H1:H1470)  =  0.001135
COVAR(F1:F1470, G1:G1470)  =  -0.000180
COVAR(F1:F1470, H1:H1470)  =  0.000453
COVAR(G1:G1470, H1:H1470)  =  0.000346
```

All values correspond closely with the values input in $OMEGA.

REFERENCES

Beal SL, Sheiner LB, Boeckmann AJ, Bauer RJ, editors. *NONMEM 7.2.0 Users Guides*. (1989–2011). Hanover: Icon Development Solutions. Available at ftp://nonmem.iconplc.com/Public/nonmem720/guides/. Accessed December 7, 2013.

Cockcroft DW, Gault MH. Prediction of creatinine clearance from serum creatinine. Nephron 1976; 16 (1):31–41.

Efron B. Bootstrap methods: another look at jackknife. Ann Statist 1979;7:1–26.

Food and Drug Administration (FDA), Guidance for Industry Population Pharmacokinetics. Food and Drug Administration: Rockville; 1999.

Karlsson MO, Savic RM. Diagnosing model diagnostics. Clin Pharmacol Therap 2007;82:17–20.

Kimko HC, Duffull SB. *Simulation for Designing Clinical Trials: A Pharmacokinetic-Pharmacodynamic Modeling Perspective*. New York: Informa Healthcare USA, Inc; 2007. p 1–130.

Poland B, Hodge FL, Khan A, Clemen RT, Wagner JA, Dykstra K, Krishna R. The clinical utility index as a practical multiattribute approach to drug development decisions. Clin Pharmacol Ther 2009; 86 (1):105–108.

Yassen A, Olofsen E, Kan J, Dahan A, Danhof M. Pharmacokinetic-pharmacodynamic modeling of the effectiveness and safety of buprenorphine and fentanyl in rats. Pharm Res 2008;25 (1):183–193.

CHAPTER 12

QUALITY CONTROL

12.1 INTRODUCTION

Enough can never be said to emphasize the importance of effective quality control (QC) and quality assurance practices throughout an entire modeling effort. It takes just one experience of identifying a fundamental problem in the analysis dataset or with a key modeling assumption moments before a regulatory deadline or before a presentation of results for senior management to convince any modeler of this truth. Sometimes in our haste to show progress or achieve some measure of results to share, we skip over or postpone steps in the process designed to prevent such stressful situations. At these times, the value of this message could not be more clear (Grasela et al. 2009; Bonate et al. 2012).

There is a myriad of process steps involved in a model development effort, from rationalization of the need for the modeling effort, to conceptualization of the data analysis plan, to creation of the analysis dataset, to performing the modeling analysis steps, to completion of the regulatory deliverable. Each step needs to be carefully checked *in parallel with* performing the step, if at all possible. Delays in completion of the QC tasks only serves to increase the amount of rework that may be required and the possible ramifications to the program due to critical error.

12.2 QC OF THE DATA ANALYSIS PLAN

In Chapter 5, the development of the analysis plan is described as perhaps the most important step of the entire data analysis effort. If the analytical plan is carefully considered and conceived, the first step in completing the modeling and simulation project according to a generally recognized quality standard will have been achieved. Even if the best model is a poor description of the data, the results are more likely to be accepted when performed according to an established plan than they would be in the absence of a well-thought-out plan.

Beyond the review of the analysis plan document itself by a senior modeler or pharmacometrician, who can carefully evaluate the appropriateness of the proposed methodology and technical details given the data, review of the analytical plan by development team members from other areas of expertise is also essential. This vetting

Introduction to Population Pharmacokinetic / Pharmacodynamic Analysis with Nonlinear Mixed Effects Models, First Edition. Joel S. Owen and Jill Fiedler-Kelly.

of the plan with team members and development team leaders not specifically expert in modeling will provide input regarding the relevance of the questions the model is intended to inform, a critical first step in assuring that the model to be developed will be of use to the team in addressing important knowledge gaps. Furthermore, input and buy-in from such team members prior to the performance of the analysis may serve to facilitate their later acceptance of the modeling results and help to forge collaborative efforts to extend the use of the model via simulation strategies.

12.3   ANALYSIS DATASET CREATION

Given a comprehensive data analysis plan, QC of the analysis dataset begins with the dataset requirements. The requirements or specifications for the analysis dataset may be in the form of a detailed specifications document detailing exactly which data are to be used and how such data are to be processed to create the required structure and content of the dataset for analysis (Chowdhury 2010). Alternatively, the requirements may be a simple bullet point list of points to consider in the creation of most NONMEM-ready datasets, updated with specific details regarding the particular data to be included or excluded for the analysis at hand.

Although dataset QC can be performed with either type of requirements document, it should be self-evident that the more detailed and specific the specifications are defined, the more precisely the data can be checked against those requirements during dataset QC. However, in either case, the mere existence of the specification provides the standard or guidance against which an independent reviewer could provide a QC review of the dataset. Without such a form, dataset QC would be an arbitrary task, relying on the instinct and experience of the QC checker. In small organizations or other situations where an independent reviewer is not available, the documentation of steps such as the dataset requirements is still necessary and perhaps even more important, especially in light of the inherent difficulties in checking one's own work and thought processes. In larger organizations or when possible, prior to implementation by the programmer, the requirements form itself may be subjected to a QC review by an independent pharmacometrician.

With regard to QC of the dataset in those situations where an analyst prepares the requirements and a programmer executes on the specifications to create the dataset, at least two levels of dataset QC should be performed. First, the programmer should verify that the code performed as expected and that the resulting output is consistent with expectations based on his/her understanding of the requirements. Second, the analyst (requestor) should verify that the dataset contents are consistent with his/her expectations based on what was intended in the request. Finally, an independent QC reviewer could be invoked to verify the analysis dataset content by checking each element of the raw data against the specifications document and the analysis dataset (this is sometimes called 100% QC or 100% inspection, although it is not typically intended to be performed on 100% of the data). Although there are many ways to approach this type of QC, one way would be to randomly select a small subset of the data on which to perform such verification. A reasonable number of patients to check might be three from each study (with study selected as the independent variable based on the assumption that different coding might be required for each study based on the individual design features of each study). Alternatively, some other significant feature of the coding may be used to (randomly) select a subset of patients for 100% QC to ensure that important variations are verified. If discrepancies are identified, additional programming or clarification of the requirements would be needed. Once such changes are complete, the new version of the analysis dataset would be subjected to this process again (Grasela et al. 2010a). Additional suggestions regarding dataset QC are provided in Chapter 5.

12.3.1   Exploratory Data Analysis and Its Role in Dataset QC

One of the objectives of the exploratory data analysis (EDA) step is to verify the content of the analysis dataset prior to modeling. If carefully planned, data displays can serve to inform the modeler about the data content as well as verify the structure and content of the dataset. For example, histograms of continuous variables can be used to facilitate the identification of possible outliers, as well as to identify potential issues with inconsistent units among studies or labs. Simple frequency tables can be used very effectively to identify unusual values for data items and to confirm the coding of NONMEM-required data items that were initialized and coded within the dataset creation programs. Scatterplots of concentration versus time since first or last dose can be used to easily identify possible errors in dates or times.

12.3.2   QC in Data Collection

Several aspects of data collection for pharmacometric analyses warrant consideration from a QC perspective. Clearly, if consideration is given to the data that will be most important to pharmacometric modeling efforts prior to finalization of the data collection device or at the very least, prior to the completion of the study, the modeling team will be better positioned to meet the development program timelines with higher quality data. Once the trial or trials have begun, it may be a very cumbersome and difficult process to make changes to the data to be collected, the data management plan (if one exists), or the process of data flow. In order to maximize the potential impact of modeling and simulation efforts, its full integration into development program timelines, including cross-department collaborative efforts regarding data flow and processing must be addressed (Collins et al. 2010; Collins and Silva 2011).

Simple checks are essential to ensure that data regarding the timing of doses prior to sample collection, as well as the amount, route, and meal status (if appropriate) of such doses, are collected with adequate detail. If the data regarding dosing and timing of sample collection are housed (databased) separately from the actual concentration results (as is typically the case), data checks can be performed and programming code set up to process these data well in advance of the close of the trial. Furthermore, even for blinded trials, this processing can be accomplished with no jeopardy to the study blind. Grasela et al. (1999), Collins et al. (2010), and Collins and Silva (2011) have discussed examples of successful programs that implemented process modifications such as these in order to facilitate and streamline the collection of high-quality data for pharmacometric modeling and simulation activities. The FDA

Guidance for Industry, Population Pharmacokinetics recognized the value of such efforts in producing higher quality data for modeling efforts in an accelerated time-frame (FDA 1999).

12.4 QC OF MODEL DEVELOPMENT

Throughout the sometimes lengthy process of model development, QC checks should be performed. Imagine the horror that one would experience following a long and challenging model development effort, if QC checking, delayed until the end of the project (when time is available), resulted in the discovery of a major error that had been initiated with the first control stream and propagated throughout the entire modeling exercise. While it may not be practical or cost-effective to perform some level of QC checking with every model that is tested, a reasonable recommendation might be to thoroughly check the first model tested, each model representing a major difference in the model structure, and each subsequent model associated with a decision-making step, and further, to do so as close in time as possible to running the model and interpreting the results.

While the use of an independent reviewer of the model code is considered optimal, if this is not possible, setting up a verification form with guidelines regarding specifically what needs to be checked for each model, is an acceptable alternative. In the absence of a form or some type of guideline to follow, it is all too easy to skip over and assume that certain portions of the code are correct. Forms that can serve as quality documents (as part of a more formal quality management system) typically require initials of the reviewer to signify completion of each specific task or at least a signature on the overall form, indicating that all tasks were completed. More extensive documentation would generally be required if any issues or inconsistencies were identified—to document the recognition of the issue and provide an explanation as to why the model is still acceptable even in the presence of the issue. Obviously, if the finding renders the model incorrect, rework would be required to address the identified issue.

Beyond the checking of model code and syntax, a perhaps bigger task lies in checking that the results and interpretation of findings are appropriate. It is for this issue that there is no substitute for an external reviewer. For modelers relatively new to modeling and the discipline of pharmacometrics, presenting the findings of a modeling exercise, whether informally or formally, as often as possible is recommended. It has been the experience of the authors that the task of explaining to someone else what you did and how you made decisions during a modeling exercise can be quite revealing. This process can serve to highlight areas of imperfect understanding—areas where perhaps more work is needed to support the findings (in the case where steps may have been skipped or recollection and documentation is lacking to support a decision) and areas where alternative approaches should be considered.

Throughout this process of discovery during model development, new understandings regarding the data are continually being formed, refined, and updated by the analyst. When findings are suddenly, noticeably inconsistent with expectations and unexpected discoveries are apparently being made, an extra level of checking is warranted. This recommendation is not meant to discredit the possibility that new findings will be generated through model development, but it is meant more as a suggestion that when an analyst's instincts tell her/him that something does not seem right, instead of accepting this new finding and moving on, the prudent course of action is to follow up on it thoroughly and immediately. Oftentimes, a data error missed during dataset QC and not easily discovered through EDA can be the source of an unexpected finding during model development. These situations that call for unscripted checking of the data and model code must be based on the particular finding at issue. For example, if the estimate of clearance is five times larger than the expected value, one could think about the problem in terms of "what in the data could make the clearance estimate very high?" or "what in the model code could make the clearance estimate very high or different from previous findings to such an extent?" This approach to thinking about what to look at may lead directly to the source of the problem or may lead to an idea for a graph to be created or code check to be performed to explore the issue a bit further, eventually leading to the source of the problem itself.

12.4.1   QC of NM-TRAN Control Streams

During model development, one of the most obvious and fundamental checks that should be done with *every* control stream run in NONMEM is to check the error file for any warnings or errors. Wasting time attempting to understand the output in the face of an unobserved error or critical warning message is a futile effort and can be avoided by always checking the error file before even opening the output file.

Establishing a program verification checklist (as recommended and discussed in Section 12.4) is not a difficult task and can be considered an evolutionary process with updates as new errors are unfortunately found even after the recommended checking is performed. The program verification checklist can be constructed to follow the typical flow and statements of most control streams to allow for the most user-friendly implementation.

Beginning with reading in the data file (and already assuming that a check has been done to ensure that the correct data file was, in fact, called), the $INPUT record in the control stream should be verified against the output statement of the program used to create the data file, against the header row of the data file. If these correspond, then a series of checks should be performed to confirm that what was read in by NONMEM is in agreement with the data content. These checks may involve confirmation of the particular columns of the dataset against the item numbers for various data items as provided in the output file as a first step. A review of the FDATA file generated by NONMEM is another means to verify the step of reading in the data correctly. Other elements that can be checked include the number of records, number of observation records, and number of individuals in the dataset against the values reported in the output file. These checks of the number of individuals and observation records are particularly important when using the IGNORE and ACCEPT options in the $DATA statement. If an error was made in the coding or interpretation of the conditional statements for data subsetting, the wrong data will be used for modeling purposes, thus invalidating the results.

The subroutines called should be verified to ensure that the appropriate model structure and parameterization are being used. Within the $PK block, confirmation should be obtained that all required variables have been defined and that appropriate compartment numbers are used in variable definitions where required. A check of the theta and eta subscripts should be made to ensure that consecutive numbers have been used and that none are reused unless intentionally so. If any new variables are created in the $PK block, each should be checked to make sure that it is initialized and that it is coded as intended. Epsilon subscripts in the $ERROR block should also be checked along with the coding of the residual variability model itself. Initial estimates in the $THETA, $OMEGA, and $SIGMA records should be checked for compatibility with the $PK and $ERROR blocks, checked for a lack of extraneous estimates, use of bounds only where intended, and that the units of the initial estimates match the units of each parameter. The $ESTIMATION record(s) should be checked to ensure that the appropriate methods and options are requested. Finally, requests for optional output, if requested, should be confirmed, along with the correct file names for the msf, table, and other files.

12.4.2 Model Diagnostic Plots and Model Evaluation Steps as QC

As described in previous chapters, there are many aspects to the typical model development process that allow for the checking and verification of results and assumptions along the way (Karlsson et al. 1998). These include model diagnostic plots, model evaluation techniques, and the various quantitative and qualitative model comparisons that can be performed. Each of these methods serves a unique purpose and can be *customized* to various extents to address particular concerns. In the end, a comprehensive QC process would be lacking if missing any of these parts.

12.5 DOCUMENTATION OF QC EFFORTS

The full integration of a QC process for pharmacometrics into an established quality management system will likely result in the generation of *quality documents* or *quality records*. Generally, tools such as verification checklists require that their use be documented and the documentation kept on file. Not only does this provide objective evidence (as for an auditor) that the established process was followed but it may also serve as a good reference for those situations when an error is discovered; the audit trail that is provided by such signed and dated documents may allow one to track down exactly, or at least approximately, when an error occurred. This is certainly useful to avoid unnecessary rework in these unfortunate situations.

A complete project file, with adequate representation of the audit trail for a modeling effort, should include the following: the signed and approved data analysis plan, dataset requirements or specifications documents; project team correspondence describing the completion of various tasks or hand-offs of project components between team members; draft and final report versions; as well as electronic copies of source data, analysis datasets, programming code and output, diagnostic plots, and other model-related output. It is often advisable to electronically archive any files related to model structures or modeling directions that were attempted and rejected; if adequately documented, these can be very helpful in addressing questions that may come from team or regulatory review later (perhaps at a time when the analyst has completely forgotten whether something was tried and if so, what the outcome was).

In addition to quality records, there are many quality-related aspects that should be documented in the technical report summarizing a modeling effort to facilitate review of the effort by a third party (Wade et al. 2005; EMEA 2007). The methods section should include a subsection detailing any deviations from the analysis plan; ideally, these should be tracked during model development to facilitate the preparation of this section after the analysis is complete. A table describing the data disposition should be included; this table tracks the data (usually in terms of counts of records and subjects) from the source (this should match that which is contained in the trial database) to the final analysis dataset used for modeling. Separate listings can be provided in a report appendix that details any exclusions of data, along with a rationale for their exclusion (Grasela et al. 2010b). If any data edits or imputations were required, these should also be reported in attached listings. Outliers identified during model development, which were excluded at any point, should not only be described, but once a final model is established, an extra step should be performed. In this extra step, the final model is re-estimated, this time including the previously identified outliers, and the results compared to the final model excluding the outliers. At times, the exclusion of the outliers is found to be necessary at a certain stage of model development, but later, once the model is expanded and refined, the inclusion of the outliers does not fundamentally change the results, with the exception of typically increasing the estimate of residual variability. In this case, the estimates of the final model including the outliers can be reported as the final parameter estimates. There are times, however, that the final model will fail to converge successfully once the outliers are included in the dataset. In these situations, this outcome can be reported and the final parameter estimates, excluding the outliers, reported as the final estimates. In some circumstances, depending on the nature of the outliers, the model will converge with very different results when the outliers are included. In this situation, a full reporting of both sets of results is recommended, along with a description of the characteristics of the data identified as outliers in comparison to the rest of the data.

12.6   SUMMARY

The practices described in this chapter are not meant to add burden to the already overwhelmed pharmacometrician. Rather, these practices represent recommendations based on lessons learned from years of doing exactly this: dealing with messy data and complicated models under intense time pressure and making plenty of mistakes along the way. The incorporation of QC processes for pharmacometric modeling can certainly be approached in a measured, ongoing way. As modeling has become an integral part of drug development, these practices are even more an expected part of the system. If the implementation of any one of these practices results in a mistake avoided, then they will be deemed well worth the effort required to perform them.

REFERENCES

Bonate PL, Strougo A, Desai A, Roy M, Yassen A, van der Walt JS, Kaibara A, Tannenbaum S. Guidelines for the quality control of population pharmacokinetic-pharmacodynamic analyses: an industry perspective. AAPS J 2012;14 (4):749–758.

Chowdhury S. Creating NONMEM datasets—how to escape the nightmare. Pharm Program 2010;3 (2):80–83.

Collins A, Peterson M, Silva G. Streamlining the PK/PD data transfer process. Pharm Program 2010;3 (1):24–28.

Collins A, Silva G. Streamlining the PK/PD data transfer process—1 year later. Pharm Program 2011;4 (1&2):28–30.

EMEA, *Guideline on Reporting the Results of Population Pharmacokinetic Analyses*, EMEA: London, 2007.

Food and Drug Administration, Guidance for Industry, Population Pharmacokinetics. Food and Drug Administration: Rockville; 1999.

Grasela TH, Antal EJ, Fiedler-Kelly J, Foit DJ, Barth B, Knuth DW, Carel BJ, Cox SR. An automated drug concentration screening and quality assurance program for clinical trials. Drug Info J 1999;33:273–279.

Grasela TH, Fiedler-Kelly J, Hitchcock DJ, Ludwig EA, Passarell JA. Forensic pharmacometrics: part 1—data assembly [abstract]. PAGE 19 (2010a) Abstr 1901. Available at www.page-meeting.org/?abstract=1901. Accessed December 14, 2013.

Grasela TH, Fiedler-Kelly J, Ludwig EA, Passarell JA, Hitchcock DJ. Forensic pharmacometrics: part 2—deliverables for regulatory submission [abstract]. PAGE 19 (2010b) Abstr 1902. Available at www.page-meeting.org/?abstract=1902. Accessed December 14, 2013.

Grasela TH, Ludwig E, Fiedler-Kelly J. Kerfuffle!. J Clin Pharmacol 2009;49 (4):386–388.

Karlsson MO, Jonsson EN, Wiltse CG, Wade JR. Assumption testing in population pharmacokinetic models: illustrated with an analysis of moxonidine data from congestive heart failure patients. J Pharmacokinet Biopharm 1998;26 (2):207–246.

Wade JR, Edholm M and Salmonson T. A guide for reporting the results of population pharmacokinetic analyses: a Swedish perspective. AAPS J 2005;7(2):E456–E460. Article 45.

INDEX

Introduction to Population Pharmacokinetic / Pharmacodynamic Analysis with Nonlinear Mixed Effects Models, First Edition. Joel S. Owen and Jill Fiedler-Kelly.
© 2014 John Wiley & Sons, Inc. Published 2014 by John Wiley & Sons, Inc.

Printed and bound by CPI Group (UK) Ltd, Croydon, CR0 4YY

16/04/2025

14658517-0002